ADVANCES IN PROSTAGLANDIN, THROMBOXANE, AND LEUKOTRIENE RESEARCH
VOLUME 20

Trends in Eicosanoid Biology

Advances in Prostaglandin, Thromboxane, and Leukotriene Research

Series Editors: Bengt Samuelsson and Rodolfo Paoletti
(Formerly *Advances in Prostaglandin and Thromboxane Research* Series)

Out of print

Advances in Prostaglandin, Thromboxane, and Leukotriene Research
Volume 20

Trends in Eicosanoid Biology

Editors

Bengt Samuelsson, M.D., Ph.D.
Department of Physiological Chemistry
Karolinska Institutet
Stockholm, Sweden

Sven-Erik Dahlén, M.D., Ph.D.
Department of Physiology
Karolinska Institutet
Stockholm, Sweden

Jürgen Fritsch, Ph.D.
Bayer AG
Health Care Group—Ethical Products
Leverkusen, F.R.G.

Per Hedqvist, M.D., Ph.D.
Department of Physiology
Karolinska Institutet
Stockholm, Sweden

Raven Press   New York

Raven Press, Ltd., 1185 Avenue of the Americas, New York, New York 10036

Made in the United States of America

ISBN 0-88167-710-8

Papers or parts thereof have been used as camera-ready copy as submitted by the authors whenever possible; when retyped, they have been edited by the editorial staff only to the extent considered necessary for the assistance of an international readership. The views expressed and the general style adopted remain, however, the responsibility of the named author. Great care has been taken to maintain the accuracy of the information contained in the volume. However, neither Raven Press nor the editors can be held responsible for errors or for any consequences arising from the use of information contained herein.

The use in this book of particular designations of countries or territories does not imply any judgment by the publisher or editors as to the legal status of such countries or territories, of their authorities or institutions, or of the delimitation of their boundaries.

Some of the names of products referred to in this book may be registered trademarks or proprietary names, although specific reference to this fact may not be made; however, the use of a name with designation is not to be construed as a representation by the publisher or editors that it is in the public domain. In addition, the mention of specific companies or of their products or proprietary names does not imply any endorsement or recommendation on the part of the publisher or editors.

The authors were responsible for obtaining the necessary permission to reproduce copyright materials from other sources. With respect to the publisher's copyright, material appearing in this book prepared by individuals as part of their official duties as government employees is only covered by this copyright to the extent permitted by the appropriate national regulations.

9 8 7 6 5 4 3 2 1

Preface

Derivatives of arachidonic acid and some closely related polyunsaturated fatty acids comprise the eicosanoid family. The members of this family—including prostaglandins, thromboxanes, leukotrienes, lipoxins, and a number of additional oxygenated metabolites—can be formed and released on demand in almost every tissue, and jointly they demonstrate an impressive range of actions which imply multiple and important regulatory functions in health and disease.

This volume of *Advances in Prostaglandin, Thromboxane, and Leukotriene Research* is based on a series of state-of-the-art lectures given at the symposium on Trends in Eicosanoid Biology held in Interlaken, Switzerland, in September 1989. It brings together the current knowledge of important areas of eicosanoid research, including biosynthesis and metabolism, cellular and molecular biology of key enzymes, receptors and receptor antagonists, signal transduction, nutritional intervention, and aspects of eicosanoids in the pulmonary and cardiovascular systems and in pathophysiological states, such as inflammation, allergy, and hypersensitivity. We are convinced that this volume, which represents a comprehensive and authoritative update of important facets of eicosanoid biology, will be a useful reference for investigators in both basic and clinical research.

We would like to express our sincere gratitude to all contributors of this volume. In particular, we would like to thank Bayer AG for extensive sponsorship and support.

The Editors

Contents

CONTENTS

Contributors

William M. Abraham
Division of Pulmonary Diseases
Mount Sinai Medical Center
4300 Alton Road
Miami Beach, Florida 33140

Stanley T. Crooke
1515, Pharmaceuticals
2280 Faraday Avenue
Carlsbad, California 92008

Sven-Erik Dahlén
Department of Physiology
Karolinska Institutet
S-10401 Stockholm, Sweden

Edward A. Dennis
Department of Chemistry
University of California at San Diego
La Jolla, California 92093-0601

Frank A. Fitzpatrick
Department of Pharmacology
University of Colorado Medical Center
4200 E. Ninth Avenue
Denver, Colorado 80262

Giancarlo Folco
Institute of Pharmacological Sciences
School of Pharmacy
University of Milano
Via Balzaretti 9
201 33 Milano, Italy

Per Hedqvist
Department of Physiology
Karolinska Institutet
S-10401 Stockholm, Sweden

Anthony W. Ford-Hutchinson
Merck Frosst Centre for Therapeutic
*   Research*
Department of Pharmacology
P.O. Box 1005
Pointe Claire-Dorval
Quebec H9R 4P8, Canada

Phillip J. Gardiner
Bayer U.K.
Research Department
Stoke Court
Stoke Poges Slough
SLZ 4 LY England

Perry V. Halushka
Department of Cell and Molecular
*   Pharmacology and Experimental*
*   Therapeutics*
Medical University of South Carolina
171 Ashley Avenue
Charleston, South Carolina 29425-2251

Dietrich Keppler
Deutsches Krebsforschungszentrum
Abteilung Tumorbiochemie
D-6900 Heidelberg 1
Federal Republic of Germany

Ruth M. Kramer
Lilly Research Laboratories
Indianapolis, Indiana 46285

Robert D. Krell
Department of Pharmacology
ICI Americas Inc.
Wilmington, Delaware 19897

James B. Lefkowith
Division of Rheumatology
Department of Medicine
Washington University Medical School
St. Louis, Missouri 63110

Robert A. Lewis
Syntex Research
3401 Hillview Avenue
P.O. Box 10850
Palo Alto, California 94304

JanÅke Lindgren
Department of Physiological Chemistry
Karolinska Institutet
S-10401 Stockholm, Sweden

Robert C. Murphy
National Jewish Center for Immunology
and Respiratory Medicine
Department of Pediatrics
1400 Jackson Street
Denver, Colorado 80206

Carlo Patrono
Department of Pharmacology
Catholic University School of Medicine
Largo F. Vito 1
00168 Rome, Italy

Priscilla J. Piper
Department of Pharmacology
Institute of Basic Medical Science
Royal College of Surgeons
33/43 Lincoln's Inn Fields
London WC21 3PN, England

Olof Rådmark
Department of Physiological Chemistry
Karolinska Institutet
S-104 01 Stockholm, Sweden

Amiram Raz
Department of Pharmacology
Washington University School of
Medicine
660 S. Euclid Avenue
St. Louis, Missouri 63110

Clive Robinson
Immunopharmacology Groups
Faculty of Medicine
Southampton General Hospital
Tremona Rd, Southampton
SO9 4XY, England

Bengt Samuelsson
Department of Physiological Chemistry
Karolinska Institutet
S-10401 Stockholm, Sweden

Michal L. Schwartzman
Department of Pharmacology
New York Medical College
Valhalla, New York 10595

Charles N. Serhan
Hematology Division
Brigham and Women's Hospital
75 Francis Street
Boston, Massachusetts 02115

Karl-Friedrich Sewing
Abteilung Allgemeine Pharmacologie
Medizinische Hochschule Hannover
Zentrum Pharmakologie und
Toxikologie
D-3000 Hannover 61
Federal Republic of Germany

Takao Shimizu
Department of Physiological Chemistry
and Nutrition
Faculty of Medicine
University of Tokyo
Bunkyo-ku, Tokyo 113, Japan

William Smith
Department of Biochemistry
Michigan State University
East Lansing, Michigan 48824-1319

Volker Ullrich
Faculty of Biology
University of Konstanz
Universitätsstrasse 10
P.O. Box 5560
D-7750 Konstanz 1
Federal Republic of Germany

Peter C. Weber
Universität München, Institut für
Prophylaxe und
Epidemiologie der
Kreislaufkrankheiten
Pettenkoferstr. 9
8000 München 2
Federal Republic of Germany

Angela Wong
Department of Cell Biology
Smith Kline and French Laboratories
King of Prussia, Pennsylvania 19479

Advances in Prostaglandin, Thromboxane,
and Leukotriene Research, Vol. 20,
edited by B. Samuelsson et al.
Raven Press, Ltd., New York © 1990.

LEUKOTRIENE B4: BIOSYNTHESIS
AND ROLE IN LYMPHOCYTES

Bengt Samuelsson and Hans-Erik Claesson

Department of Physiological Chemistry
Karolinska Institutet
S-104 01 Stockholm, Sweden

Studies on the metabolism of arachidonic acid in leukocytes ten years ago led to the discovery of leukotrienes
(1,2). Although considerable progress has been made during
the past decade regarding the biological and pharmacological
actions of leukotrienes, our knowledge about the regulation
of leukotriene biosynthesis is still very limited. The enzymes involved in leukotriene $(LT)B_4$ biosynthesis, the 5-lipo-
xygenase and the LTA_4 hydrolase, appear to be unequally
distributed. The 5-lipoxygenase gene is primarily expressed
in cells of myeloid lineage (1). In contrast, the LTA_4
hydrolase gene is expressed in many different types of cells
such as leukocytes (1), erythrocytes (3), endothelial cells
(4), fibroblasts (5) and lymphocytes (6,7). This differential expression of the two genes controlling LTB_4 formation
indicates that transcellular metabolism of LTA_4 into LTB_4
(3,4,8) might be physiologically important.

Leukotriene B_4 augments human natural cytotoxic cell
activity (9,10) and influences the activity of human suppressor and helper T lymphocytes (11,12). Since monocytes
and lymphocytes interact in certain immunological reactions,
we have studied the effects of monocyte-lymphocyte interactions on LTB_4 synthesis and the role of this compound in
human B lymphocyte activation. This review deals with the
molecular biology of LTB_4 formation and our studies on the
formation and effects of LTB_4 in B lymphocytes.

1

5-LIPOXYGENASE

The 5-lipoxygenase is the key enzyme in leukotriene biosynthesis. The enzyme possesses two enzymatic activities, conversion of arachidonic acid into 5-hydroperoxy-eicosatetraenoic acid (5-HPETE) and the subsequent formation of LTA_4. That these enzymatic activities reside in a single protein was first demonstrated by using 5-lipoxygenase isolated from potato tubers, and later confirmed for the mammalian enzymes (13). The human leukocyte 5-lipoxygenase constitutes a multicomponent system which activity is regulated by several factors. Calcium and ATP were shown to be required for maximal enzymatic activity and different cytosolic and membrane-associated protein fractions stimulated the activity (13). Studies on the subcellular localization of the 5-lipoxygenase demonstrated that the enzyme was cytosolic in resting cells. In contrast, after homogenization and subcellular fractionation, in the presence of calcium, part of the 5-lipoxygenase was membrane-associated. The membrane binding was suggested to be involved in the activation of 5-lipoxygenase (Fig.1).

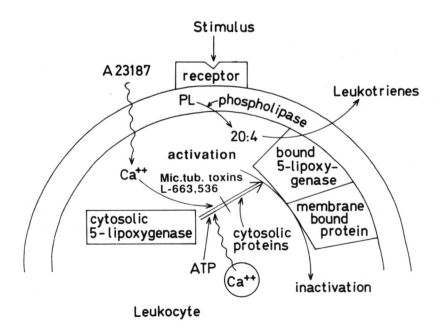

Fig. 1 Translocation of 5-lipoxygenase

Cloning of the cDNA for 5-lipoxygenase from human placenta (14) and differentiated HL-60 cells (15) predicts an enzyme of 673 amino acid residues with a calculated molecular weight of 78000. There are, however, no easily predicted domains for ATP-binding and calcium-dependent membrane binding proteins. Homology to "E-F hand calcium binding domain" found in many calcium-binding proteins was also lacking. Therefore, the precise mechanism of action of ATP and calcium on 5-lipoxygenase activity remains to be elucidated.

Based on the predicted structure of 5-lipoxygenase, the enzyme is hydrophilic but exhibits rather hydrophobic properties during chromatographic procedures. The most hydrophobic region of the enzyme is encoded by exon 7 (amino acids 278-326) and might constitute an important structural region associated with the catalytic site and arachidonic acid binding (14,15).

The human 5-lipoxygenase displays extensive homologies to rat 5-lipoxygenase (93 % identity), human 15-lipoxygenase (61% identity) and shares 40% homology with the known plant lipoxygenases from soybean and pea seeds (13). One sequence, containing 12 or 13 amino acids, are identical in all enzymes. The amino-terminal part of these lipoxygenases appears to be quite divergent in structure but the middle and carboxyl-terminal regions are quite related. These results suggest that all lipoxygenases may have diverged from a common ancestral gene.

Recombinant 5-lipoxygenase has been expressed in a mammalian osteosarcoma cell line (16) and a baculovirus/ insect cell line (17). The enzyme produced by the transfected osteosarcoma cell line, appears to be identical to the human leukocyte 5-lipoxygenase in terms of its subcellular localization, molecular weight, antigenicity and requirement for stimulatory factors. The recombinant 5-lipoxygenase, overexpressed in the transfected Spodoptera frugiperda insect cell line, was able to synthesize large amounts of 5-HPETE (Fig. 2), together with smaller amounts of the non-enzymatic products of LTA_4. These results confirmed the earlier observation with native purified leukocyte enzyme that the protein possesses both 5-lipoxygenase and LTA_4 synthase activities.

In vitro mutagenesis experiments were performed on recombinant 5-lipoxygenase, produced by the baculovirus/ insect cell system, in an initial attempt to elucidate regions of importance for catalytic activity (17). Since the iron atom is intricately involved in the catalytic mechanism of the related enzyme from soybean, two of the potential iron-atom ligands within a putative iron-binding domain, histidine-362 and histidine-372, were exchanged to serine residues. However, the activity of the mutant 5-lipoxygenase enzyme was not substantially altered (Fig.2), indicating that neither of these histidines were essential in iron coordination.

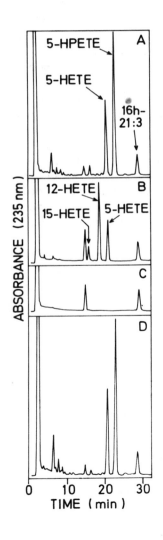

Fig. 2
HPLC profiles (UV detection at 235 nm) of products formed from arachidonic acid by 10,000 X g supernatants.
(A) Recombinant baculovirus-infected cells.
(B) Human leukocytes plus some platelet contamination.
(C) Wild-type baculovirus-infected cells.
(D) Mutant recombinant 4D-324 (His-372 → Ser-372) baculovirus-infected cells.

In order to get a better understanding of the regulation of leukotriene biosynthesis, efforts have been made to characterize the 5-lipoxygenase gene. The organization of this gene was recently deduced from several overlapping bacteriophage and cosmid clones, obtained from four different genomic libraries (18). The gene, which appears to be a single copy, span > 82 kb of DNA and is organized into 14 exons divided by 13 introns. The putative promotor region is GC-rich and contains eight potential sites (GGGCGGG or CCGCCC) for binding of the Spl transcription factor but is lacking typical TATA and CCAAT boxes in close proximity to the major transcription initiation site (Fig. 3).

The putative promotor region of the 5-lipoxygenase gene seems to share common characteristics (multiple Spl binding sites, lack of TATA and CCAAT boxes, GC-rich) with the promotors of housekeeping genes which are usually constitutively expressed in multiple tissues. This is rather surprising since the 5-lipoxygenase gene is primarily expressed in cells of myeloid lineage. However, these characteristics of the promotor region is not only restricted to housekeeping genes since several genes involved in growth control, such as the gene for human EGF receptor (19) and human Ha-ras (20), have similarly organized 5' flanking sequences. Studies with HL-60 cells and chicken myelomonocytic cells, transformed by a temperature-sensitive mutant of avian leukemia virus, indicate that differentiation of these cells is associated with an up-regulation of the 5-lipoxygenase pathway (13). Clues to the control of tissue specific 5-lipoxygenase expression whether at the transcriptional, translational, or may be, posttranslational level will certainly become more evident in the near future.

LEUKOTRIENE A$_4$ HYDROLASE

The unstable epoxide intermediate LTA$_4$ is enzymatically hydrolyzed into LTB$_4$ by the enzyme LTA$_4$ hydrolase. The enzyme, a cytosolic monomeric protein of molecular weight of about 690000, has been purified from peripheral leukocytes, rat neutrophils, human erythrocytes, human lung, guinea pig liver and guinea pig lung (13). Leukotriene A$_4$ hydrolase displayed strict substrate specificity, including a free acid moiety, 5,6-epoxide and the tetraene structure with the 7,9-trans-11,14-cis configuration (13). The enzyme appeared

distinct from the previously described cytosolic and microsomal epoxide hydrolases found in liver (13). In fact, incubation of cytosolic epoxide hydrolase from mouse liver with
LTA_4 led to the formation of 5(S), 6(R)-dihydroxy-7,9-trans-
11,14-cis-eicosatetraenoic acid and the enzyme also accepted
the 14,15-isomer of LTA_4 as a substrate (13).

```
CTGCAGACTCCCGGAGCACCCCCTGCTCCAAGTACCGCAAGTGGCACTGAGAACTTGGGGAGAGCAGAGG  -463

CTGTGCCTAGATTTGTAGGGAGTCCCCGCAGCTCCACCCCAGGGCCTACAGGAGCCTGGCCTTGGGCGAA  -393

GCCGAGGCAGGCAGGCAGGGCAAAGGGTGGAAGCAATTCAGGAGAGAACGAGTGAACGAATGGATGAGGG  -323

GTGGCAGCCGAGGTTGCCCCAGTCCCCTGGCTGCAGGAACAGACACCTCGCTGAGGAGAGACCCAGGAGC  -253

GAGGCCCCTGCCCCGCCCGAGGCGAGGTCCCGCCCAGTCGGCGCCGCGCGTGAAGAGTGGGAGAGAAGTA  -183

CTGCGGGGGCGGGGGCGGGGGCGGGGGCGGGGGCGGGGGCAGCCGGGAGCCTGGAGCCAGACCGGGGCGG  -113

GGCCGGGACCGGGGCCAGGGACCAGTGGTGGGAGGAGGCTGCGGCGCTAGATGCGGACACCTGGACCGCC  -43

GCGCCGAGGCTCCCGGCGCTCGCTGCTCCCGCGGCCCGCGCC ATGCCCTCCTACACGGTCACCGTGGCC   27
                                           MetProSerTyrThrValThrValAla

ACTGGCAGCCAGTGGTTCGCCGGCACTGACGACTACATCTACCTCAGCCTCGTGGGCTCGGCGGGCTGCA   97
ThrGlySerGlnTrpPheAlaGlyThrAspAspTyrIleTyrLeuSerLeuValGlySerAlaGlyCysS

GCGAGAAGCACCTGCTGGACAAGCCCTTCTACAACGACTTCGAGCGTGGCGCGGTGAGCGCGGGCGGGGC  167
erGluLysHisLeuLeuAspLysProPheTyrAsnAspPheGluArgGlyAla

ACGGGTGGAGCGCGGGCTGAGGTGCGTCCGGGACCCGGTTTGGACGGCAGAGGCCTGGGCGGGGGCGCCG  237

AGGGCCCGTCGGGGCGGCCCGGACAGGACTGGGGGTGTCCAGGACCCTGTCAGGGAGGGCAGAACTGCGG  307

TGGGGCGTGCCCTGGGCTCCCAGTGGCCGGTGGGTACC                                  345
```

Fig. 3

DNA sequence of the 5' end of the human 5-lipoxygenase gene.
The first base of the ATG initiation codon is designated +1.
The 5' ends of fragments protected by S1 nuclease digestion
and generated by primer extension are indicated by open and
closed circles, respectively. The major transcription initiation site is indicated by ↓. Sites corresponding to the
core consensus for Sp1 binding are boxed. An 11-bp inverted
repeat is underlined. The DNA was sequenced entirerly on
both strands.

A characteristic feature of LTA_4 hydrolase is the inactivation by its substrate. This irreversible inactivation may be linked to the covalent binding of LTA_4 to the enzyme (13).

Polyclonal antiserum raised against LTA_4 hydrolase was used in the immunoscreening of a human lung λgt11 expression library to isolate a cDNA clone corresponding to LTA_4 hydrolase (21). By using this isolated clone as a probe, several additional clones were isolated from lung and placenta cDNA libraries. LTA_4 hydrolase has also been cloned from a human spleen cDNA library using an oligonucleotide probe (48 bases), based on the sequence of a peptide from the human leukocyte enzyme (22). From the predicted primary structures, the mature enzyme contains 610 amino acids and shares no apparent homology with the liver microsomal epoxide hydrolases, or in fact to any other known protein. Predictions of secondary structure and calculations of hydropathy revealed mixed pattern but a region centered around position 200 might be related to the catalytic activity of LTA_4 hydrolase. Thus, segment 170-185 was the most hydrophilic in the enzyme, segment 190-205 the most hydrophobic and in between those two was one of two strong predictions for a reverse turn (followed by a prediction for β-strand). In addition, short internal repeat segment is located adjacent to this segment (residues 209-238) and has a prediction for a long α-helix (residues 220-240).

LTA_4 hydrolase has been expressed in E. coli as a fusion protein containing the first 10 amino acids of the β-galactosidase gene (23). The recombinant enzyme exhibited comparable characteristics to the human neutrophil enzyme including reaction kinetics, Km and Vmax values, suicide inactivation and susceptibility to thiol-modifying reagents.

LTA_4 hydrolase activity has been detected in leukocytes (1), erythrocytes (3), endothelial cells (4), fibroblasts (5), human epithelial cells (H.-E. Claesson, to be published) and lymphocytes (6,7). This is surprising since 5-lipoxygenase expression appears primarily to be restricted for cells of myeloid lineage. This differential expression of two genes controlling LTB_4 synthesis suggests that transcellular metabolism LTA_4, as demonstrated for granulocytes and erythrocytes or endothelial cells (3,4,8), might be an important mechanism for biosynthesis of LTB_4.

FORMATION AND EFFECTS OF LTB$_4$ IN B LYMPHOCYTES

LTB$_4$ has been described as a modulator of various T lymphocyte functions. It augments natural cytotoxic cell activity, induces suppressor T cell activity and inhibits the proliferation of helper-inducer T cells (9-12). The expression of 5-lipoxygenase in human lymphocytes has been a matter of controversy for several years. However, studies with highly purified T cells, B cells and monoclonal lymphocytic cells have demonstrated that these cells lack an active 5-lipoxygenase (6,24,25). In contrast, isolated peripheral T cells and tonsillar B cells as well as a number of monoclonal lymphocytic cell lines possess LTA$_4$ hydrolase activity (6,7). The expression of LTA$_4$ hydrolase, but not of 5-lipoxygenase, was also demonstrated at transcriptional and translational level in Raji cells, a Burkitt lymphoma derived B-cell line (26). Several transformed B- and T-cell lines expressed more LTA$_4$ hydrolase activity than normal B and T cells (6). Similarly, transformation of fibroblasts with simian virus-40 has also been shown to be associated with an increased LTA$_4$ hydrolase activity (5).

Monocytes/macrophages interact with lymphocytes in certain immunological reactions. To elucidate the relevance of LTA$_4$ hydrolase in lymphocytes, we investigated if monocytes could supply lymphocytes with LTA$_4$. Human monocytes, isolated from peripheral blood, were stimulated with the ionophore A 23187 in buffer containing albumin. Five min after the activation, considerable amounts of extracellular LTA$_4$ were detected by trapping of the epoxide with methanol followed by RP-HPLC analysis (27). Transcellular metabolism of LTA$_4$ was investigated between monocytes and Raji cells, which possessed high LTA$_4$ hydrolase activity (6). Human monocytes either alone or together with Raji cells were incubated with the ionophore A 23187 for 10 min. Fig.4 A shows a typical RP-HPLC chromatogram of the products formed by monocytes alone. In the presence of Raji cells, at a ratio of Raji cells versus monocytes of 3:1, the levels of LTB$_4$ increased about 2-fold (Fig.4 B). The non-enzymatic hydrolysis products of LTA$_4$ did not increase in parallel with the increament in LTB$_4$ levels. Donation of arachidonic acid from activated Raji cells to monocytes might also contribute to the increased formation of LTB$_4$ in mixed cell

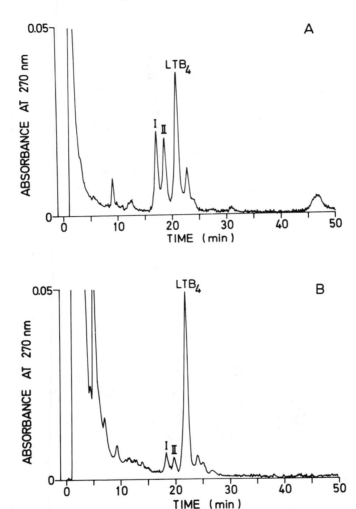

Fig. 4 HPLC chromatograms of the products formed by (A) Monocytes (10^7 cells) alone or (B) in the presence of Raji cells (3×10^7 cells) after stimulation with the ionophore A23187 (5 μm) for 10 min. Peaks designated I and II are the non-enzymatic isomers of LTB_4, Δ^6-trans-LTB_4 and 12-epi-Δ^6 trans-LTB_4, respectively.

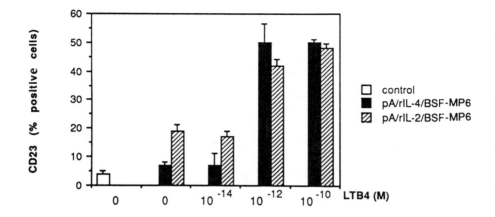

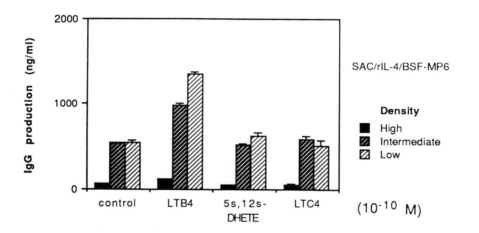

Fig. 5. Upper panel: Expression of CD 23 antigen in high
density B cells, preincubated for three hours with
indicated concentrations of LTB₄, or vehicle only,
followed by 12 hours incubation with protein A(pA)/
B cell stimulating factor from MP-6 cells (BSF-MP6)
and recombinant interleukin 2 or 4, (rIL-2 and
rIL-4, respectively). The expression of CD 23 antigen was determined by immunofluorescence. Lower
panel: Production of IgG in B cells of various cell
density after treatment with indicated compound and
SAC (Staphylococcus aureus Cowan 1)/rIL-4/BSF-MP6.
IgG production was measured by using a micro-ELISA
technique.

incubations. However, this mechanism solely would presumably lead to an increase also in the levels of the non-enzymatic isomers of LTB$_4$. Thus, transfer of LTA$_4$ from stimulated monocytes to Raji cells is likely to be, at least in part, responsible for the increased synthesis of LTB$_4$ observed in coincubations of these cells. At a ratio of Raji cells versus monocytes of 9:1, up to a 10-fold increase of LTB$_4$ levels was found (27).

The involvement of B cells in the biosynthesis of LTB$_4$ initiated studies on the role of this compound on various B cell functions. Highly purified human tonsillar B lymphocytes at different stages of activation were incubated with LTB$_4$ (28). As a key marker for B cell activation, the CD23 antigen was used. Strong evidence has been mounting to implicate CD23 as an important molecule in B cell growth regulation. LTB$_4$ enhanced the CD23 expression on resting B cells in synergy with B cell stimulating factors, such as interleukin-2 and -4, and maximal effect was observed at a concentration of 10^{-10} and 10^{-12} M (Fig. 5A). LTB$_4$, in the presence of lymphokines, also augmented initiation of DNA synthesis and cellular replication in intermediate density B cells. Low and intermediate density B cells responded to treatment with LTB$_4$ (10^{-10} M) with an about 2-fold increased production of immunoglobulins (Fig. 5B). Neither 5S, 12S-DHETE nor LTC$_4$ stimulated the secretion of immunoglobulins at the same concentration. In the absence of lymphokines, LTB$_4$ did not exert any potentiating effects on these B cell functions. Thus, transcellular metabolism of monocyte-derived LTA$_4$ into LTB$_4$ by lymphocytes leads to an increased biosynthesis of LTB$_4$, which might act as a fine tuning modulator of certain B cell functions.

ACKNOWLEDGEMENTS

The work from the authors laboratory was supported by grants from the Swedish Medical Research Council (project 03X-217 and 03X-07135), the Wallenberg Foundation and the Swedish Cancer Society (project 2801-B90-01XA).

REFERENCES

1. Samuelsson, B. (1983) Science 220:568-575.
2. Samuelsson, B., Dahlen, S.-E., Lindgren, J.A., Rouzer, C.A. and Serhan, C. N. (1987) Science 237:1171-1176.
3. McGee, J.E. and Fitzpatrick, F.A. (1986) Proc. Natl. Acad. Sci. USA 83:1349-1353.
4. Claesson, H.-E. and Haeggström, J. (1988) Eur.J. Biochem. 173:93-100.
5. Medina, J., Barrios, C., Funk, C.D., Larsson, O., Haeggström, J. and Rådmark, O. (1990) Eur. J. Biochem., in press.
6. Odlander, B., Jakobsson, P.-J., Rosen, A. and Claesson, H.-E. (1988) Biochem. Biophys. Res. Comm. 153:203-208.
7. Fu, J.Y., Medina, J.F., Funk, C.D., Wetterholm, A. and Rådmark, O. (1988) Prostaglandins 36:241-248.
8. Dahinden, C.A., Clancy, R.M., Gross, M., Chiller, J.M. and Hugli, T.E. (1985) Proc. Natl. Acad. Sci. USA 83:1349-1353.
9. Rola-Pleszczynski, M., Gagnon, L. and Sirois, P. (1983) Biochem. Biophys. Res. Commun. 113:531-537.
10. Rola-Pleszczynski, M., Gagnon, L., Rudzinski, M., Borgeat, P. and Sirois, P. (1984) Prostaglandins Leukotrienes Med. 13:113-117.
11. Payan, D.G., Missirian-Bastian, A. and Goetzl, E.J. (1984) Proc. Natl. Acad. Sci. USA 81:3501-3505.
12. Rola-Pleszczynski, M. (1985) J. Immun. 135:1357-1360.
13. Samuelsson, B. and Funk, C.D. (1989) J. Biol. Chem. 264, 19469-72.
14. Matsumoto, T., Funk, C.D., Rådmark, O., Höög, J.-O., Jörnvall, H. and Samuelsson, B. (1988) Proc. Natl. Acad. Sci. USA 85:26-30, and correction (1988) 85:3406.
15. Dixon, R.A.F., Jones, R.E., Diehl, R.E., Bennett, C.D., Kargman, S. and Rouzer, C.A. (1988) Proc. Natl. Acad. Sci. USA 85:416-420.
16. Rouzer, C.A., Rands, E., Kargman, S., Jones, R.E., Register, R.B. and Dixon, R.A.F. (1988) J. Biol. Chem. 263:10135-10140.
17. Funk, C.D., Gunne, H., Steiner, H., Izumi, T. and Samuelsson, B. (1989) Proc. Natl. Sci. USA 86:2592-2596.

18. Funk, C.D., Hoshiko, S., Matsumoto, T., Rådmark, O. and Samuelsson, B. (1989) Proc. Natl. Acad. Sci. USA 86:2587-2591.
19. Ishii, S., Xu, Y.-H., Stratton, R.H., Roe, B. A. Merlino, G.T. and Pastan, I. (1985) Proc. Natl. Sci. USA 82:4920-4924.
20. Ishii, S., Merlino, G.T. and Pastan, I. (1985) Science 230:1378-1381.
21. Funk, C.D., Rådmark, O., Fu, J.Y., Matsumoto, T., Jörnvall, H., Shimizu, T. and Samuelsson, B. (1987) Proc. Natl. Acad. Sci. USA 84:6677-6681.
22. Minami, M., Ohno, S., Kawasaki, H., Rådmark, O., Samuelsson, B., Jörnvall, H., Shimizu, T., Seyama, Y. and Suzuki, K. (1987) J. Biol. Chem. 262: 13873-13876.
23. Minami, M., Minami, Y., Emori, Y., Kawasaki, H. Ohno, S., Suzuki, K., Ohishi, N., Shimizu, T. and Seyama, Y. (1988) FEBS Lett. 229: 279-282.
24. Poubelle, P.E., Borgeat, P. and Rola-Pleszczynski, M. (1987) J. Immunol. 139:1273-1277.
25. Goldyne, M.E. and Rea, L. (1987) Prostaglandins 34:783-795.
26. Medina, J.F., Odlander, B., Funk, C.D., Fu, J.Y., Claesson, H.-E. and Rådmark, O. (1989) Biochem. Biophys. Res. Comm. 161:740-745.
27. Jakobsson, P.-J., Odlander,B. and Claesson, H.-E. (1989) Submitted for publication.
28. Yamaoka, K.A., Claesson, H.-E. and Rosen, A. (1989) J. Immunol. 143: in press.

Advances in Prostaglandin, Thromboxane, and Leukotriene Research, Vol. 20,
edited by B. Samuelsson et al.
Raven Press, Ltd., New York © 1990.

STRUCTURE--FUNCTION RELATIONSHIPS IN SHEEP, MOUSE, AND HUMAN

PROSTAGLANDIN ENDOPEROXIDE G/H SYNTHASES

W.L. Smith, D.L. DeWitt, S.A. Kraemer, M.J. Andrews,
*T. Hla, *T. Maciag, T. Shimokawa

Department of Biochemistry, Michigan State University,
East Lansing, Michigan, U.S.A. 48824, and *Laboratory
of Molecular Biology, American Red Cross,
Rockville, Maryland, U.S.A. 20855

ABSTRACT

Our studies are designed to determine which amino acid residues are involved in catalyzing the cyclooxygenase and hydroperoxidase activities of prostaglandin endoperoxide (PGG/H) synthase. We have deduced from complementary (c)DNAs the amino acid sequences of the sheep and mouse PGG/H synthases, and a portion of the human PGG/H synthase. These enzymes have amino acid sequences which are about 90% identical. Sequence similarities with putative heme binding regions of myeloperoxidase and thyroid peroxidase suggest that the sequence TI(L)WLREHNRV of PGG/H synthase contains the histidine (His309) which is the proximal heme ligand; the distal heme ligand may be His226 which is found in the sequence 222-KALGH-226. Using site-directed mutagenesis, we have replaced Ser530, the serine residue which is acetylated by aspirin, with Ala530 and with Asn530; the Ala530 mutant has both cyclooxygenase and hydroperoxidase activity, while the Asn530 mutant lacks cyclooxygenase activity but retains hydroperoxidase activity. These results establish that the hydroxyl group of Ser530 is not essential for catalysis or substrate binding and suggest that a bulky group at position 530, such as that introduced by aspirin acetylation, prevents arachidonate binding to the cyclooxygenase active site. Finally, we have found that tetranitromethane causes irreversible inactivation of cyclooxygenase activity and that the enzyme is protected from inactivation when ibuprofen is included in the reaction mixture. These results suggest that there is an essential tyrosine at the active site of PGG/H synthase.

INTRODUCTION

PGG/H synthase catalyzes the formation of PGH_2 from arachidonic acid. The enzyme exhibits two independent activities including a <u>bis</u>-oxygenase activity which facilitates PGG_2 formation and a hydroperoxidase activity involved in converting PGG_2 to PGH_2 (19,20,25). Current evidence suggests that the following sequence of events occurs during cyclooxygenase catalysis (Fig. 1 (4,8,12,14)): (a) interaction of a lipid hydroperoxide with the heme group of PGG/H synthase and subsequent formation of a ferryl-oxo compound I-like intermediate and an alcohol; (b) oxidation of a tyrosyl sidechain to a radical cation; (c) abstraction of the 13-proS hydrogen atom from arachidonate (5); (d) sequential oxygen addition reactions; (e) reformation of the tryosine radical cation and dissociation of PGG_2 from the enzyme. The hydroperoxidase reaction (Fig. 1) also appears to involve formation of the Compound I-like intermediate and two sequential one electron reductions to regenerate the native enzyme (4,8,14). Although there is now a good model for explaining various facets of the cyclooxygenase and hydroperoxidase reactions, little is known about how the protein molecule itself is involved in facilitating these reactions. The goal of studies reported here has been to determine which amino acid residues are involved in heme binding and catalysis.

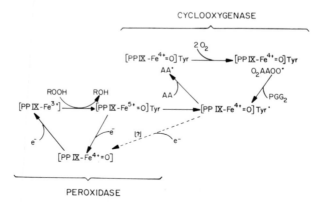

FIG. 1. Mechanism of cyclooxygenase and hydroperoxidase reactions of PGG/H synthase (adapted from Karthein et al. (8)). PPIX, protoporphyrin IX; ROOH, alkylhydroperoxide; ROH, alcohol; AA, arachidonic acid.

RESULTS AND DISCUSSION

Comparison of Deduced Amino Acid Sequences of Sheep, Mouse, and Human PGG/H Synthases

We have sequenced cDNAs which contain the coding regions of sheep (2,3) and mouse (1) PGG/H synthases; these cDNAs were isolated from sheep vesicular gland and mouse 3T3 cell λgt10 cDNA libraries, respectively. We have also determined the sequence of a cDNA derived from a human umbilical cord endothelial cell library and containing an estimated 55% of the coding region for the human PGG/H synthase.

The deduced amino acid sequences of the sheep, mouse, and human PGG/H synthases are compared in Fig 2. The numbers refer to the location of amino acids in the sheep enzyme, which, including the signal peptide, contains 600 amino acids. The mouse PGG/H synthase contains 602 amino acids; the two additional amino acids are found in the signal peptide. The human umbilical cord cDNA for PGG/H synthase codes for 341 amino acids. The sheep and mouse sequences exhibit 87% sequence identity over 600 amino acids; there is 90% identity between the sheep and human sequences over the 341 amino acid sequence. Taking into account conservative substitutions, the sequence similarities are 98%.

The two longest regions of identity among the sequences of the three PGG/H synthases include: (a) residues 198 to 242 and (b) residues 514 to 546. The sequence KALGH (residues 222-226) containing His226, which, as discussed below, may be the distal heme ligand, lies within the first of these regions. The "active site" Ser530 is at the midpoint of the second of these regions.

The Proximal and Distal Histidine Ligands of the Heme

Sequence comparisons using the GenBank database identified human myeloperoxidase (7,18) and thyroid peroxidase (10) as proteins with sequence similarities to PGG/H synthase. The sequence identities between the sheep PGG/H synthase and myeloperoxidase and thyroid peroxidase are less than 25%. However, there is a highly homologous region containing the sequence TI(L)WLREHNRV (residues 303-312 of the sheep) which is present in the sheep, mouse, and human PGG/H synthases and in thyroid peroxidase (residues 408-417 (10)) and myeloperoxidase (residues 417-426 (7,18)). The histidine in these latter sequences is the putative axial heme ligand of these mammalian peroxidases (9). By analogy, we suggest that the histidine present in the TIWLREHRV sequence (His309) is the proximal heme ligand of PGG/H synthases (Fig. 3).

The location of the distal histidine residue is not obvious. In plant and mammalian peroxidases, the distal histidine is present in a sequence RXXXH (9,21,26). There is no histidine present in PGG/H synthase in a sequence of this type. However, one sequence, KALGH (residues 222-226), has a basic amino acid four residues distant from a histidine and, thus, is analogous to the RXXXH of other peroxidases. The KALGH sequence is found in a highly conserved region (residues 198-242) of sheep, mouse, and human PGG/H synthases. We suggest that His226 is the distal heme ligand of PGG/H synthase (Fig. 3). Because there are only 13 conserved histidines in PGG/H synthases (Fig. 3), it should be feasible to prepare mutations of all histidines to determine which ones are essential for heme binding.

```
1         10        20        30        40        50
MSRRSLSLWFPLLLLLLLPPTPSVLLADPGVPSPVNPCCYYPCQNQGVCVRFGLDNYQCD   mouse
:::.:.::..::^:::::::.:.:^:..::::.:.::::::::::.::.:::::::::.:::
MSRQSISLRFP-LLLLLLSPSP-VFSADPGAPAPVNPCCYYPCQHQGICVRFGLDRYQCD   sheep


60        70        80        90        100       110
CTRTGYSGPNCTIPEIWTWLRNSLRPSPSFTHFLLTHGYWLWEFVNATFIREVLMRLVLT   mouse
::::::::::::::::::::::.::::::.:::::::.:::.::::::::...:::::::
CTRTGYSGPNCTIPEIWTWLRTTLRPSPSFIHFLLTHGRWLWDFVNATFIRDTLMRLVLT   sheep
          :::::::::::::::::::.:::::::::.::..:::::::.  :::::::
          LRPSPSFTHLLLLTHGRWFWEFVNATFIRHMLMRLVLT   human


120       130       140       150       160       170
VRSNLIPSPPTYNSAHDYISWESFSNVSYYTRILPSVPKDCPTPMGTKGKKQLPDVQLLA   mouse
:::::::::::::::.:::::::::::::::::::::::::.:::::::::::::::...:.
VRSNLIPSPPTYNIAHDYISWESFSNVSYYTRILPSVPRDCPTPMGTKGKKQLPDAEFLS   sheep
::::::: :::: .:::::::::::::::.::.:.::::.::::::::::::::::::...:.
VRSNLIPVPPTYNSAHDYISWESFSNVSYHTRILPCVPKDCPTPMGTKGKKQLPDAQLLA   human


180       190       200       210       220       230
QQLLLRREFIPAPQGTNILFAFFAQHFTHQFFKTSGKMGPGFTKALGHGVDLGHIYGDNL   mouse
...:::::.:::.:::::..::::::::::::::::::::::::::::::::::::::::::
RRFLLRRKFIPDPQGTNLMFAFFAQHFTHQFFKTSGKMGPGFTKALGHGVDLGHIYGDNL   sheep
:::::::::::::::::::::.::::::::::::::::::::::::::::::::::::::::
RRFLLRRKFIPDPQGTNLMFALFAQHFTHQFFKTSGKMGPGFTKALGHGVDLGHIYGDNL   human


240       250       260       270       280       290
ERQYHLRLFKDGKLKYQVLDGEVYPPSVEQ-ASVLMRYPPGVPPERQMAVGQEVFGLLPG   mouse
:::::.::::::::::::.:::::::::::.  :.:::.:.:.:..:::::::::::::::
ERQYQLRLFKDGKLKYQMLNGEVYPPSVEE-APVLMHYPRGIPPQSQMAVGQEVFGLLPG   sheep
:::::::::::::::::::.:::::.:::::::::::::::::::::::::::::::::::::
ERQYQLRLFKDGKLKYQVLDGEMYPPSVEEPAPVLMHYPRGIPPQSQMAVGQEVFGLLPG   human


300       310       320       330       340       350
LMLFSTIWLREHNRVCDLLKEEHPTWDDEQLFQTTRLILIGETIKIVIEEYVQHLSGYFL   mouse
:::::.::::::::::::::::.:::::.:::::::.:::::::::::::::::.:::::::
LMLYATIWLREHNRVCDLLKAEHPTWGDEQLFQTARLILIGETIKIVIEEYVQQLSGYFL   sheep
:::::::.:::::::::.::.:::::::.::::::::.::::::::::::::::.:::::::
LMLYATLWLREHNRVCEVLKAEHPTWGDQQLFQTTRLILIGETIKIVIEEYVQQLSGYFL   human


360       370       380       390       400       410
QLKFDPELLFRAQFQYRNRIAMEFNHLYHWHPLMPNSFQVGSQEYSYEQFLFNTSMLVDY   mouse
::::::::::::.:::::::::::::.:::::::::::.:::.:::..:::::::::::::::
QLKFDPELLFGAQFQYRNRIAMEFNQLYHWHPLMPDSFRVGPQDYSYEQFLFNTSMLVDY   sheep
::::::::::::.:::::::::.:::::::::::::::.:::..:.:::.::::::::::::
QLKFDPELLFGVQFQYRNRIQMEFNHLYHWHPLMPDSFKVGSQEYSYEHFLFNTSMLVDY   human


420       430       440       450       460       470
GVEALVDAFSRQRAGRIGGGRNFDYHVLHVAVDVIKESREMRLQPFNEYRKRFGLKPYTS   mouse
:::::::::::::.::::::::::.:::::::::::::::::.:..:::::::::::.::::
GVEALVDAFSRQPAGRIGGGRNIDHHILHVAVDVIKESRVLRLQPFNEYRKRFGMKPYTS   sheep
::::
GVEA                                                          human


480       490       500       510       520       530
FQELTGEKEMAAELEELYGDIDALEFYPGLLLEKCQPNSIFGESMIEMGAPFSLKGLLGN   mouse
:::::::::::::::::::::::::::::::::::::.:::::::::::::::::::::::::
FQELTGEKEMAAELEELYGDIDALEFYPGLLLEKCHPNSIFGESMIEMGAPFSLKGLLGN   sheep


540       550       560       570       580       590
PICSPEYWKPSTFGGDVGFNLVNTASLKKLVCLNTKTCPYVSFRVPDYPGDDGSVLVRRS   mouse
:::::::::.:::::.:::::::.::.:::::::::::::::::.  . .: . . . :..
PICSPEYWKASTFGGEVGFNLVKTATLKKLVCLNTKTCPYVSFHVPDPRQEDRPGVERPP   sheep


600
TEL   mouse
:::
TEL   sheep
```

FIG. 2. Comparison of deduced amino acid sequences of sheep (2,3,16,27), mouse (1), and human PGG/H synthases.

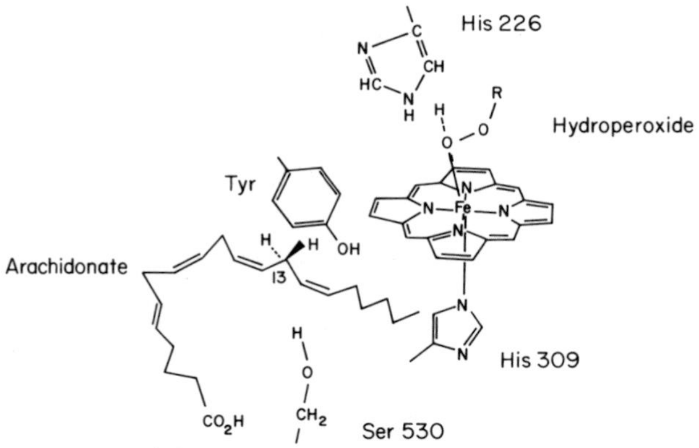

FIG. 3. Model of the active site of PGG/H synthase.

The sequence which includes residues 274-277 (HYPR) of sheep PGG/H synthase was proposed by Marnett and coworkers to contain the distal histidine (15). However, the corresponding sequence in the mouse enzyme (RYPP) is different than that of the sheep and includes an arginine at the position occupied by the histidine in the sheep sequence (Fig. 2). Thus, the HYPR sequence cannot represent a consensus distal heme binding site for PGG/H synthases. Furthermore, as shown in Table 1 below, replacement of Tyr275 with Phe275 in sheep PGG/H synthase had no major effect on either cyclooxygenase or peroxidase activities.

TABLE 1. Cyclooxygenase and hydroperoxidase activities in membranes of cos-1 cells transfected with pSVT7 expression vectors coding for native and mutant PGG/H synthases[a]

cos-1 cells transfected with:	Cyclooxygenase (nmoles/min/mg)	Hydroperoxidase (nmoles/min/mg)	ASA $t_{1/2}$ (min)
sham transfected	0	4.6	--
$pSVT7-PGHS_{OV}$ (native)	450	70	30
$pSVT7-PGHS_{OV}$-ASA-acetylated	0	70	ND
$pSVT7-PGHS_{OV}$-Ala530	388	79	stable
$pSVT7-PGHS_{OV}$-Phe275	435	67	ND
$pSVT7-PGHS_{OV}$-Asn530	0	222	ND

[a]PGG/H synthase enzyme activities were measured as detailed elsewhere (1). The half-life for cyclooxygenase activity in the presence of aspirin was determined at 37° with 0.1 mM aspirin. ND, not determined; ASA, aspirin.

Site-Directed Mutagenesis of Active Site Ser530

Using a Muta-Gene kit (Bio-Rad) based on the method developed by Kunkel (13), we prepared a mutant of the sheep PGG/H synthase in which Ser530 (the "active site" serine which is acetylated by aspirin (3,16,23,27)) was replaced with Ala530; a pSVT7 expression vector was constructed which contained the cDNA for the mutant protein (1,2). The vector coding for the native enzyme is designated pSVT7-PGHS$_{OV}$, while the vector coding for the mutant enzyme is designated pSVT7-PGHS$_{OV}$-A530. Populations of cos-1 cells were transfected with either pSVT7-PGHS$_{OV}$ or pCD-PGHS$_{OV}$-A530, and microsomal membrane preparations from the two cell populations were assayed for cyclooxygenase and hydroperoxidase activities; in addition, the sensitivities toward aspirin and flurbiprofen of native and mutant cyclooxygenases were examined. As shown in Table 1, native and mutant PGG/H synthases were both able to catalyze both cyclooxygenase and peroxidase reactions and the specific activities of the two preparations were comparable. Both enzymes were inhibited by flurbiprofen at similar concentrations (ID$_{50}$ = 5 μM). In addition, the K$_m$ for arachidonate was 7 μM and 8 μM for the native and alanine-containing mutants, respectively. In fact, the only difference we have detected between the native and mutant enzymes is that the native, but not the mutant enzyme is irreversibly inactivated by aspirin (Table 1).

Our results clearly establish that Ser530 is not essential for catalysis and suggest, when analyzed in conjunction with studies on salicylate binding (6), that acetylation of Ser530 causes steric interference with arachidonic acid binding. To test this concept, we replaced Ser530 with Asn530, an uncharged amino acid similar in size to an acetylated serine. As seen in Table 1, the Asn530 mutant lacked cyclooxygenase activity but retained hydroperoxidase activity. Western transfer blotting indicated that the Asn530 mutant protein was expressed at about the same levels as the native enzyme in transfected cells (data not shown). The results of studies with the Asn530 mutant support the concept that acetylation of Ser530 causes a loss of cyclooxygenase activity because it places a bulky group in the protein which interferes with arachidonate binding (Fig. 3). Kulmacz (11) has recently presented data which also suggest that acetylation of Ser530 interferes with arachidonate binding.

Active Site Tyrosine of PGG/H Synthase

Karthein et al. (4,8) have presented spectral evidence that a tyrosine radical cation is formed upon interaction of PGG$_2$ with sheep PGG/H synthase. As noted earlier (Fig. 1; (4,8)), this tyrosine radical cation may be the reactive species which removes the 13-proS-hydrogen from arachidonate to initiate the cyclooxygenase reaction. Accordingly, we performed an experiment to determine if the cyclooxygenase was sensitive to inactivation by the tyrosine-specific reagent tetranitromethane (24).

Microsomal preparations of PGG/H synthase from sheep vesicular gland were incubated with 4.2 mM tetranitromethane for 30 min at room temperature in the presence or absence of two stereoisomers of ibuprofen, a nonsteroidal anti-inflammatory drug which is a reversible inhibitor of cyclooxygenase activity (22); ibuprofen competes with arachidonate for binding to the active site of the cyclooxygenase (22). The d-ibuprofen is 10-50 times more active than the l-isomer as a cyclooxygenase inhibitor. As shown in Table 2, cyclooxygenase activity was lost following treatment with tetranitromethane for 30 min in the absence of ibuprofen; however, d-ibuprofen (10^{-4} M) protected the cyclooxygenase from inactivation,while l-ibuprofen at the same concentration provided little or no protection. At pH 8.0, tetranitromethane can modify both tyrosine and cysteine residues (22). However, in confirmation of earlier results using sulfhydryl reagents (17), p-chloromercuribenzoate (1 mM for 10 min at room temperature) was found to have no effect on cyclooxygenase activity. These results suggest that there is a tyrosine(s) located at the ibuprofen (i.e. arachidonate) binding site which is essential for cyclooxygenase activity.

TABLE 2. Inactivation of Cyclooxygenase by Tetranitromethane[a]

Treatment	Cyclooxygenase Activity (nmoles 20:4/min/mg protein)
No treatment	168
Tetranitromethane	0
Tetranitromethane + l-ibuprofen	5
Tetranitromethane + d-ibuprofen	176
l-ibuprofen	150
d-ibuprofen	164

[a]Sheep vesicular gland microsomal suspensions were treated with tetranitromethane (TNM) and assayed for cyclooxygenase activity (1). The concentration of ibuprofen was 10^{-4} M in the preincubation mixtures, and ibuprofen was added prior to TNM. When the cyclooxygenase assays are performed, ibuprofen is diluted 100-fold and, at this concentration, d-ibuprofen does not inhibit cyclooxygenase activity.

ACKNOWLEDGMENTS

    This work was supported in part by National Institutes of Health Grants DK22042 and GM40713, by a Grant-In-Aid from the American Heart Association of Michigan, and by a National Heart, Lung, and Blood Institute Predoctoral Training Grant HL07404.

REFERENCES

1. DeWitt, D.L., El-Harith, E.A., Kraemer, S.A., Yao, E.F., Armstrong, R.L., and Smith, W.L. (1989): J. Biol. Chem. (in press).
2. DeWitt, D.L., Meade, E.A., El-Harith, E.A., and Smith, W.L. (1989): In Platelets and Vascular Occlusion, Vol. 54, edited by C. Patrono and G.A. FitzGerald, pp. 109-118, Raven Press, New York.
3. DeWitt, D.L., and Smith, W. L. (1988): Proc. Natl. Acad. Sci. U.S.A., 85:1412-1416.

4. Dietz, R., Nastainczyk, W., and Ruf, H.H. (1988): Eur. J. Biochem., 171:321-328.
5. Hamberg, M., and Samuelsson, B. (1967): J. Biol. Chem., 242:5336-5343.
6. Humes, J.L., Winter, C.A., Sadowski, S.J., and Kuehl, F.A., Jr. (1981): Proc. Natl. Acad. Sci. U.S.A., 78:2053-2056.
7. Johnson, K.R., Nauseef, W.M., Care, A., Weelock, J.J., Shane, S., Hudson, S., Koeffler, H.P., Selsted, M., Miller, C., and Rovera, G. (1987): Nucleic Acids Res., 15:2013-2028.
8. Karthein, R., Dietz, R., Nastainczyk, W., and Ruf, H.H. (1988): Eur. J. Biochem., 171:313-320.
9. Kimura, S., and Ikeda-Saito, M. (1988): Proteins: Struc. Func. Gene., 3:113-120.
10. Kimura, S., Kotani, T., McBride, O.W., Umeki, K., Hirai, K., Nakayama, T., and Ohtaki, S. (1987): Proc. Natl. Acad. Sci. U.S.A., 84:5555-5559.
11. Kulmacz, R.J. (1989): J. Biol. Chem., 264:14136-14144.
12. Kulmacz, R.J., Tsai, A-L., and Palmer, G. (1987): J. Biol. Chem., 262:10524-10531.
13. Kunkel, T.A., Roberts, J.D., and Zakour, R.A. (1987): Meth. Enz., 154:9149-9154.
14. Lambeir, A-M., Markey, C.M., Dunford, H.B., and Marnett, L.J. (1985): J. Biol. Chem., 260:14894-14896.
15. Marnett, L.J., Chen, Y-N.P., Maddipati, K.R., Pie, P., and Labeque, R. (1988): J. Biol. Chem., 263:16532-16535.
16. Merlie, J.P., Fagan, D., Mudd, J., and Needleman, P. (1988): J. Biol. Chem., 263:3550-3553.
17. Miyamoto, T., Ogino, N., Yamamoto, S., and Hayaishi, O. (1976): J. Biol. Chem., 251:2629-2636.
18. Morishita, K., Kubota, N., Asono, S., Kaziro, Y., and Nagata, S. (1987): J. Biol. Chem., 262:3844-3851.
19. Ohki, S., Ogino, N., Yamamoto, S., and Hayaishi, O. (1979): J. Biol. Chem., 254:829-836.
20. Pagels, W.R., Sachs, R.J., Marnett, L.J., DeWitt, D.L., Day, J.A., and Smith, W.L. (1983): J. Biol. Chem., 258:6517-6523.
21. Poulos, T.L., Freer, S.T., Alden, R.A., Edwards, S.L., Skogland, U., Takio, K., Eriksson, B., Xuong, N-H. Yonetani, T., and Kraut, J. (1980): J. Biol. Chem., 255:575-580.
22. Rome, L.H., and Lands, W.E.M. (1975): Proc. Natl. Acad. Sci. U.S.A., 72:4863-4865.
23. Roth, G.J., Machuga, E.T., and Ozols, J. (1983): Biochemistry, 22:4672-4675.
24. Sokolowsky, M., Riordan, J.F., and Vallee, B.L. (1966): Biochemistry, 4, 1758-1764.
25. Van der Ouderaa, F.J., Buytenhek, M., Nugteren, D.H., and van Dorp, D.A. (1977): Biochim. Biophys. Acta, 487:315-331.
26. Welinder, K.G., and Mazza, G. (1977): Eur. J. Biochem., 73:353-358.
27. Yokoyama, C., Takai, T., and Tanabe, T. (1988): FEBS Lett., 231:347-351.

Advances in Prostaglandin, Thromboxane, and Leukotriene Research, Vol. 20, edited by B. Samuelsson et al. Raven Press, Ltd., New York © 1990.

REGULATION OF PROSTANOIDS SYNTHESIS IN HUMAN FIBROBLASTS AND HUMAN BLOOD MONOCYTES BY INTERLEUKIN-1, ENDOTOXIN, AND GLUCOCORTICOIDS

Amiram Raz, Angela Wyche, Jiyi Fu, Karen Seibert and Philip Needleman

Department of Pharmacology, Washington University School of Medicine, 660 S. Euclid Ave., St. Louis, MO 63110 USA

Modulation of prostaglandin production occurs either at the release of arachidonic acid from cellular phospholipids or during the cyclooxygenase-mediated conversion of arachidonate into prostaglandins. The Mϕ-derived monokine interleukin-1 (IL-1) stimulates formation of PGE_2 in fibroblasts (1,2) as well as formation of PGE_2 and other cyclooxygenase (COX) products in other cells. Fibroblast-produced PGE_2 may in turn feedback suppress Mϕ release of IL-1 (3-5) as well as Mϕ immune competency as judged by Ia antigen expression (6). Studies with human synovial cells (7) and rabbit chondrocytes (8) have indicated that IL-1 induced PGE_2 production is mediated via stimulation of phospholipase(s). Our studies with human dermal fibroblasts (9) have demonstrated that monocyte-conditioned media (which contains IL-1) produced increased V_{max} of COX that appeared to be dependent on new protein synthesis.

We employed a polyclonal antisera against sheep COX that cross-reacted with the human COX and permitted the selective and quantitative immunoprecipitation of [^{35}S]methionine COX from fibroblast cell sonicates, thus enabling us to quantitate changes in the turnover of COX (1).

Effect of IL-1 on Fibroblast Cyclooxygenase - The time-dependent IL-1 induction of fibroblast PGE_2 production and of new cyclooxygenase enzyme synthesis was assessed by assaying in parallel three different parameters: (a) PGE_2 released into the media; (b) cellular COX activity in the solubilized cell sonicate; and (c) the radioactivity in the COX band following [^{35}S]methionine labeling, immunoprecipitation, and SDS-PAGE electrophoresis. Within 6 hr of IL-1 addition, there is a 3-fold increase in the rate of COX synthesized as indicated by the increased [^{35}S]methionine incorporation into the COX band and parallel stimulation of COX activity. As little as 0.03 unit/ml of Il-1 caused significant stimulation of COX synthesis, half-maximal stimulation being at approximately 0.1 unit/ml, with maximal stimulation at 0.3 unit/ml (1). To estimate the COX turnover, cells preincubated with IL-1 for 16 hrs, were then labeled with [^{35}S]methionine for varying periods after which they were processed for immunoprecipitation and SDS-PAGE electrophoresis. Synthesis of [^{35}S]methionine COX increased gradually during 3 hr of labeling and was maximal at 6 hr (1). A theoretical half-life of 1 hr would yield 87.5% of maximal steady state labeling level after 3 hr (i.e., 3 half-lives). Contrasting this with the observed 85% of the maximal, steady state radioactivity after a three hour labeling period indicates that the half-life of fibroblast cyclooxygenase is approximately 1 hr. This conclusion is supported by our results from pulse-chase experiments (1).

TABLE 1. Effect of mRNA and protein synthesis inhibitors
on IL-1 stimulation of fibroblasts cyclooxygenase activity

Addition during first incubation (0-4 hrs)	Addition during second incubation (4-8 hrs)	COX activity pg PGE$_2$/μg protein/min (n=4)
(control)	- -	4.5 ± 0.4
IL-1 (0.3 unit/ml)	- -	29.6 ± 2.3*
IL-1	actinomycin D (1μM)	34.4 ± 4.5*
IL-1	cycloheximide (10 μM)	3.0 ± 0.6
IL-1 + actin. D	- -	2.4 ± 0.4

* Significantly different from control (p<0.01, t-test).

We next attempted to resolve the temporal sequence for IL-1 stimulation of COX synthesis into transcription and translation phases by the use of selective inhibitors. When fibroblasts were incubated for 3-4 hr with IL-1, only a small increase (30-40%) in PGE$_2$ production was observed. Cellular COX activity at the end of this initial incubation was increased by only 50-100% in the IL-1-treated cells. However, following further incubation for 4 hr in the absence of IL-1, a dramatic 5-fold increase in COX activity is observed (Table 1). Inhibition of transcription with actinomycin D during the initial 4 hr blocked subsequent induction of COX activity, as well as [^{35}S]COX production (Fig. 4), whereas the presence of actinomycin D during the second incubation period (4-8 hr) did not affect COX induction or PGE$_2$ synthesis (Table 1). Addition of the translation inhibitor cycloheximide during the second incubation period produced total inhibition.

IL-1 Induction of COX Synthesis is Mediated via Activation of Protein Kinase C. Phorbol myristate acetate (PMA), a tumor promoter and potent protein kinase C (PKC) activator, was found to produce a significant, albeit modest, increase in COX activity (Table 2) and in the synthetic rate of newly formed ^{35}S-labeled enzyme (10). This PMA effect was dose-dependent in the 1-100 nM range and blocked by cycloheximide or actinomycin D if added together with PMA. Addition of PMA together with IL-1 produced a marked synergistic stimulation of COX induction (Table 2). We employed protein kinase inhibitors to evaluate the possible role of PKC in mediating IL-1 stimulation of COX. We used the PKC inhibitor H-7 and compared its effect to that of the non-PKC inhibitor HA1004. The results (Fig. 1) showed that H-7, but not HA1004, totally inhibited the stimulatory effect of IL-1 on COX activity and mass. Similar effects to those of H-7 were also observed with 25 nM staurosporine, a highly potent inhibitor of PKC. H-7 was found to exert its inhibition of COX when added during the initial 4 hr incubation (presumed transcription phase) but to have no effect if added during the presumed translation phase (Fig. 1). Therefore, we conclude that the IL-1 signal transduction mechanism to induce COX synthesis involves a critical step in which activation of PKC is required.

TABLE 2. IL-1 Induction of Fibroblast Cyclooxygenase: Effect of PMA

Agent	Cyclooxygenase Activity Pg PGE_2/μg protein/10 min
IL-1 (1 unit/ml)	58 ± 8*
PMA (10^{-7} M)	355 ± 36
IL-1 + PMA	99 ± 16
	765 ± 113

* Mean ± SEM (n=4)

Anti-inflammatory Glucocorticoids Inhibit COX Synthesis. Following the initial report by Pash and Bailey (11) on the apparent dexamethasone (DEX) blockade of COX synthesis in vascular smooth muscle cells, we carried out detailed studies on the effect of glucocorticoids on fibroblast COX. Addition of DEX (2 μM) throughout the entire transcription-translation sequence produced a marked inhibition of IL-1-stimulated COX activity (Fig. 2). In subsequent experiments, we found that the full inhibitory effect of the steroid was obtained when it was added only during the presumed translational period (i.e., 4-8 hr). DEX is a highly potent inhibitor of COX synthesis (>92% inhibition at 20 nM; IC_{50} of ≈1 nM) (10). Non-glucocorticoid steroids do not affect COX synthesis. The DEX-induced effect was completely reversed by actinomycin D (Fig. 3, panel A), suggesting that it involves the synthesis of one or more new proteins.

Can the stimulatory effect of IL-1 and the inhibitory effect of dexamethasone be demonstrated at the level of cellular mRNA? To answer this, we prepared total RNA from FB pretreated with IL-1 with or without DEX and used the RNA for *in vitro* translation experiments employing a rabbit reticulocyte lysate kit. The results of these studies (Fig. 3, Panel B) are in complete agreement with those obtained for ^{35}S-COX synthesized by intact cells (Fig. 3, Panel A). Thus both the stimulatory effect of IL-1 and the suppressing effect by DEX appears to be due to up-regulation or down-regulation, respectively, of COX mRNA.

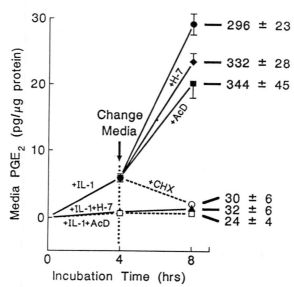

FIG. 1. <u>PKC inhibitors block IL-1-induction of COX synthesis.</u> Fibroblasts were initially incubated for 4 hrs with IL-1 (0.3 μ/ml) in the absence or presence of actinomycin (1 μM), H-7 (15 μM) or HA 1004 (15 μM). The cells were then washed and fresh DMEM media added with or without the same agents, as indicated in the figure, and the cells incubated for additional 4 hrs. PGE_2 released into the media is plotted on the Y axis and values for COX activity at the 8 hr time point are given for each sample. Modified figure from ref. 10.

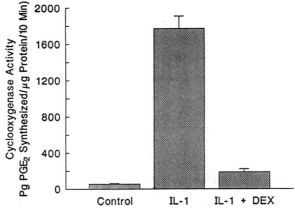

FIG. 2. <u>Dexamethasone (DEX) inhibition of COX synthesis.</u> Cells were first incubated for 4 hrs with either no DEX or IL-1 ("control"); with IL-1 (0.3 unit/ml) ("IL-1") or with both IL-1 and DEX (2 μM) ("IL-1 + DEX"). The cells were then washed with DMEM and incubated for 10 hrs without DEX ("control", "IL-1") or with DEX ("IL-1 + DEX") and COX activity of cell sonicate samples was then determined.

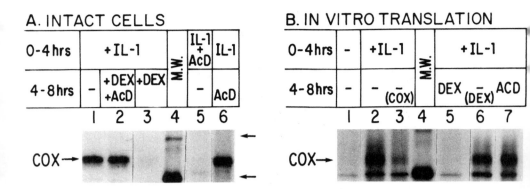

FIG. 3. <u>IL-1 and DEX regulation of COX synthesis: In vitro translation experiments.</u> Fibroblasts were incubated according to a two period protocol in the absence or presence of IL-1 (0.3 u/ml); DEX (40 nM), and actinomycin D (AcD, 1 μM). Some of the cells were then labelled with ^{35}S-methionine and cell sonicates then subjected to immunoprecipitation and SDS-PAGE electrophoresis (Panel A, from ref. 10). In parallel cell samples, total RNA was isolated by standard methods and used together with rabbit reticulocytes lysate kit for *in vitro* translation incubation (Panel B).

We have recently begun studies on the regulation of COX synthesis in monocytes/Mϕ. Studies by others have shown that bacterial lipopolysaccharide (LPS) can stimulate PGE$_2$ and TxB$_2$ production by blood monocytes and peritoneal Mϕ. In studies we performed, LPS dose-dependently (0.01-1 μg/ml) stimulated the COX activity and the rate of ^{35}S-COX synthesis. DEX inhibited monocytes COX activity but did not affect Tx-synthase activity (Table 3) or prostacyclin synthase (not shown).

The inhibitory effect of DEX on COX activity and thus prostanoid synthesis is novel and distinct from other inhibitory effects of DEX on eicosanoids production which are mediated very acylhydrolase(s) blockade. The relative contribution of the COX inhibition vs. acylhydrolase inhibition to the overall blockade of prostanoid generation by glucocorticoids under physiological and pathophysiological situations remains to be elucidated.

TABLE 3.   DEX inhibits COX synthesis in human blood monocytes.*

Sample	Media PGE$_2$ pg/μg protein	COX Activity pg/min PGE$_2$/ μg protein	Media TxA$_2$ pg/μg protein	Tx-Synthase Activity pg TxB$_2$/μg protein/min
Control	8 ± 2	24 ± 6	30 ± 10	185 ± 24
LPS	255 ± 52	110 ± 12	2850 ± 180	149 ± 88
LPS + DEX	30 ± 4	23 ± 4	630 ± 65	205 ± 18

*Human blood monocytes fraction was allowed to adhere for 2 hrs in DME containing 1% FBS. Non-adherent cells were then removed and adhering cells incubated for 24 hrs with LPS in the absence or presence of DEX (40 nM). At the end of the incubation, COX activity was assayed by adding arachidonic acid (30 μM) plus BSA (1 mg/ml) for 10 min and determining PGE$_2$ produced. Tx synthase activity was assayed by incubating parallel samples with PGH$_2$ (5 μM) for 1 min and assaying for TxB$_2$ generated. Values are Mean ± SEM (n=3).

ACKNOWLEDGEMENT

This work was supported by National Institutes of Health Grants PO1-DK3811 and RO1-HL20787.

REFERENCES

1.   Raz A, Wyche A, Needleman P. J. Biol. Chem. 1988; 263:3022-3028.
2.   Albrightson CR, Baenziger NL, Needleman P. J. Immunol. 1985; 135:1872-1877.
3.   Boraschi D, Censini S, and Tagliabue A. J. Immunol. 1984; 133:764-768.
4.   Zucali JR, Dinarello CA, Oblon DJ, Gross MA, Anderson L, Wiener RS. J. Clin. Invest. 1986: 77:1857-1863.
5.   Kunkel SL, Chensue SW, and Phan SH. J. Immunol. 1986: 136:186-190.
6.   Snyder DS, Beller DI, and Unanue ER. Nature 1982: 299:163-165.
7.   Godfrey RW, Johnson WJ, Hoffstein ST. 1987; Biochem. Biophys. Res. Commun. 142:235-241.
8.   Chang J, Gilman SC, Lewis AJ. J. Immunol. 1986; 136:1283-1287.
9.   Jonas-Whitely PE, Needleman P. J. Clin. Invest. 1984; 74:2249-2253.
10.   Raz A, Wyche A, and Needleman P. Proc. Natl. Acad. Sci. USA 1989: 86:1657-1661.
11.   Pash JH, and Bailey JM. FASEB J. 2:2613-2618, 1988.

Advances in Prostaglandin, Thromboxane,
and Leukotriene Research, Vol. 20,
edited by B. Samuelsson et al.
Raven Press, Ltd., New York © 1990.

The Regulation of 5-Lipoxygenase Activity in Rat Basophilic Leukemia Cells

Angela Wong, Shing Mei Hwang and Michael N. Cook

Department of Cell Biology, Smith Kline & French Laboratories,
King of Prussia, PA 19406

INTRODUCTION

5-Lipoxygenase catalyzes the first two steps in the biosynthesis of the leukotrienes. These include the oxygenation of free arachidonic acid (AA) to form 5-hydroperoxy-6,8,11,14-eicosatetrenoic acid (5HPETE) followed by the subsequent conversion of 5HPETE to 5,6-oxido-7,9,11,14-eicosatetraenoic acid (LTA_4) (1,2,3). The LTA_4 is in turn converted to a variety of products including leukotriene B_4 and the peptidoleukotrienes (LTC_4, LTD_4 and LTE_4) (4,5). In addition, the enzyme is involved in the biosynthesis of the lipoxins through the oxidation of 15HPETE (6). Because of their biological activities, leukotrienes and lipoxins are believed to have an important role in the pathophysiology of a variety of inflammatory and allergic responses (7).

For many years, regulation of 5-lipoxygenase activity in intact cells remains an interesting topic. It is known that cellular activation by calcium ionophore A23187 induces the synthesis of leukotriene. This implies that a Ca^{2+}-sensitive component(s) initiates leukotriene synthesis. Since the cytosolic 5-lipoxygenase is activated *in vitro* by Ca^{2+} (8,9), it is likely that the ionophore effect is mediated at least in part, by an activation of the enzyme. Parallel to the leukotriene synthesis is the changes in subcellular localization of 5-lipoxygenase: the enzyme translocates from cytosol to membranes (10,11). The nature of the membrane translocation and its physiological relevance are not yet understood. Considering the abundance of arachidonic acid in the membranes, the binding of 5-lipoxygenase to membranes may facilitate the access of the enzyme to substrate that is being released from phospholipid stores. Furthermore, the product of the 5-lipoxygenase catalyzed reaction, LTA_4, is in close proximity to the next enzyme of the pathway, LTC_4 synthetase, which is also membrane bound.

In this chapter, we shall summarize our recent results on the regulation of membrane-association of the enzyme. Possible mechanisms that may account for the enzyme translocation in intact cells will be discussed.

METHODS

Cell Culture. Rat basophilic leukemia cells (RBL-2H3) were maintained as monolayer cultures in Eagle's essential medium supplemented with 16% fetal calf serum as described. To obtain spinner cultures, cells were harvested by trypsinization and diluted with the culture medium to 0.2×10^6 cells/ml. Cell were grown for 2 days to reach a density of $0.7-1.0 \times 10^6$ cells/ml.

Cell Activation and Preparation of Subcellular Fractions. Cells were centrifuged (200 x g, 10 min), washed once with 5 mM Hepes, pH 7.4, 140 mM NaCl, 5 mM KCl, 0.6 mM $MgCl_2$, 5 mM glucose, 1 mM Ca^{2+} (buffer A), and was resuspended in the same medium at 1.0×10^6 cells/ml. Six milliliter of the cell suspension was treated with calcium ionophore A23187 (0, 10, 30, 100, 300 and 1000 nM) at 37 °C for various times. The cells were then harvested by centrifugation (200 x g, 10 min). The supernatant was removed and set aside for assaying the synthesis of 5-lipoxygenase products using RP-HPLC. Cells were resuspended in 0.3 ml of 10 mM Hepes, pH 7.4, 150 mM NaCl, 1 mM EDTA (Buffer B) and lysed by sonication. The cell homogenate was centrifuged at 800 x g for 10 min and the resulting supernatant was recentrifuged at 35,000 x g for 20 min. The pellet was rinsed on the surface with 3 ml of ice cold buffer B. The 35,000 x g supernatant and pellet obtained were described as the soluble and particulate fraction, respectively. The 5-lipoxygenase present in the two fractions were examined with both activity assays and western blots. A polyclonal antibody raised against the purified RBL-5-lipoxygenase was used. Preparation of the antibody and western blots were described in previous studies (11). Quantitation of the amount of 5-lipoxygenase in the fractions was performed as described (10) with some modifications.

RESULTS and DISCUSSION

We have selected the RBL-2H3 cells as our model system to study the cellular regulation process that takes place during leukotriene biosynthesis. The cell shares many of the properties of mast cells and responds to the crosslinking of immunoglobulin E receptors (12). Unstimulated RBL-2H3 cells produce undetectable amount of leukotriene. Addition of the calcium ionophore A23187 to cells induces the production and release of 5-lipoxygenase metabolites in a dose and time-dependent manner. The 5-lipoxygenase products include LTC_4, LTD_4, LTB_4, Δ^6-transLTB$_4$ and $5S, 12S$-DiHETE (Table 1). Maximal 5-lipoxygenase product formation (74 ± 9 pmols/10^6 cells, n= 4) was obtained at 100 nM ionophore. The products were detected within 2 min and reached peak level at 7.5 min.

Table1. <u>5-Lipoxygenase products synthesized from calcium ionophore
A23187-stimulated RBL-2H3 cells</u>[a]

5LO Products	pmols[b]
LTC_4	11.7 ± 1.2
LTD_4	19.3 ± 7.5
Δ^6 transLTB$_4$	76.0 ± 12.3
DiHETE	22.3 ± 2.1

[a] RBL-2H3 cells (6×10^6 cells) were incubated 20 min at 37 °C with 100 nM calcium ionophore. The cells were then harvested by centrifugation. The supernatant was mixed with equal volume of ice-cold acetonitrile. The samples were dried and analyzed by RP-HPLC (column: Radial-Pak C18).
[b] $n = 3$.

Accompanying the synthesis of leukotrienes was the translocation of enzyme from soluble to particulate fraction (Fig. 1). In unstimulated cells, 5-lipoxygenase presents in the soluble fraction. Upon stimulation by the ionophore (100 nM), there was a 65% loss of enzyme activity from the soluble fraction. Approximately 80% of the decrease in soluble 5-lipoxygenase activity was due to a loss of 5-lipoxygenase protein (as determined by western blot) and, to a small extent (20%), enzyme inactivation. The particulate enzyme obtained from ionophore treated cells was catalytically inactive and could not be extracted by EDTA or KCl. In view of the magnitude of the translocation and the tightness of the 5-lipoxygenase-membrane binding, it is likely that the membrane association is not an artifact of cell homogenization.

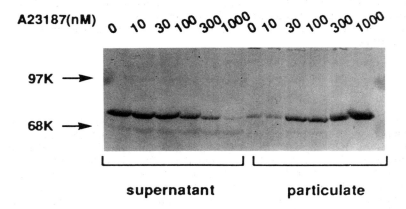

FIG. 1. Dose dependency of calcium ionophore A23187 on the translocation of 5-lipoxygenase. Cells (10^6 cells/ml) were incubated 20 min at 37 °C with various concentrations of A23187. 5-Lipoxygenase present in the soluble (35,000 x g supernatant) and the particulate fractions (35,000 x g pellet) were determined by western blot. The results shown were representative of at least three experiments.

Identification of the Regulatory Factors of Membrane Translocation

Calcium. As enzyme translocation requires stimulation by the calcium ionophore, we have examined the effect of Ca^{2+} on stimulating membrane binding of 5-lipoxygenase. When cells were lysed in buffers containing increasing concentrations of free Ca^{2+} (0.05-10 μM), there was a gradual decrease in soluble 5-lipoxygenase (Fig. 2). At 10 μM of Ca^{2+}, there was an approximately 80% decrease in the soluble enzyme protein which is similar to the percentage of enzyme activity loss (data not shown). These changes are paralleled with an increase in the amount of particulate associated 5-lipoxygenase protein (Fig. 2). The particulate-associated enzyme is active and behaves similarly to the cytosolic enzyme in exhibiting suicidal inactivation and requirement for Ca^{2+} and ATP for maximal activity (data not shown).

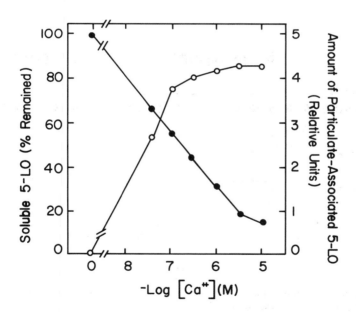

FIG.2. Relative distribution of 5-lipoxygenase when cells were lysed in Ca^{2+}-containing media. Cells(20 x 10^6 cells/ml) were lysed in 5 mM Hepes buffer, pH 7.6, containing various concentrations of free Ca^{2+} (0.05-10 μM). The apparent free Ca^{2+} concentrations in solutions containing EGTA were calculated as described by Bartfai (13), using a K_a value of 8.04 x 10^7 M^{-1} for Ca-EGTA at pH 7.6. 5-Lipoxygenase was determined in the soluble (35,000 x g supernatant) (-●-) and particulate fractions (35,000 x g pellet) (-0-) by western blot.

Therefore, although the membrane-binding of 5-lipoxygenase obtained in the ionophore-treated cells and in cell free system are both Ca^{2+}-mediated, differences exist between their particulate-associated enzymes. It is possible that in intact cells, the ionophore stimulates other component(s) in addition to an increase in cytosolic free Ca^{2+} to produce an inactivated, EDTA-nonextractable membrane-bound enzyme.

Arachidonic Acid. Among the intracellular activities that are sensitive to the cytosolic Ca^{2+} concentration and might, therefore, transduce the Ca^{2+} with a functional response is the phospholipase(s). When cells are stimulated with calcium ionophore, the activated phospholipase liberates arachidonic acid (AA) from the membrane phospholipid stores which may be utilized by the 5-lipoxygenase. The enzyme undergoes suicide inactivation and becomes tightly bound to the membranes.

AA is not effective in inducing membrane association of 5-lipoxygenase when added in cell homogenate containing 1 mM EDTA (Fig. 3B, EDTA, 10 and 20 μM AA). However, it stabilizes the Ca^{2+}-induced, EDTA-reversible membrane association of the enzyme. This is illustrated by the following experiment.

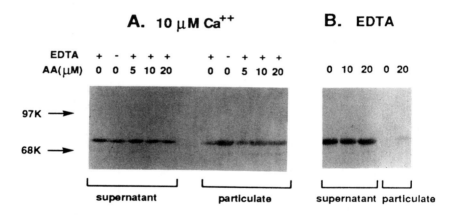

FIG. 3. Effects of arachidonic acid on the membrane-association of 5-lipoxygenase. **A.** Arachidonic acid (0, 5, 10, 20 μM) was added into cell homogenate (20 x 10^6 cells/ml) containing 10 μM Ca^{2+}. Samples were incubated 10 min at 20 °C before the addition of 5 mM EDTA. The homogenate was centrifuged (35,000 x g, 20 min) and the relative distribution of 5-lipoxygenase between the soluble and particulate fractions was examined by western blot. **B.** Cell homogenate (20 x 10^6 cells/ml) containing 1 mM EDTA was incubated with various concentrations of arachidonic acid (0, 10, 20 μM). 5-Lipoxygenase was determined in the resulting soluble and particulate fractions.

Cells were lysed in the presence of 10 µM Ca^{2+}. The cell homogenate was incubated (20 °C, 10 min) with various concentrations of AA (0, 5, 10 and 20 µM). EDTA (5 mM) was then added. The samples were centrifuged (35,000 x g, 20 min) and the relative distribution of 5-lipoxygenase between the soluble and particulate fractions were examined by western blots. Fig. 3A shows that when cells were lysed in 10 µM Ca^{2+}, 60% of their cellular 5-lipoxygenase protein became particulate-associated (lane: -EDTA; 0 AA; supernatant and particulate). To maintain this association, the continued presence of Ca^{2+} is required, since addition of EDTA to the cell homogenate inhibit the particulate-association of the enzyme (lane: +EDTA; 0 AA; supernatant and particulate). However, if the cell homogenate was incubated with 10 or 20 µM AA before the addition of EDTA, increased 5-lipoxygenase protein was recovered in the particulate fraction (lane: +EDTA; 10 and 20 AA; particulate). Parallel to this change is the decrease of enzyme protein in the supernatant (lane: +EDTA; 10 and 20 AA; supernatant). This suggests that AA acts complementarily with Ca^{2+} to induce an irreversible membrane-binding of the enzyme.

In summary, the results presented here suggest that stimulation of RBL-2H3 cells with calcium ionophore results in leukotriene synthesis and membrane translocation of 5-lipoxygenase. The particulate associated enzyme is inactive and cannot be extracted by EDTA. Two factors may be involved in mediating this process. Firstly, Ca^{2+} at 0.5-10 µM, induces reversible binding of active 5-lipoxygenase to the membranes. Secondly, AA stabilizes the Ca^{2+}-induced membrane association.

Acknowledgement

The authors like to thank Dr. Paul Marshall for critically reviewing the manuscript.

REFERENCES

1. Borgeat, P., and Samuelsson, B. (1979): *Proc. Natl. Acad. Sci. USA,* 76: 3213-3217.
2. Hammarstrom, S., Murphy, R. C., Samuelsson, B., Clark, D. A., Mioskowski, C., and Corey, E. J. (1979): *Biochem. Biophys. Res. Commun.,* 91: 1266-1272.
3. Radmark, O., Malmsten, C., Samuelsson, B., Goto, G., Marfat, A., and Corey, E. J. (1980): *J. Biol. Chem.,* 255: 11828-11831.
4. Maycock, A. L., Anderson, M. S., Desousa, D. M., and Kuehl, F. A., Jr. (1982): *J. Biol. Chem.,* 257: 13911-13914.
5. Maas, R. L., Ingram, C. D., Taker, D. F., Oates, F. A., and Brash, A. R. (1982): *J. Biol. Chem.,* 257: 13515-13519.
6. Serhan, C. N., Hamberg, M., and Samuelsson, B. (1984): *Proc. Natl. Acad. Sci. USA,* 81: 5335-5339.
7. Samuelsson, B. (1983): *Science,* 220: 568-575.
8. Jakschik, B. A., Sun, F. F., and Steinhoff, M. M. (1980): *Biochem. Biophys. Res. Commun.,* 95: 103-110.

9. Ochi, K., Yoshimoto, T., and Yammamoto, S. (1983): *J. Biol. Chem.*, 258: 5754-5758.
10. Rouzer, C. A., and Kargman, S. (1988): *J. Biol. Chem.*, 263: 10980-10988.
11. Wong, A., Hwang, S. M., Cook, M. N., Hogaboom, G. K., and Crooke, S. T. (1988): *Biochemistry*, 27: 6763-6769.
12. Barsumian, E. L., Isersky, C., Petrino, M. G., and Siraganian, R. P. (1981): *Eur. J. Immunol.*, 11: 317-323.
13. Bartfai, T. (1979): *Adv. Cyclic Nucleotide Res.*, 10: 219-242.

Advances in Prostaglandin, Thromboxane, and Leukotriene Research, Vol. 20,
edited by B. Samuelsson et al.
Raven Press, Ltd., New York © 1990.

PROPERTIES OF LEUKOTRIENE A_4-HYDROLASE

Olof Rådmark and Jesper Haeggström

Department of Physiological Chemistry
Karolinska Institutet
S-10401 Stockholm, Sweden

Leukotriene A_4-hydrolase (LTA_4-hydrolase) catalyzes the enzymatic hydrolysis of the allylic epoxide LTA_4 (5(S)6(R)-oxido-7,9-trans11,14-cis-eicosatetraenoic acid) to the chemotactic 5,12-dihydroxyacid leukotriene B_4 (LTB_4, 5(S),12(R)-dihydroxy-6,14-cis-8,10-trans-eicosatetraenoic acid) (1). Previously characterized epoxide hydrolases, primarily connected with detoxification of xenobiotics, produce vicinal diols. Thus already the nature of the reaction catalyzed separates LTA_4-hydrolase from other epoxide hydrolases.

Physical properties.

LTA_4-hydrolase, a stable soluble protein with a M_r close close to 70.000 was originally purified by relatively simple procedures from human leukocytes (2) and rat neutrophils (3). Subsequently this enzyme has been isolated also from human erythrocytes (4), human lung (5), guinea pig liver (6), and guinea pig lung (7). LTA_4-hydrolases from the different sources appear to be similar both regarding physical and catalytic properties, see table 1. Thus, also the enzyme in human erythrocytes appeared to have a M_r close to 70.000, as judged from Western blots. Erythrocyte LTA_4-hydrolase was previously reported to have a M_r of 54.000. This could be a product of proteolysis (8), possibly with retained enzymatic activity.

In addition, the existence of a heat-labile factor in human liver microsomes, capable of converting LTA_4 to LTB_4 has been described (9). The possible similarity between this factor and cytosolic LTA_4 hydrolase is unclear.

TABLE 1

Properties of LTA$_4$-hydrolase

	Human leukocyte	Rat neutrophils	Human erythrocyte	Human lung	Guinea pig liver	Guinea pig lung
M_r kD SDS-PAGE	68-70	68	54±1[1]	68-71	67-70	70
M_r kD gelfiltr.	48-49	50		49-51	42-46	42-45
pI	5.1-5.7		4.9±0.2	5.1-5.3	6.2[2]	5.7[2]
pH-opt.	8-9	7-8	7-8		8	7.6-8.9
K_m µM	20-30	20-30	7-36	13-14	7(27)[3]	17
V_{max} µmol/mg/min	1.7	0.3		2-3	10(68)[3]	4.3
Inact. by LTA$_4$	+	+	+	+	+	

The data in this table was from refs 2-7 and 11.

[1] In Western blots M_r was the same as for human leukocyte LTA$_4$-hydrolase (Rådmark, Haeggström and Fitzpatrick, unpublished).

[2] pI values for DTT-treated guinea pig enzymes. Without DTT, several forms exist (6,7).

[3] Data within parentheses were obtained from Arrhenius plots (7).

Catalytic properties

Cytosolic LTA$_4$-hydrolase is active as a monomer and there is no cofactor requirement. The time course of the hydrolysis of LTA$_4$ to LTB$_4$ displays some distinct features. As shown in Fig. 1 it is characterized by a steep initial rise in product which levels off within 30 seconds, after which no more LTB_4 appears. The instability of LTA_4 in aqueous solution (the half-life at pH 7 at 37° C is less than 10 sec (10)) is certainly a major reason for this phenomenon. The observed self-inactivation of LTA_4-hydrolase (4,11) could also contribute. Thus, after a sufficiently high initial dose of LTA_4, a second dose is converted much less efficiently (Fig 1). However, this self-inactivation did not occur to the same extent when low doses of LTA_4 were given repeatedly to a batch of enzyme.

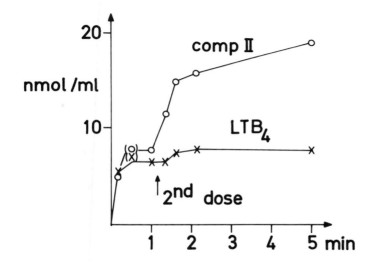

Fig 1
Time course of LTA_4-hydrolase. LTA_4 was added twice (to give 85 µM at zero and 1.1 min) to a semipurified batch of human leukocyte LTA_4-hydrolase (85 µg/ml, 2 ml). Aliquots of the incubation mixture (250 µl) was removed at the indicated time intervals and analyzed by HPLC for the hydrolysis products of LTA_4.

The result of such an experiment is shown in Fig 2. After the first and second doses of LTA_4 equal amounts of LTB_4 were formed, hereafter the amounts gradually decreased, but the appearance of product was never completely abolished in this series of incubations. Whether the self-inactivation of LTA_4-hydrolase could have any regulatory function regarding

LTB$_4$ formation in vivo would thus depend on the LTA$_4$ concentrations reached in living cells. An interesting finding in this context was the demonstration of covalent binding of LTA$_4$ to the enzyme (11,12). This irreversible reaction between enzyme and part of the substrate has been suggested to account for the self-inactivation of LTA$_4$-hydrolase.

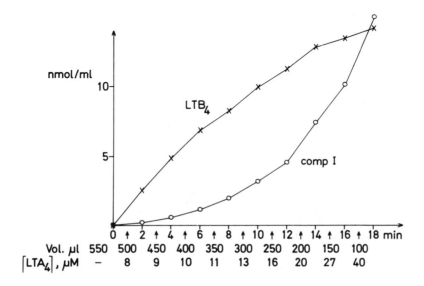

Fig 2
Time course of LTA$_4$-hydrolase at 37^{0}C. LTA$_4$ was added repeatedly (4 nmol at each arrow) to a purified batch of LTA$_4$ hydrolase (5 µg/ml, 550 µl). Between the substrate additions aliquots (50 µl) were removed and analyzed by HPLC for the hydrolysis products of LTA$_4$. The LTA$_4$ concentrations on the x-axis are the concentrations reached after each single addition of 4 nmol LTA$_4$. Since the volume decreased gradually, these concentrations increased succesively.

5-lipoxygenase which provides the substrate for LTA$_4$-hydrolase has been shown to associate with the microsomal fraction upon stimulation of human neutrophils (14,15) or rat basophilic leukaemia cells (16) with the calcium ionophore A23187. We have tried the possible association also of LTA$_4$-hydrolase with the membrane fraction of human leukocytes, either after incubation of intact cells with ionophore A23187, or following homogenization in buffers containing calcium. No membrane association was detectable, either by screening for LTA$_4$-hydrolase activity or using immunochemical methods.

Activation of LTA$_4$-hydrolase by phosphorylation was suggested since phorbol-12-myristate-13-acetate doubled the LTB$_4$-production in human neutrophils stimulated by fMLP (17). This could not be confirmed in vitro however, since LTA$_4$-hydrolase was a poor substrate for protein kinase C purified from human placenta (Haeggström, J. and Hansson, A., unpublished).

The LTA$_4$-hydrolase catalysis apparently conforms to Michaelis & Menten kinetics and K$_m$ and v$_{max}$ have been determined. However, correct analysis of these constants depends on accurate determinations of the initial linear reaction velocities, which is difficult in the case of LTA$_4$-hydrolase because of the instability of the substrate and selfinactivation of the enzyme. This could explain the distribution of K$_m$- (7-36 µM) and v$_{max}$-values (0.3 - 3 µmol/ /mg/min) which have been published for the human enzyme preparations.

Specific properties of guinea pig LTA$_4$-hydrolase

LTA$_4$ is more stable at lower temperatures and this was utilized when the kinetics of LTA$_4$-hydrolase from guinea pig liver were analyzed (6). In this case incubation series were performed at -10°C, ±0°C and 10°C. Extrapolation according to Arrhenius gave a K$_m$ of 27 µM and a v$_{max}$ of 68 µmol/mg/min. Also conventional v$_{max}$ determination for the guinea pig enzyme gave a high value (10 µmol/mg/min) compared to the human enzyme. This higher activity of the guinea pig enzyme is assumed to depend on structural differencies between the enzymes from different species. Thus, the pI was higher for guinea pig LTA$_4$-hydrolases, and the presence of a reducing agent was required in order to obtain homogeneous proteins in the purifications which could indicate a different number and distribution of cys-residues (6,7). Nevertheless, LTA$_4$-hydrolases from the two different species (human and guinea pig) probably display considerable homology, since only two amino acids of 20 in the aminoterminal sequences were different. Also, both proteins reacted similarly to an antiserum raised to human leukocyte LTA$_4$-hydrolase (8).

Substrate specificity

A number of other substrates have been tried with LTA$_4$-hydrolase, mostly eicosanoid-epoxides but also some xenobiotics, see Fig 3. Only LTA$_5$ was hydrolyzed with a velocity comparable to that of LTA$_4$ (about 40%). However, the enzyme was less discriminative regarding inactivation. Here, several of the substances that were not accepted as substrates could inhibit subsequent hydrolysis of LTA$_4$. An allylic epoxide moiety appeared sufficient for this inhibition. However, the relationship between the epoxide and the carboxylic acid function, or if the carboxylic acid was methylated, seemed less important.

Distribution

The distribution of LTA$_4$-hydrolase in different cells and tissues is much wider than for 5-lipoxygenase. Besides in leukocytes, LTA$_4$ - hydrolase was first demonstrated in plasma (18), and subsequently it has been found almost in all tissues tested from guinea pig, rat and human (8, 19-27). In studies of cultured cells, LTA$_4$-hydrolase was found in lymphocytes (28-30), endothelial cells (31) and in fibroblasts (32). Interestingly, the LTA$_4$-hydrolase content of SV-40 transformed fibroblasts was three-fold higher as compared to normal diploid cells. 5-lipoxygenase was undetectable in all cases. Since other functions for LTA$_4$-hydrolase are unknown this can be taken as additional evidence for the occurrence of transcellular metabolism of LTA$_4$ in vivo. The significance of the wide occurrence of LTA$_4$-hydrolase should be to increase the overall LTB$_4$ formation within, and thus the recruitment of more leukocytes to, sites of recently initiated acute inflammation. However, it is also possible that formation of LTB$_4$ in lymphocytes is of relevance for these particular cells, since LTB$_4$ augments activation and differentiation of human B-cells (33). Regarding fibroblasts, the growth of human diploid fibroblasts in culture was stimulated by LTB$_4$ (Larsson, O. personal communication), and LTB$_4$ also stimulates fibroblast chemotaxis (34).

		Substrate	Inhibitor
	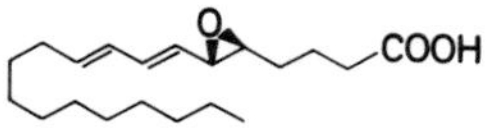 ~~~O~~ COOH	−	+ + +
LTA₃	~~~O~~ COOH	(+)	+ + +
LTA₄	~~~O~~ COOH	+ + +	+ + +
LTA₅	~~~O~~ COOH	+	+ + +
	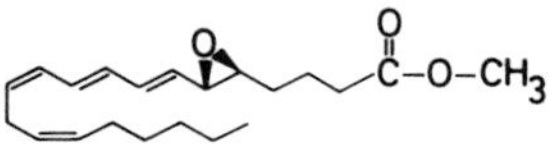 ~~~O~~ C-O-CH₃	−	+ + +
	~~O~~ COOH	−	+ + +
	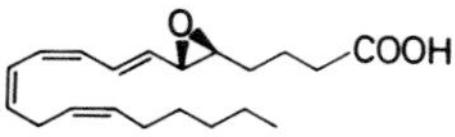 ~~~O~~ COOH	−	+ + +
	~~O~~ COOH	−	−
14,15-LTA₄	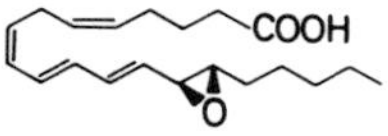 ~~~O~~ COOH	−	+ + +
11,12-EET	~~~O~~ COOH	−	−
14,15-EET	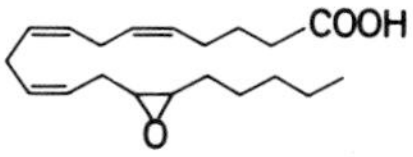 ~~~O~~ COOH	−	−
trans-stilbene oxide	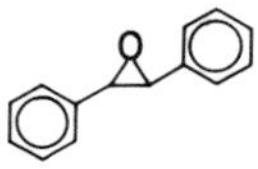	−	(+)
styrene oxide	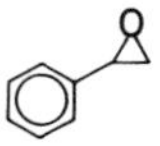	−	−

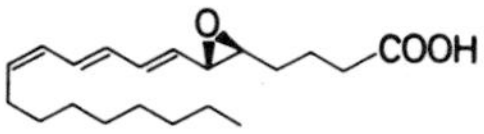

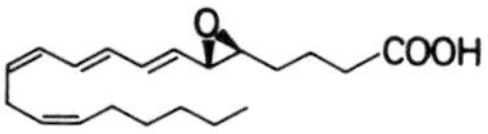

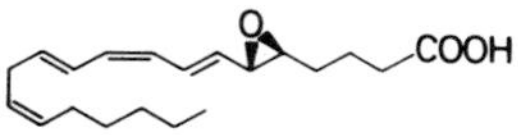

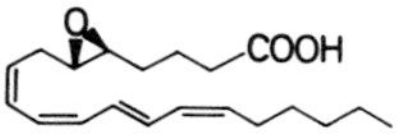

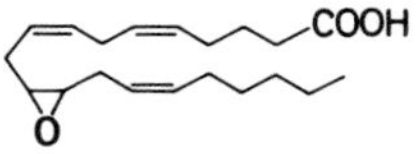

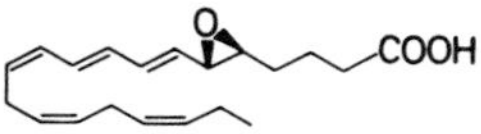

Fig 3

Substrate specificity of LTA₄-hydrolase. The conversion of various compounds, as well as their ability to inactivate LTA₄ hydrolase are indicated. The data were collected from references 11-13, 2, 5 and 4.

Cloning of cDNA

Clones corresponding to human LTA_4-hydrolase have been isolated from placenta and spleen cDNA libraries (35,36). In both cases a mature protein of 610 amino acids could be deduced. Secondary structure predictions and calculations of hydropathy revealed mixed patterns as for most proteins. A segment between residues 165-240 was of particular interest. Within this stretch, both the most hydrophilic part (170-185) and the most hydrophobic part (190-205) were located. Between these, one of two strong predictions for a reverse turn was found, followed by a predicted β-strand. Also an α-helix was predicted between residues 220-240. These, plus some additional features thus focus on the segment 165-240 which could be related to the structure and function of LTA_4-hydrolase. A cys-residue at pos 199, within the most hydrophobic part of the protein, was of particular interest, since its thiol group could mediate the covalent binding of LTA_4, which has been suggested to account for the self-inactivation of LTA_4 hydrolase. Expression of recombinant LTA_4-hydrolase (37) combined with in vitro mutagenesis should clarify such speculations.

The predicted protein sequence of human LTA_4-hydrolase did not display any homologies with microsomal epoxide hydrolases from rat or rabbit liver, or any other known proteins. Cytosolic epoxide hydrolase has not been sequenced, but this enzyme converts LTA_4 to another product, i.e 5(S),6(R)-dihydroxy-7,9-trans-11,14-cis-eicosatetraenoic acid (38) and there was no immunologic cross-reactivity with LTA_4 hydrolase (8). In addition, these liver epoxide hydrolases have wide substrate specificities and act on several, both endogeneous and xenobiotic, epoxides to give vicinal diols, while LTA_4-hydrolase only catalyzes the hydrolysis of LTA_4 to the chemotactic 5,12-dihydroxyacid LTB_4.

Acknowledgements. These studies were supported by grants from the Swedish Medical Research Council (03X-217, 03X-7467), from the Konung Gustaf V 80-årsfond, from Hedlunds Stiftelse, from Magnus Bergwalls Stiftelse and from O.E. and Edla Johanssons Stiftelse.

References

1. Samuelsson, B. (1983) Science 220, 568-575.
2. Rådmark,O., Shimizu, T., Jörnvall, H. and Samuelsson, B. (1984) J. Biol. Chem. 259, 12339-12345.
3. Evans, J.F., Dupuis, P. and Ford-Hutchinson, A.W. (1985) Biochim. Biophys. Acta 840, 43-50.
4. McGee, J. and Fitzpatrick, F. (1985) J. Biol. Chem. 260, 12832-12837.
5. Ohishi, N., Izumi, T., Minami, M., Kitamura, S., Seyama, Y., Ohkawa, S., Terao, S., Yotsumoto, H., Takaku, F. and Shimizu, T. (1987) J. Biol. Chem. 262, 10200-10205.
6. Haeggström, J., Bergman, T., Jörnvall, H. and Rådmark, O. (1988) Eur. J. Biochem. 174, 717-724.
7. Bito, H., Ohishi, N., Miki, I., Minami, M., Tanabe, T., Shimizu, T. and Seyama, Y. (1989) J. Biochem. 105, 261-264.
8. Fu, Ji Yi, Haeggström, J., Collins, P. Meijer, J. and Rådmark, O. (1989) Biochim. Biophys. Acta., 1006, 121-126.
9. Gut, J., Goldman, D.W., Jamieson, G.C. and Trudell, J.R. (1987) Arch. Biochem. Biophys. 259, 497-509.
10. Fitzpatrick, F.A., Morton, D.R. and Wynalda, M.A. (1982) J. Biol. Chem. 257, 4680-4683.
11. Evans, J.F., Nathaniel, D.J., Zamboni,R.J. and Ford-Hutchinson, A.W. (1985) J. Biol. Chem. 260, 10966-10970.
12. Nathaniel, D.J., Evans, J.F., Leblanc, Y., Leveille, C., Fitzsimmons, B.J. and Ford-Hutchinson, A.W. (1985) Biochem. Biophys. Res. Commun. 131, 827-835.
13. Evans, J., Nathaniel, D., Charleson, S., Leveille, C., Zamboni, R., Leblanc, Y., Frenette, R., Fitzsimmons, B.J., Leger, S., Hamel, P. and Ford-Hutchinson, A.W. (1986) Prostaglandins, Leukotrienes and Medicine 23, 167-171.
14. Rouzer, C.A. and Samuelsson, B. (1987) Proc. Natl. Acad. Sci. USA 84, 7393-7397.
15. Rouzer, C.A. and Kargman, S. (1988) J. Biol. Chem. 263, 1098010988.
16. Wong, A., Hwang, S.H., Cook, M.N., Hogaboom, K. and Crooke, S.T. (1988) Biochemistry 27, 6763-6769.
17. McColl, S.R., Hurst, N.P., Betts, W.H. and Cleland, L.G. (1987) Biocem. Biophys. Res. Comm. 147, 622-626.

18. Fitzpatrick, F., Haeggström, J., Granström, E. and Samuelsson, B. (1983) Proc. Natl. Acad. Sci. USA 80, 5425-5429.
19. Fitzpatrick, F, Liggett, W., McGee, J., Bunting, S., Morton, D. and Samuelsson, B. (1984) J. Biol. Chem. 259, 114003-114007.
20. Haeggström, J., Rådmark, O. and Fitzpatrick, F. (1985) Biochim. Biophys. Acta 835,. 378-384.
21. Sirois, P., Brosseau, Y., Chagnon, M., Gentile, J., Gladu, M., Salari, H. and Borgeat, P. (1985) Experimental Lung Research 9, 17-30.
22. Wong, P.Y.K., Chao, P.H.W. and Spokas, E.G. (1985) Adv. in Prostaglandin, Thromboxane and Leukotriene Research 15, 423-426.
23. Pace-Asciak, C.R., Klein, J., Lombard, S., Torchia, J. and Rokach, J. (1985) Biochim. Biophys. Acta 836, 153-156.
24. Izumi, T., Shimizu, T., Seyama, Y., Ohishi, N. and Takaku, F. (1986) Biochem. Biophys. Res. Commun. 135, 139-145.
25. Shimizu, T., Takusagawa, Y., Izumi, T., Ohishi, N. and Seyama, Y. (1987) J. Neurochemistry 48, 1541-1546.
26. Medina ,J.F., Haeggström, J., Wetterholm, A., Wallin, A. and Rådmark, O. (1987) Biochem. Biophys. Res. Commun. 143, 697-703.
27. Medina, J.F., Haeggström, J., Kumlin, M. and Rådmark, O. (1988) Biochim. Biophys. Acta 961, 203-212.
28. Odlander, B., Jakobsson, P.-J., Rosen, A. and Claesson, H.-E. (1988) Biochem. Biophys. Res. Commun. 153, 203-208.
29. Fu, Ji Yi, Medina, J.F., Funk, C.D., Wetterholm, A. and Rådmark, O. (1988) Prostaglandins 36, 241-248.
30. Medina, J.F., Odlander, B., Funk, C.D., Ji-Yi Fu, Claesson, H.-E. and Rådmark, O. (1989) Biochem. Biophys. Res. Commun. 161, 740-745.
31. Claesson, H.-E. and Haeggström, J. (1988) Eur. J. Biochem. 173, 93-100.
32. Medina, J.F., Barrios, C., Funk, C.D., Larsson, O., Haeggström, J. and Rådmark, O. (1989) Submitted for publication.
33. Yamaoka, K.A., Claesson, H.-E. and Rosen, A. (1989) J. of Immunology, 143, 1996-2000.

34. Mensing, H. and Czarnetzki, B.M. (1984) J. Invest. Derm. 82, 9-12.
35. Funk, C.D., Rådmark, O., Fu, Ji Yi, Matsumoto, T., Jörnvall, H., Shimizu, T. and Samuelsson, B. (1987) Proc. Natl. Acad. Sci. USA 84, 6677-6681.
36. Minami, M., Ohno, S., Kawasaki, H., Rådmark, O., Samuelsson, B., Jörnvall, H., Shimizu, T., Seyama, Y. and Suzuki, K. (1987) J. Biol. Chem. 262, 13873-13876.
37. Minami, M., Minami, Y., Emori, Y., Kawasaki, H., Ohno, S., Suzuki, K., Ohishi, N., Shimizu, T. and Seyama, Y. (1988) FEBS-Letters 229, 279-282.
38. Haeggström, J., Meijer, J. and Rådmark, O. (1986) J. Biol. Chem. 261, 6332-6337.

Advances in Prostaglandin, Thromboxane, and Leukotriene Research, Vol. 20,
edited by B. Samuelsson et al.
Raven Press, Ltd., New York © 1990.

BIOSYNTHESIS AND FUNCTIONS OF LEUKOTRIENE C$_4$

Takao Shimizu, Takashi Izumi, Zen-ichiro Honda, Yousuke Seyama,
Yoshihisa Kurachi* and Tsuneaki Sugimoto*

Department of Physiological Chemistry and Nutrition,
and *Department of Internal Medicine, Faculty of
Medicine, University of Tokyo, Tokyo 113, Japan

Arachidonic acid is converted to 5-hydroperoxyeicosatetraeno-
ic acid (5-HPETE), and subsequently to leukotriene A$_4$ (LTA$_4$) by
the action of 5-lipoxygenase (4, 23, 25, 26, 32). LTA$_4$ is
further metabolized to LTB$_4$, a potent chemotactic compound by
LTA$_4$ hydrolase (3, 17, 22). Alternatively, this labile epoxide
enzymically conjugates reduced glutathione (GSH) to yield LTC$_4$,
a spasmogenic compound (FIG. 1) (see reviews; 5, 12, 15, 24,
27). In the last several years, two important enzymes (5-lipox-
ygenase and LTA$_4$ hydrolase) were purified to homogeneity and
complete primary structures were determined by molecular cloning
(refer to other chapters in this Volume). LTC$_4$ synthase has yet
to be purified, mostly because of its instability of the enzyme
(7, 30, 31). Described herein are: (A) biosynthesis of leukotriene C$_4$ with special attention directed to guinea pig lung
LTC$_4$ synthase and rat brain glutathione S-transferases (GSTs),
and (B) a novel function of LTC$_4$ as an intracellular messenger,
as demonstrated in guinea pig atrial cells.

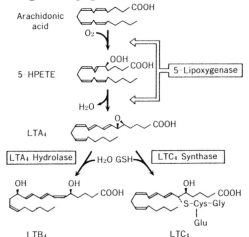

FIG. 1. Arachidonate 5-Lipoxygenase Pathway.

BIOSYNTHESIS OF LEUKOTRIENE C_4

Partial purification of LTC_4 synthase from guinea pig lung

Tissue distribution of enzymes.
Enzymic conversion of LTA_4 to LTC_4 was originally noted in rat basophilic leukemia (RBL) cells (2, 8), mouse macrophages (1) and human platelets (18). The enzyme was first solubilized by Yoshimoto *et al.*, using RBL cells (30). In systemic surveys of guinea pig and rat tissues, we found that LTC_4 synthase was rich in the microsomal fractions of the guinea pig spleen and lung, whereas the microsomal GST activity is highest in the guinea pig liver (7). Obviously, there is no correlation of activities between LTC_4 synthase and GST. In both species, LTA_4 hydrolase is ubiquitously distributed with a relatively high activity in lung, spleen and alimentary tract. In the guinea pig, these activities are higher than those in rats (Table 1).

Table 1. **Tissue distribution of LTC_4 synthase, GST and LTA_4 hydrolase in guinea pig and rat (6, 7, 13)**

Tissues	LTC_4 synthase (nmol/mg · 5 min)	GST (μmol/mg·min)	LTA_4 hydrolase (nmol/mg·min)
guinea pig		microsomes	cytosol
brain	0.40 ± 0.15	n. d.	0.47 ± 0.12
heart	0.55 ± 0.45	n. d.	0.56 ± 0.06
lung	11.0 ± 2.50	0.01 ± 0.01	1.14 ± 0.14
liver	0.75 ± 0.65	0.33 ± 0.30	0.28 ± 0.04
spleen	29.8 ± 14.4	n. d.	0.72 ± 0.09
kidney	2.80 ± 1.90	0.06 ± 0.07	0.63 ± 0.11
adrenal gland	1.20 ± 0.40	0.05 ± 0.04	0.67 ± 0.06
stomach	0.25 ± 0.25	n. d.	0.60 ± 0.17
small intestine	0.85 ± 0.35	n. d.	1.59 ± 0.33
colon	0.65 ± 0.35	n. d.	0.86 ± 0.17
rat		microsomes	cytosol [a]
brain	0.90 ± 0.40	n. d.	0.17
heart	n. d.	n. d.	n. d.
lung	3.20 ± 1.55	n. d.	0.46
liver	0.25 ± 0.20	0.09 ± 0.06	0.04
spleen	1.15 ± 0.40	n. d.	0.26
kidney	n. d.	n. d.	0.07
adrenal gland	0.85 ± 0.50	0.05 ± 0.02	–
stomach	0.50 ± 0.45	n. d.	0.07
small intestine	0.25 ± 0.25	0.01 ± 0.004	0.27
colon	n. d.	n. d.	0.20

n. d. less than 0.2 nmol/mg·5 min for LTC_4 synthase and 0.01 μmol/mg·min for GST.
[a] Data are from Ref. 13 (n. d. not detectable).

Solubilization and purification of LTC4 synthase from guinea pig lung

The guinea pig microsomes were mixed with 1.5% CHAPS (3-[(cholamidopropyl)dimethylammonio]-1-propanesulfonate/0.75% digitonin/1 M KCl/5% glycerol/1 mM EDTA/0.5 mM dithiothreitol/1 mM GSH for 1h at $4^{\circ}C$. By this treatment, approximately 110% of the total activity and 70% of the protein were recovered. The solubilized sample was purified by successive column chromatography (Superose 12 and DEAE-5PW), which resulted in a complete separation of LTC4 synthase from GST, also present in the microsomal fraction of the guinea pig lung (7). The specific activity of the purified enzyme is 40 nmol/mg·min, when LTA4 is used as a substrate. The Km values for LTA4 and GSH are 35 μM, and 1.6 mM, respectively. LTA4 (5,6-epoxide) proves to be the best substrate, in terms of both Km and Vmax values. In contrast, rat liver cytosolic GSTs (3-3, 4-4) act on various positional isomers of epoxide LTs and their methyl esters. LTC4 synthase has no GST activity (1-Cl-2,4-dinitrobenzene). Thus, LTC4 synthase in the guinea pig lung is unique and specific (7).

Purification and properties of glutathione S-transferase (GST) from rat brain

Purification of two types of GST from rat brain

Various types of GST play an important role in detoxification by catalyzing the conjugation of various hydrophobic substances with GSH. The cytosolic GST also catalyzes the conversion of PGH_2 to PGE_2 (16) and LTA4 to LTC4 (28). Recent studies from the Karolinska group demonstrated that LTC4 is produced in the rat median eminence, and exhibits a luteinizing hormone (LH)-releasing activity (24). We isolated two types of GST from rat brain (29). A new acidic form of GST was purified from rat brain by S-hexylglutathione affinity chromatography, followed by chromatofocusing. The pI is 6.2. The enzyme is a homodimer (Mr of subunit, 26 KDa). This GST, as termed GST Yn_1Yn_1, occupies about 20% of the total activity. A major GST in the brain, constituting about 40% of the total activity is identical to GST-P (7-7), originally purified from human placenta and hepatoma cells. GST-P is a homodimer (Mr of subunit, 24 KDa) with pI of 7.0.

LTC4 synthase activity of various GSTs

Table 2 summarizes LTC4 synthase activity of rat cytosolic GSTs. Among them, a new GST found in the brain, Yn_1n_1, is the most efficient in catalyzing LTA4 to C4. The Km values for LTA4 and GSH are 26 μM, and 3.5 mM, respectively. It is possible that the production of LTC4 in the rat brain is mostly due to the GST. In contrast to LTC4 synthase in the guinea pig lung, these enzymes act on various isomers of LT epoxide including 11,12-LTA4 (14), 14,15-LTA4. In all cases the enzymes prefer methyl ester forms rather than free acids.

Table 2. LTC$_4$ synthase activity of various GST isozymes

Enzyme	LTC$_4$ synthase [a]
	nmol/mg of protein
GST 1-1	5.34
1-2	7.59
2-2	2.94
3-3	3.02
3-4	22.8
4-4	140
Yn$_1$n$_1$	496
6-6 (M$_T$)	310
7-7 (P)	67.2

[a] The activity is measured in the presence of 70 μM LTA$_4$ and 10 mM GSH (29). The activity is expressed as nmol LTC$_4$ produced/mg of enzyme in 5 min.

NOVEL FUNCTION OF LEUKOTRIENE C$_4$

A Second Messenger Role of Lipoxygenase Metabolites

in *Aplysia* Sensory Neurons

In 1987, Piomelli *et al.* demonstrated that 12-lipoxygenase products serve as a second messenger in *Aplysia* sensory neurons (19-21), as based on the following evidence. (a) The inhibitory effect of FMRF amide (a mollusk tetrapeptide) is mimicked by arachidonic acid. (b) 12-HPETE is formed in the neuron by the action of FMRF amide. (c) The action of FMRF amide or arachidonic acid is blocked by lipoxygenase inhibitors, but not by indomethacin. (d) 12-HPETE, but not 12-HETE mimics the action (opening K$^+$ channel) by FMRF amide.

These results appear to substantiate the second messenger role of 12-HPETE or its metabolites in synaptic transmission.

LTC$_4$ as an Intracellular Messenger in Guinea Pig Atrium

The concept that lipoxygenase products act as intracellular messengers was further supported by our group (10, 11) and Kim *et al.* (9), by a patch clamp method using atrial cells. In these cells, opening of the muscarinic potassium channel (termed I$_{K.ACh}$) is regulated by acetylcholine via pertussis-toxin sensitive G protein (termed G$_K$). A similar chronotropic action by phenylephrine, an α1-adrenergic agonist is probably mediated by an arachidonate lipoxygenase metabolite, LTC$_4$ (11). Guinea pig atrial cells have LTC$_4$ synthesizing capacity.

Patch-clamp of single cells
Single atrial cells are dispersed from the guinea pig heart with collagenase. The patch-clamp technique is used to record currents flowing through $I_{K.ACh}$ in cell-attached and inside-out patch modes. The pipette solution contains 145 mM KCl, 1 mM $MgCl_2$, 5 mM HEPES-KOH (pH 7.4), 10 μM atropine and 100 μM theophylline. Arachidonic acid (50 μM) activates the potassium channel in atrial myocytes. This level of channel opening persists for more than 10 min after washing of arachidonic acid. The arachidonate-activated channel has the same conductance (45-50 pS) and kinetic properties (time constant 1 msec) as $I_{K.ACh}$ (10).

A cyclooxygenase inhibitor, indomethacin (5-10 μM) enhances the activation of the channel by arachidonic acid. In contrast, NDGA (nordihydroguaiaretic acid, 10 μM) and AA-861 (3 μM) prevents activation of the channel. Neither 12-HPETE nor 12-HETE (8-40 μM) stimulates the opening of the channel. Among various lipoxygenase products examined, 5-HPETE (4 μM), LTA_4 (4.5 μM) and LTC_4 (1.6 μM) increases the channel opening. Neither LTB_4 (10 μM) nor LTD_4 (10 μM) activates $I_{K.ACh}$, under the present conditions.

Effects of α 1-agonist on the channel opening
Phenylephrine, another negative chronotropic agent stimulates the potassium channel ($I_{K.ACh}$) in the cell-attached patch. Channel activation is completely blocked by prazosin, an α 1-adrenergic antagonist, thereby indicating that the response is mediated by the α 1-adrenergic receptor. Phenylephrine-induced activation is prevented by NDGA and AA-861, but not by indomethacin or baicalein (12-lipoxygenase inhibitor). Taken together, these observations suggest that LTC_4 may be involved in the α 1-adrenergic activation of $I_{K.ACh}$.

Possible mechanism of LTC_4 action
The activation of $I_{K.ACh}$ by arachidonic acid or LTC_4 disappears quickly in inside-out patches, but reappears on application of GTP. When LTC_4 or arachidonic acid is applied to inside-out patches, the potassium channel ($I_{K.ACh}$) is not activated, but the addition of GTPγS does activate the same preparations. Furthermore, LTC_4 activates $I_{K.ACh}$ in pertussis toxin-treated atrial cells, where G_K is uncoupled, under these conditions. These results can be interpreted to mean that arachidonate metabolites might stimulate GDP/GTP exchange of G_K, by binding to receptors coupled to $I_{K.ACh}$ through pertussis toxin-insensitive G proteins. Kim et al. further state that the $\beta\gamma$-subunit of G-proteins activates phospholipase A_2, which releases arachidonic acid for further metabolism.

The proposed mechanism of LTC_4 action on $I_{K.ACh}$ is illustrated in FIG. 2.

Whether LTC_4 acts as a messenger under physiological conditions remains to be clarified.

SUMMARY

1. The LTC$_4$ synthase activity is rich in the microsomal fraction of the guinea pig spleen and lung. The enzyme was partially purified from the guinea pig lung and separated from the microsomal glutathione S-transferase (GST), by column chromatography. The enzyme has a specific activity of 40 nmol/min•mg, and acts preferentially on 5, 6-LTA$_4$. Various types of cytosolic GSTs utilize all types of LTA$_4$ isomers (5,6-, 11,12- and 14,15-LTA$_4$) almost to the same extent, and methyl ester forms are better substrates for GST.

2. Two different types of GSTs (Yn$_1$n$_1$ and P) were purified from rat brain cytosol, to homogeneity. Because both types have a high LTC$_4$ synthase activity, they may participate in the LTC$_4$ production in the *rat brain*.

3. LTC$_4$, produced in the guinea pig atrium, stimulates pertussis toxin (IAP)-sensitive muscarinic K$^+$ channel ($I_{K.ACh}$). The negative chronotropic action of α1-adrenergic agonist might relate to the production of arachidonate lipoxygenase metabolites.

    These results together with the findings in *Aplysia* sensory neurons, suggest a novel mode of eicosanoid actions.

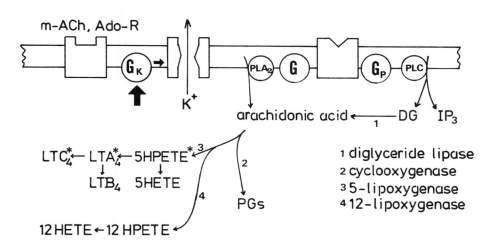

FIG. 2. Proposed Model of LTC4 Action in Atrial Myocytes. Metabolites (*) activate $I_{K.ACh}$ (10).

REFERENCES

1. Abe, M.,Kawazoe, Y., Tsunematsu, H., and Shigematsu, N: (1985) *Biochem. Biophys. Res. Commun.* 127: 15-23

2. Bach, M. K., Brashler, J. R., and Morton, D. R., Jr.: (1984) *Arch. Biochem. Biophys.* 230: 455-465

3. Evans, J. F., Dupuis, P., and Ford-Hutchinson, A. W: (1985) *Biochim. Biophys. Acta* 840: 43-50

4. Goetze, A. W., Fayer, L., Bouska, J., Bornemeier, D., and Carter, G. W: (1985) *Prostaglandins* 29: 689-701

5. Hammarström, S: (1983) *Annu. Rev. Biochem.* 52: 355-377

6. Izumi, T, Shimizu, T., Seyama, Y., Ohishi, N., and Takaku, F: (1986) *Biochem. Biophys. Res. Commun.* 135: 139-145

7. Izumi, T., Honda, Z., Ohishi, N., Kitamura, S., Tsuchida, S., Sato, K., Shimizu, T., and Seyama, Y: (1988) *Biochim. Biophys. Acta* 959: 305-315

8. Jakschik, B. A., Harper, T., and Murphy, R. C: (1982) *J. Biol. Chem.* 257: 5346-5349.

9. Kim, D., Lewis, D. L., Graziadei, L., Neer, E. J., Bar-Sagi, D., and Clapham, D. E: (1989) *Nature* 337: 557-560

10. Kurachi, Y., Ito, H., Sugimoto, T., Shimizu, T., Miki, I., and Ui, M: (1989) *Nature* 337: 555-557

11. Kurachi, Y., Ito, H., Sugimoto, T., Shimizu, T., Miki, I., and Ui, M: (1989) *Pflugers Arch.* 414: 102-104

12. Lewis, R. A., and Austen, K. F: (1983) *J. Clin. Invest.* 73: 889-897

13. Medina, J. F., Haeggström, J., Kumlin, M., and Rådmark, O: (1988) *Biochim. Biophys. Acta* 961: 203-212

14. Miki, I., Shimizu, T., Seyama, Y., Kitamura, S., Yamaguchi, K., Sano, H., Ueno, H., Hiratsuka, A., and Watabe, T: (1989) *J. Biol. Chem.* 264: 5799-5805

15. Needleman, P., Turk, J., Jakschik, B. A., Morrison, A. R., and Lefkowith, J. B: (1986) *Ann. Rev. Biochem.* 55: 69-102

16. Ogorochi, T., Ujihara, M., and Narumiya, S: (1987) *J. Neurochem.* 48: 900-909

17. Ohishi, N., Izumi, T., Minami, M., Kitamura, S., Seyama, Y., Ohkawa, S., Terao, S., Yotsumoto, H., Takaku, F., and Shimizu, T: (1987) *J. Biol. Chem.* 262: 10200-10205

18. Pace-Asciak, C. R., Klein, J., and Spielberg, S. P: (1986) *Biochem. Biophys. Res. Commun.* 140: 857-860

19. Piomelli, D., Volterra, A., Dale, N., Siegelbaum, S. A., Kandel, E. R., Schwartz, J. H., and Belardetti, F: (1987) *Nature* 328: 38-43

20. Piomelli, D., Feinmark, S., Shapiro, E., and Schwartz, J. H: (1988) *J. Biol. Chem.* 263: 16591-16596

21. Piomelli, D., Shapiro, E., Zipkin, R., Schwartz, J. H., and Feinmark, S. (1989) *Proc. Natl. Acad. Sci. U. S. A.* 86: 1721-1725

22. Rådmark, O., Shimizu, T., Jörnvall, H., and Samuelsson, B: (1984) *J. Biol. Chem.* 259: 12339-12345

23. Rouzer, C. A., and Samuelsson, B: (1985) *Proc. Natl. Acad. Sci. U. S. A.* 82: 6040-6044

24. Samuelsson, B., Dahlén, S-É., Lindgren, J-Å., Rouzer, C. A., and Serhan, C. N: (1987) *Science* 237: 1171-1176

25. Shimizu, T., Rådmark, O., and Samuelsson, B: (1984) *Proc. Natl. Acad. Sci. U. S. A.* 81: 689-693

26. Shimizu, T., Izumi, T., Seyama, Y., Tadokoro, K., Rådmark, O., and Samuelsson, B: (1986) *Proc. Natl. Acad. Sci. U. S. A.* 83: 4175-4179

27. Shimizu, T: (1988) *Int. J. Biochem.* 20: 661-666

28. Söderström, M., Mannervik, B., Örning, L., and Hammarström, S: (1985) *Biochem. Biophys. Res. Commun.* 128: 265-270

29. Tsuchida, S., Izumi, T., Shimizu, T., Ishikawa, T., Hatayama, I., Satoh, K., and Sato, K: (1987) *Eur. J. Biochem.* 170: 159-164

30. Yoshimoto, T., Soberman, r. J., Lewis, R. A., and Austen, K. F: (1985) *Proc. Natl. Acad. Sci. U. S. A.* 82: 8399-8403

31. Yoshimoto, T., Soberman, R. J., Spur, B., and Austen, K. F: (1988) *J. Clin. Invest.* 81: 866-871

32. Ueda, N., Kaneko, S., Yoshimoto, T., and Yamamoto, S: (1986) *J. Biol. Chem.* 261: 7982-7988

Advances in Prostaglandin, Thromboxane, and Leukotriene Research, Vol. 20, edited by B. Samuelsson et al. Raven Press, Ltd., New York © 1990.

LIPOXIN FORMATION: EVALUATION OF THE ROLE AND ACTIONS OF LEUKOTRIENE A$_4$

Charles N. Serhan, Kelly-Ann Sheppard and Stefano Fiore

Hematology Division, Department of Medicine, Brigham and Women's Hospital and Harvard Medical School, Boston, MA 02115

INTRODUCTION

The lipoxins are a series of biologically active, eicosanoids which contain a conjugated tetraene structure as a characteristic feature (reviewed in ref. 15). The two main compounds which carry biological activities are positional isomers: one designated lipoxin A$_4$ (5S,6R,15S-trihydroxy-7,9,13-trans-11-cis-eicosatetraenoic acid) and the other lipoxin B$_4$ (5S,14R,15S,trihydroxy-6,10,12-trans-8-cis-eicosatetraenoic acid). Multiple pathways have been documented in vitro which can lead to the formation of lipoxins (7,15,17,18). It appears, at present, that the biosynthetic pathways utilized to generate either LXA$_4$ or LXB$_4$ are species-, cell type- and substrate-specific. One route, which has been demonstrated with results from both isotopic oxygen studies as well as the identification of alcohol trapping products, involves the transformation of 15-HETE to a 5(6)-epoxytetraene by human leukocytes (15). When this putative intermediate (15S-hydroxy-5,6-epoxy-7,9,13-trans-11-cis-eicosatetraenoic acid) was synthesized and incubated with purified cytosolic epoxide hydrolase, it was quantitatively converted into LXA$_4$ (11). During the formation of lipoxins from exogenous 15-HETE by human neutrophils (an event which may occur in cell-cell interactions), an inverse relationship is observed between leukotriene and lipoxin production (14). Thus, the generation of epoxide-containing intermediates by human neutrophils appears to play pivotal roles in the biosynthesis of both leukotrienes and lipoxins.

Aside from its role as an intermediate in the

formation of leukotrienes within its cell type of origin, it is now recognized from the studies of Dahinden et al. (2) that the epoxide LTA_4 can also be released by or escape from cells to be transformed via transcellular routes. In general, lipoxygenases catalyze the oxygenation of 1,4-cis-pentadiene structures of polyunsaturated fatty acids (6). Since LTA_4 also contains a 1,4-cis-pentadiene which is not within its conjugated triene structure (see insert, Figure 1), it was of interest to determine whether LTA_4 could play a role in the biosynthesis of lipoxins. Here, evidence is presented for: (a) the conversion of LTA_4 by 15-LO to a 5(6)epoxytetraene; (b) Ca^{2+} mobilizing actions of LTA_4 in human neutrophils; (c) the lack of LTA_4 conversion to lipoxins by human neutrophils; and (d) the transformation of LTA_4 to lipoxins by the 12-LO of human platelets.

MATERIALS AND METHODS

Soybean LO (EC.1.13.11.12) and methyl formate were from Sigma Chemical Company, St. Louis, MO. Synthetic LTA_4, LXA_4 and LXB_4 were from Biomol Research Laboratories, Inc. (Philadelphia, PA). Other eicosanoids used as reference materials were prepared as in (14). The free acid of LTA_4-methyl ester was prepared by saponification in tetrahydrofurane with LiOH at 4°C for ~24h. Prior to each experiment, the UV spectrum of LTA_4 was examined and the products formed from hydrolysis of the epoxide were analyzed by RP-HPLC (12) to assess the purity and stability of the free acid.

Human neutrophils and platelets were prepared (10,16) from fresh venous blood of healthy volunteers who had not taken aspirin or other medications for at least 7 days. Incubation conditions are as described (16) and eicosanoids were extracted and analyzed as in (14).

RESULTS AND DISCUSSION

LTA₄ and SB 15-LO. Before examining whether LTA_4 could be converted to lipoxins by individual cell types, we first tested if LTA_4 could serve as a substrate for the soybean 15-LO (in vitro). The time course of this conversion is shown in Figure 1. Here, LTA_4 was added to 1 ml sodium borate buffer (0.1 M, pH 8.5) at 4°C, and the UV spectrum recorded (left

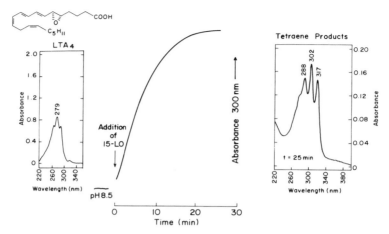

Figure 1.   <u>Transformation of LTA₄ by soybean 15-LO.</u>

insert). Upon addition of HCl to an aliquot of this sample in MeOH, the λ_{max} shifted from 279 nm to 269 nm, indicating that the 5(6)-epoxide was intact. (The shift in λ_{max} to 269 nm upon addition of acid indicates the opening of the epoxide with the formation of hydrolysis products of LTA₄.) Upon addition of ~4 μg of the 15-lipoxygenase to LTA₄, a rapid increase in absorbance at 300 nm observed which increased with time. This increase at 300 nm suggested the formation of a conjugated tetraene chromophore (i.e., conversion of the triene to a tetraene structure). The insert at the right of Figure 1 shows the UV spectrum (220-400 nm) at 25 min of an aliquot of this material. The UV spectrum shows a triplet of absorption at 288, 302 and 317 nm indicative of conjugated tetraenes. When this sample was treated with NaBH₄ and analyzed by RP-HPLC, the products formed co-eluted with the aqueous hydrolysis products of authentic 5(6)-epoxytetraene [15(S)-hydroxy-5,6-oxido-7,9,13-<u>trans</u>-11-<u>cis</u>-eicosatetraenoic acid]. Neither the aqueous hydrolysis products of LTA₄ (i.e., 6-trans-LTB₄ and 12 epi-6-trans-LTB₄) nor LTA₃ were converted to tetraenes by the SB 15-LO under similar conditions. Thus, these findings indicate that LTA₄ can serve as a substrate for the 15-lipoxygenase <u>in vitro</u> to give a 5(6)-epoxytetraene.

<u>Exogenous LTA₄ and human neutrophils.</u> Since human neutrophils possess a 15-lipoxygenase, it is possible that extracellular LTA₄ could be transported and converted to its 15-hydroperoxy derivative (i.e., 5,6-epoxytetraene). To test this hypothesis, human neutrophils (30 x 10⁶ cells/ml) were incubated with

either exogenous LTA_4 (30 nmol) or exogenous LTA_4 with A23187 (2.5 μM). In neither case did neutrophils generate lipoxins from exogenous LTA_4 (n=3 different donors). Dose-response studies with LTA_4 (0.1, 1, 10, 50 and 100 nmol LTA_4) incubated with neutrophils (20 min, 37°C) were also negative for lipoxin production from LTA_4 (n=2). Further experiments were performed with 100,000 g supernatants prepared from purified neutrophils which converted LTA_4 to LTB_4. However, in these incubations, neither lipoxins nor the ω-oxidation products of LTB_4 were detected. Together, these findings suggest that extracellular LTA_4 is not converted to the 5(6)-epoxytetraene upon exposure to human neutrophils (16).

Transcellular metabolism of LTA_4 implies that during this event: (i) LTA_4 must first "exit" the neutrophil; (ii) come in contact with the plasma membrane of the "acceptor cell"; and (iii) traverse or gain access to intracellular compartments prior to its enzymatic conversion. Within this temporal framework, several cellular responses may be affected by LTA_4. To test this, Ca^{2+} mobilization was monitored as an early and sensitive signal involved in neutrophil activation (9). When added to fura-2-loaded neutrophils, LTA_4 provoked a rapid and transient increase in $[Ca^{2+}]_i$ (maximum within 8-10 seconds) which returned to baseline within 60-90 seconds. Ca^{2+} mobilization was dose-dependent (10^{-12} - 10^{-6}M and evident at concentrations as low as 10^{-11}M. At 1 μM, LTB_4 and LTA_4 were quantitatively similar while within the range of 10^{-10} - 10^{-8}M LTB_4 proved to be more effective than its precursor LTA_4. Prior exposure to EGTA (3 mM) did not diminish either the amplitude or extent of $[Ca^{2+}]_i$ mobilization by LTA_4. Results from alcohol trapping studies revealed that LTA_4 was intact during the initial phase of Ca^{2+} mobilization (t_o - 10 seconds) stimulated by LTA_4 and that neither LTB_4 nor its ω-oxidation products were detected within this time interval (9). Their formation from extracellular ^{3}H label LTA_4/cold LTA_4 was observed only at intervals >30 seconds of exposure to neutrophils. This finding, along with those obtained with 5(6)- and 14(15)-epoxytetraenes, suggest that these eicosanoid epoxides possess intrinsic activities (9).

The ability of eicosanoid epoxides to mobilize $[Ca^{2+}]_i$ may serve to amplify cellular responses either within their cells of origin or by acting upon

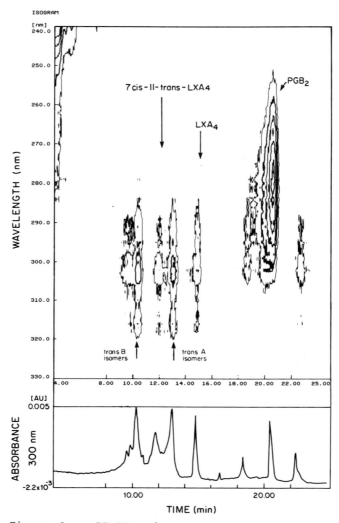

Figure 2. <u>RP-HPLC isogram and chromatogram of products obtained from human platelets incubated with leukotriene A₄.</u>

Human platelets (1.5 x 10⁹ cells) suspended in PBS (1 ml) containing albumin (0.1%) were incubated for 5 min at 37°C prior to addition of LTA₄ (50 nmol) plus ionophore A23187 (0.1 μM) for 20 min. The upper plot shows an isogram display of the stored spectral data (240-330 nm). Arrows indicate the retention time of synthetic standards. The lower plot shows the same spectral data recalled as a single wavelength chromatogram (300 nm). Post-HPLC analyses were performed with a Wavescan 2140-002 program and Nelson Analytical data system.

adjacent cells during transcellular metabolism. Along these lines, we have recently found that phospholipid bilayers can enhance the stability of LTA_4 as well as the epoxytetraenes by protecting the epoxides from non-enzymatic aqueous hydrolysis (4). Thus, the biological half-life of these intermediates as well as the response they evoke may be increased during their association with membranes. Together, these results indicate that although LTA_4 can be converted by the SB-15-LO to an epoxytetraene, exogenous LTA_4 is not transformed to lipoxins by human neutrophils. In this case, exogenous LTA_4 appears to serve as a signal to mobilize Ca^{2+} which may, in turn, amplify the generation of LTB_4.

Transformation of LTA_4 to Lipoxins. Platelets can utilize and transform neutrophil-derived eicosanoids (10). To determine if neutrophil-derived LTA_4 can be transformed to lipoxins by platelets, exogenous LTA_4 was incubated with isolated human platelets (Figure 2). Following extraction, products were analyzed with a gradient, RP-HPLC equipped with a rapid spectral detector and chromatographic software (14). When the stored spectral data were recalled at 300 nm, several prominent peaks displaying strong absorbance at 300 nm were revealed (Figure 2; lower panel). An isogram plot of these spectral data (240-330 nm; upper panel) showed that each product carried a conjugated tetraene chromophore. Materials beneath the major peaks co-eluted with the all-trans-isomers of LXA_4 and LXB_4 as well as both the synthetic and neutrophil-derived LXA_4 (16). In addition, platelets also generated the recently identified 7-cis-11-trans-LXA_4 (14) from exogenous LTA_4. The identity of the platelet-derived LXA_4 was further substantiated by GC/MS analysis of its C value and prominent ions present in the mass spectrum of its trimethylsilyl derivative (16).

The conversion of LTA_4 to lipoxins was enhanced by platelet agonists (Table 1). Cyclooxygenase inhibitors (indomethacin, aspirin) did not significantly alter lipoxin generation by platelets. In contrast, esculetin, an LO inhibitor (13), completely blocked the formation of lipoxins. Further studies with platelet-derived 100,000 g supernatants, which displayed 12-LO activity with C20:4 and no detectable 15-LO activity, provide a role for the human platelet 12-LO and its ω-6-oxygenase activity in converting LTA_4 to lipoxins (16). These results suggest a direct action on LTA_4 by the 12-LO to generate lipoxins via a delocalized cation

TABLE 1.　Conversion of LTA$_4$ to lipoxins by platelets: Effects of agonists and inhibitors*

Incubation	LXA$_4$	7-cis-11-trans LXA$_4$	trans-LXA$_4$	trans-LXB$_4$
LTA$_4$	21.7 ± 7.8	6.7 ± 3.6	52.5 ± 25.0	35.7 ± 18.0
LTA$_4$ + A23187 (0.1 μM)	64.0 ± 23.2	19.4 ± 10.9	157.1 ± 74.8	106.9 ± 44.1
LTA$_4$ + thrombin (1 U)	48.0 ± 16.4	2.6 ± 1.4	32.0 ± 15.2	136.5 ± 68.0
ASA-treated cells plus LTA$_4$ + A23187	44.8 ± 16.5[NS]	13.1 ± 6.3[NS]	71.4 ± 34.1[NS]	36.8 ± 15.2[NS]
Esculetin-treated cells plus LTA$_4$ + A23187	0.0 ± 0.0	0.0 ± 0.0	0.0 ± 0.0	0.0 ± 0.0

*Platelets (1.5 x 10^9 cells) in 1 ml buffer were incubated 5 min at 37°C before addition of either LTA$_4$ (30 μM) or LTA$_4$ plus stimuli. All incubations were performed with cells in PBS with 0.1% albumin at 37°C for 20 min. Cells were treated with either esculetin (100 μM), indomethacin (100 μM), or acetylsalicylic acid for 20-30 min at 37°C prior to incubation with LTA$_4$ (30 μM) and A23187 (0.1 μM). The P values show NS difference in the conversion of LTA$_4$ in the presence of ASA. Results are presented in ng of product/1 ml; mean ± S.E. with between 3-8 separate experiments.

intermediate. A similar intermediate has been proposed in the biosynthesis of lipoxins from a common substrate (1).

CONCLUSIONS

Although LTA$_4$ is converted to an epoxytetraene by soybean 15-LO _in vitro_ (Figure 1) results obtained with both intact human neutrophils and platelets as well as their respective 100,000 g supernatants revealed a differential profile of LTA$_4$ utilization. Neutrophils which contain an active 15-LO did not transform exogenous LTA$_4$ to lipoxins, while results with platelets as well as their 100,000 g supernatants which display 12-LO activity transform LTA$_4$ to lipoxins (16). These findings suggest that within cells the human 12-LO rather than 15-LO can act upon LTA$_4$ to generate lipoxins. During the course of the present investigation, Edenius et al. (3) reported that LTA$_4$ is converted to lipoxins by platelets, and Garrick et al. (5) showed that LTA$_4$ is converted to lipoxins by mesangial cells. Our results are consistent with these observations and provide evidence for a novel biosynthesis route for the formation of lipoxins, namely the conversion of LTA$_4$ by the human 12-LO. In addition, we have found that costimulation of neutrophils and platelets via receptor-mediated routes can lead to the generation of lipoxins <u>in vitro</u> (16). Since LXA$_4$ is found in the bronchoaveolar lavage of patients with selected pulmonary diseases (8), this new route of lipoxin formation may contribute, at least in part, to their production <u>in vivo</u>.

ACKNOWLEDGMENTS

The authors wish to thank Paula McColgan for skillful preparation of this manuscript.
This work was supported in part by NIH grants #AI26714 and GM38765 (CNS). CNS is a recipient of the J.V. Satterfield Arthritis Investigator Award from the National Arthritis Foundation and is a Pew Scholar in the Biomedical Sciences.

REFERENCES

1. Corey, E.J., and Mehrotra, M.M. (1986): Tetrahedron Lett. 27:5173-5176.
2. Dahinden, C.A., Clancy, R.M., Gross, M., Chiller, J.M., and Hugli, T.E. (1985): Proc. Natl. Acad. Sci. USA 82:6632-6636.
3. Edenius, C., Haeggström, J., and Lindgren, J.A. (1988) Biochem. Biophys. Res. Commun. 157:801-807.
4. Fiore, S., and Serhan, C.N. (1989): Biochem. Biophys. Res. Commun. 159:477-481.
5. Garrick, R., Shen, S.-Y., Ogunc, S., and Wong, P.Y.-K. (1989): Biochem. Biophys. Res. Commun. 162:626-633.
6. Hamberg, M. (1983): Biochem. Biophys. Res. Commun. 117:593-600.
7. Kühn, H., Wiesner, R., Alder, L., Fitzsimmons, B.J., Rokach, J., and Brash, A.R. (1987): Eur. J. Biochem. 169:593-601.
8. Lee, T.H., Crea, A.E.G., Gant, V., Spur, B.W., Marron, B.E., Nicolaou, K.C., Reardon, E., Brezinski, M., and Serhan, C.N. (Submitted).
9. Luscinskas, F.W., Nicolaou, K.C., Webber, S.E., Veale, C.A., Gimbrone, M.A., Jr., and Serhan, C.N. (In Press): Biochem. Pharm.
10. Marcus, A.J., Broekman, M.J., Safier, L.B., Ullman, H.L., and Islam, N. (1982): Biochem. Biophys. Res. Commun. 109:130-137.
11. Puustinen, T., Webber, S.E., Nicolaou, K.C., Haeggström, J., Serhan, C.N., and Samuelsson, B. (1986): FEBS Lett. 207:127.

12. Rådmark, O., Malmsten, C., Samuelsson, B., Goto, G., Marfat, A., and Corey, E.J. (1980): J. Biol. Chem. 255:11828-11831.
13. Sekiya, K., Okuda, H., and Arichi, S. (1982): Biochim. Biophys. Acta 713:68-72.
14. Serhan, C.N. (1989): Biochim. Biophys. Acta 1004:158-168.
15. Serhan, C.N., and Samuelsson, B. (1988): Adv. Exp. Med. Biol. 229:1-14.
16. Serhan, C.N., and Sheppard, K.A. (Submitted).
17. Ueda, N., Yokoyama, C., Yamamoto, S., Fitzsimmons, B.J., Rokach, J., Oates, J.A., and Brash, A.R. (1987): Biochem. Biophys. Res. Commun. 149:1063-1069.
18. Walstra, P., Verhagen, J., Vermeer, M.A., Klerks, J.P.M., Veldink, G.A., and Vliegenthart, J.F.G. (1988): FEBS Lett. 228:167-171.

Advances in Prostaglandin, Thromboxane, and Leukotriene Research, Vol. 20, edited by B. Samuelsson et al. Raven Press, Ltd., New York © 1990.

PLATELET-GRANULOCYTE INTERACTIONS AND THE PRODUCTION OF LEUKOTRIENES AND LIPOXINS

JAN ÅKE LINDGREN AND CHARLOTTE EDENIUS

Department of Physiological Chemistry, Karolinska Institutet, Box 60 400, S-104 01 Stockholm, SWEDEN

Leukotriene (LT)A_4 is not only an intracellular intermediate in leukotriene biosynthesis but may also be released to the environment by activated granulocytes (1). As a consequence, the control of leukotriene synthesis is not exclusively restricted to cells expressing 5-lipoxygenase (mainly leukocytes with the exception of lymphocytes), but can also be exerted by other cell types equipped with LTA_4-metabolizing enzymes. Thus, LTA_4, released by 5-lipoxygenase expressing cells, can be converted to LTB_4 by surrounding erythrocytes (2), endothelial cells (3) and lymphocytes (4), all possessing LTA_4 hydrolase activity. Similarly, mast cells (1), endothelial cells (3,5) and smooth muscle cells (6) may convert released LTA_4 to cysteinyl-containing leukotrienes.

Transcellular interactions between platelets and granulocytes have earlier been demonstrated to generate unique lipoxygenase products that neither cell type alone can produce. Thus, 5(S),12(S)-DHETE is formed via interaction of the platelet 12-lipoxygenase and the granulocyte 5-lipoxygenase (7). In addition, 5(S),20-DHETE is synthesized via neutrophil specific ω-oxidation of platelet-derived 12-HETE (8). However, although these compounds have been described as an LTB_4 antagonist (9) and weak chemotaxin (8), respectively, their biological significance have not been secured. In light of the increasing evidence that platelets are important inflammatory cells (10,11), and interact with many aspects of leukocyte function, it was of interest to investigate if platelet-granulocyte co-operation could lead to formation of other biologically active eicosanoids.

The present report describes interactions between these cell types leading to increased formation of the cysteinyl-containing leukotrienes, LTC_4, D_4 and E_4 (12). Furthermore, transcellular lipoxin (LX) production from endogenous substrate due to co-operation between granulocytes and platelets is demonstrated (13).

METHODS

Preparation of platelet and granulocyte suspensions from peripheral human blood, incubation of intact cells and subcellular fractions, sample purification, leukotriene and lipoxin determination using reversed-phase high-performance liquid chromatography (RP-HPLC) and gas chromatography-mass spectrometry (GC/MS) were carried out as described (12,13,14).

RESULTS AND DISCUSSION

Addition of autologous platelets to human granulocyte suspensions (platelet/granulocyte ratio 100:1), caused a significant increase in ionophore A23187-induced LTC_4 formation. The levels obtained in the presence of platelets were 1.4-3.4 times higher than in control incubations (mean values 225 and 117 pmol/ml, respectively). In contrast, LTB_4 levels decreased to 12-72% (mean values 263 and 487 pmol/ml, respectively) of control levels. As expected, extremely high levels (2650 ± 602 pmol/ml) of the double dioxygenation product 5(S),12(S)-DHETE were observed in mixed cell incubations. The formation of this product was negligible (11 ± 5 pmol/ml) in the absence of added platelets, excluding significant contamination of platelets in the granulocyte suspensions.

The mechanism leading to increased LTC_4 formation in the presence of platelets was investigated in experiments using suspensions of [35S]-cysteine-prelabeled platelets and unlabeled granulocytes. Isolation of radiolabeled LTC_4 from these incubations indicated transcellular LTC_4 synthesis via release of granulocyte-derived LTA_4, followed by platelet-dependent conjugation of glutathione to this intermediate.

As judged by the increased formation of LTC_4 in mixed cell incubations (containing 1.5×10^7 granulocytes), it can be calculated, that the platelets metabolized 64-137 pmol granulocyte-derived LTA_4 to LTC_4. This is in good agreement with the reported release of 40-300 pmol LTA_4 per 10 milj human neutrophils after ionophore A23187 stimulation (1).

In contrast to the elevated LTC_4 synthesis, the production of LTB_4 gradually decreased in the presence of increasing number of platelets. This suggests that released LTA_4 can either be converted by the platelet to LTC_4 or re-enter into granulocytes and be further metabolized to LTB_4.

Ionophore stimulation of mixed platelet/granulocyte suspensions also led to the formation of several lipoxin isomers as judged by UV spectroscopy and cochromatography with authentic standards in several RP-HPLC systems. The compounds eluted as five major peaks, all showing typical UV spectra of conjugated tetraenes with maximal absorbance at 302 nm (Fig. 1). The major metabolite (peak IV), coeluted with synthetic LXA_4. The structure was confirmed by GC/MS analysis. Peaks I, II, and III coeluted with synthetic 8-*trans*-LXB_4, LXB_4 and 11-*trans*-LXA_4, respectively. In the absence of added platelets, no significant lipoxin formation could be observed.

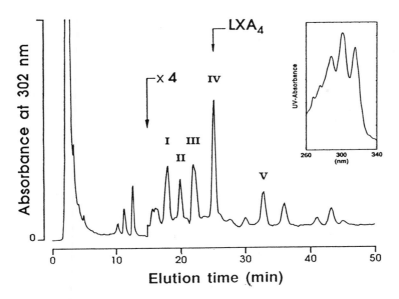

FIG. 1. Reversed-phase HPLC chromatography of lipoxins. Mixed platelet/granulocyte (100:1) suspensions were incubated in the presence of ionophore A23187 (1µM) for 30 min at 37 °C. The retention time of LXA_4 is indicated. Inserted: On-line UV-spectrum of the material eluted in peak IV.

The effects of platelets on leukotriene and lipoxin synthesis in granulocyte suspensions were platelet-concentration dependent. Production of lipoxins was observed already at a platelet/granulocyte ratio of 3:1 and was maximal (137 pmol LXA_4/ml) at the highest ratio (Fig. 2). At 10 platelets per granulocyte a substantial elevation of LTC_4 levels was observed together with a slight decrease in LTB_4 production. At higher platelet/granulocyte ratios these effects were more pronounced.

To further investigate the mechanism of platelet dependent formation of cysteinyl-containing leukotrienes, human platelet suspensions were incubated

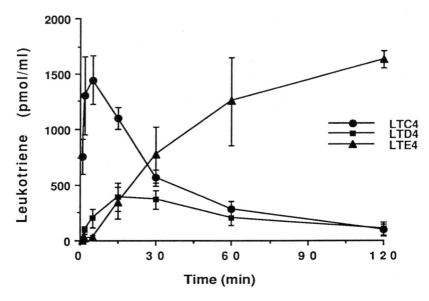

FIG. 2. Time course of the metabolism of LTA$_4$ in platelets. Human platelets were incubated with LTA$_4$ (4µM) at 37 °C in the presence of human serum albumin (0.3 mg/ml).

with exogenous LTA$_4$. The platelets converted this compound to leukotrienes C$_4$, D$_4$ and E$_4$. Control incubations, performed in the absence of platelets, or with heat-inactivated platelets, contained no measurable amounts of cysteinyl-containing leukotrienes, whereas high levels of the non-enzymatic hydrolysis products of LTA$_4$, 6-trans-LTB$_4$ and 12-epi-6-trans-LTB$_4$ were observed.

The platelet-dependent conversion of LTA$_4$ to LTC$_4$ was rapid with maximal levels of LTC$_4$ after 5 min (Fig 3). Thereafter, a pronounced catabolism of LTC$_4$ together with increasing amounts of LTD$_4$ and LTE$_4$ were observed. After 30 min, LTE$_4$ was the major metabolite. In agreement, platelet suspensions almost totally metabolized exogenous LTC$_4$ (400 pmol/ml) within 60 min. This degradation of LTC$_4$ by platelets may be of importance *in vivo* since granulocytes possessed a low LTC$_4$-metabolizing capacity. Thus, in granulocyte suspensions a slow conversion of LTC$_4$ was observed with around 55% of added LTC$_4$ still remaining after 60 min.

In experiments with subcellular platelet preparations, only the particulate fraction (100.000 x g pellet) converted LTA$_4$ to LTC$_4$. The production of LTC$_4$ was linearly correlated to the amounts of added protein. In contrast, GSH S-

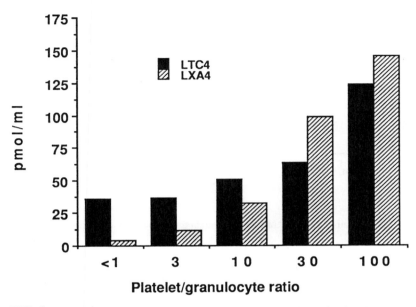

FIG. 3. Effect of platelet concentration on LTC_4 and LXA_4 formation in mixed platelet/granulocyte suspensions incubated with ionophore A23187 (1µM) for 30 min at 37°C.

transferase activity, measured as conjugation of GSH to 1-chloro-2,4-dinitrobenzene, was almost exclusively found in the soluble fraction. The results suggest the presence of a specific LTC_4 synthase (15) in human platelets.

The platelets also converted exogenous LTA_4 to LXA_4, 11-trans-LXA_4 and 8-trans-LXB_4, while no LXB_4 formation was observed. In this context, it is of interest that non-enzymatic hydrolysis of synthetic 5,6-epoxy-15-HETE led to the formation of LXA_4, 6(S)-LXA_4 and the all-trans isomers of LXA_4 and LXB_4, but not to lipoxin B_4 (16). However in the presence of leukocytes, LXB_4 was formed from this intermediate in addition to the non-enzymatically formed isomers. In agreement, LXB_4 was a prominent product in our ionophore stimulated mixed platelet/granulocyte suspensions. Taken together, the results suggest platelet-dependent conversion of LTA_4 to 5,6-epoxy-15-HETE, which is either hydrolyzed to lipoxin A_4 or further converted, possibly by a granulocyte-dependent epoxide hydrolase, to lipoxin B_4 (Fig. 4). Furthermore, the conversion of LTA_4 to lipoxins was stimulated by the presence of ionophore A23187, indicating a correlation between lipoxin formation by platelets and

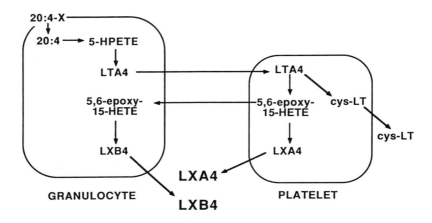

FIG. 4. Transcellular leukotriene and lipoxin formation (hypothetical scheme).

platelet activation. Thus, a pronounced increase in LXA_4 formation was observed already at 0.1 µM ionophore A23187 and maximal stimulation was obtained at 1 µM. At this ionophore concentration, the amounts of LXA_4 reached 228 ± 57 pmol/ml as compared to 41 ± 16 pmol/ml in the absence of ionophore. Human platelets incubated with ionophore A23187 did not produce detectable amounts of lipoxins or cysteinyl-containing leukotrienes, indicating the lack of 5-lipoxygenase in these cells.

Based on isolation of lipoxins from leukocyte suspensions incubated with 15-H(P)ETE and ionophore A23187, it has been postulated that the lipoxins are formed via interactions between the 5- and the 15-lipoxygenase (17,18). In addition, the present findings indicate a role of platelets in the synthesis of lipoxins. Furthermore, the 12-lipoxygenase is the principal lipoxygenase in human platelets (19), while granulocytes mainly possess 5- and 15-lipoxygenase activities (20). Therefore, the results suggest a role of the 12-lipoxygenase in lipoxin formation. Such a function was further indicated by the findings obtained with 12-lipoxygenase deficient platelets derived from a patient with chronic myelogenous leukemia (CML). In agreement with earlier reports (21), these platelets were unable to produce 12-HETE after stimulation with arachidonic acid. In contrast, normal levels of the cyclo-oxygenase products HHT and TXB_2 were formed. Granulocytes from the patient possessed active 5- and 15-lipoxygenases, producing both 5-HETE and 15-HETE after incubation with exogenous arachidonic acid plus ionophore. Furthermore, leukotrienes C_4 and B_4 were formed after ionophore A23187 stimulation of granulocytes from the patient.

Mixed platelet/granulocyte suspensions from this patient did not produce measurable amounts of lipoxins or the double dioxygenation product 5(S),12(S)-DHETE. However, when granulocytes from the patient were mixed with platelets from a healthy donor, the formation of lipoxins was normalized, demonstrating release of LTA_4 from the CML granulocytes. Furthermore, CML platelets completely lacked the ability to transform exogenous LTA_4 to lipoxins.

The formation of lipoxins from LTA_4 involves a lipoxygenation at C-15. A minor ω6-lipoxygenase activity has been demonstrated in platelets using arachidonic acid as substrate (22). Incubation of platelets with 6,9,12-octadecatrienoic acid led to the formation of both 10-hydroxy- and 13-hydroxy-γ-linolenic acid in a ratio of 2:1 (23). Although the involvement of a minor platelet ω6-lipoxygenase can not be excluded, it is probable that these reactions is catalysed by the 12-lipoxygenase. Furthermore, multiple actions of several lipoxygenases, catalyzing dioxygenation at different sites of the substrate, has been reported.

In summary, the results demonstrate that human platelets efficiently convert released LTA_4 to cysteinyl-containing leukotrienes. Similar results have also been reported by others (24). Furthermore, the present observations show that co-operation between granulocytes and platelets leads to formation of lipoxins from endogenous substrate. These findings may be of importance since platelet accumulation and activation has been indicated in non-allergic and allergic inflammation (10,11). Thus, increased amounts of platelets in e.g. the asthmatic lung may direct the conversion of leukocyte-derived LTA_4 towards elevated formation of the potent bronchoconstrictors, leukotrienes C_4, D_4 and E_4 and biologically active lipoxins.

ACKNOWLEDGEMENTS

We thank Ms Barbro Näsman-Glaser and Ms Inger Forsberg for excellent technical assistance. This project was supported by the Swedish National Association against Heart and Chest Disease, The Swedish Medical Research Council, The Swedish Cancer Society, King Gustav V 80-years Funds, Magnus Bergvalls Foundation and Karolinska Institutet´s Research Funds.

REFERENCES

1. Dahinden, C.A., Clancy, R M., Gross, M., Chiller, J.M. and Hugli, T. E.(1985) Proc. Natl. Acad. Sci. USA 82, 6632-6636.
2. McGee, J.E. and Fitzpatrick, F.A. (1986) Proc. Natl. Acad. Sci. USA 83, 1349-1353.
3. Claesson, H.-E. and Haeggström, J. (1988) Eur. J. Biochem. 173, 93-100.
4. Odlander, B., Jakobsson, P-J., Rosén, A. and Claesson, H-E. (1988) Biochem. Biophys. Res. Commun. 153, 203-208.
5. Feinmark, S.J. and Cannon, P.J. (1986) J. Biol. Chem. 261, 16466-16472.
6. Feinmark, S.J. and Cannon, P.J. (1987) Biochim. Biophys. Acta 922, 125-135.
7. Lindgren, J.Å., Hansson, G. and Samuelsson, B. (1981) FEBS Lett. 128, 329-335.
8. Marcus, A.J., Safier, L.B., Ullman, H.L., Broeckman, M.J., Islam, N.,Oglesby, T.D. and Gorman, R.R. (1984) Proc. Natl. Acad. Sci. USA 81, 903-907.
9. Claesson, H-E. and Feinmark, S.J. (1984) Biochim,. Biophys. Acta 804, 52-57.
10. Page, C.P. (1989) Immunopharmacology 17, 51-59.
11. Weksler, B.B. (1988) In: Platelet Membrane Receptors: Molecular Biology, Immunology, Biochemistry, and Pathology. pp 611-638, Alan R. Liss Inc.
12. Edenius, C., Heidvall, K. and Lindgren, J.Å. (1988) Eur. J. Biochem. 178, 81-86.
13. Edenius, C., Haeggström, J. and Lindgren, J.Å. (1988) Biochem,. Biophys.Res. Commun. 157, 801-807.
14. Edenius, C., Stenke, L. and Lindgren, J.Å. (1989) Submitted
15. Bach, M.K., Brashler, J.R. and Morton, Jr. D.R. (1984) Arch. Biochem. Biophys. 230, 455-465.
16. Rokach, J., Fitzsimmons, B.J., Leblanc, Y., Ueda, N. and Yamamoto, S. (1987) In: Advances in Prostaglandin, Thromboxane and Leukotriene Research. Eds B. Samuelsson, R. Paoletti and P. W. Ramwell, Raven Press, New York, vol 17, 761-767.
17. Serhan, C. N., Hamberg, M. and Samuelsson, B. (1984) Proc. Natl. Acad. Sci. USA 81, 5335-5339.
18. Samuelsson, B., Dahlén, S.-E., Lindgren, J.Å., Rouzer, C.A. and Serhan, C. N. (1987) Science 220, 568-575.
19. Hamberg, M. and Samuelsson, B. (1974) Proc. Natl. Acad. Sci. USA 71, 3400-3404.
20. Borgeat, P. and Samuelsson, B. (1979) Proc. Natl. Acad. Sci. USA 76, 2148-2152.
21. Okuma, M. and Uchino, H. (1979) Blood 54, 1258-1271.
22. Wong, P.Y.-K., Westlund, P. Hamberg, M. Granström. E., Chao, P.H.-W. and Samuelsson, B. (1985) J. Biol. Chem. 260, 9162-9165.
23. Hamberg, M. (1983) Biochem. Biophys. Res. Commun. 117, 593-600.
24. Maclouf, J. and Murphy, R.C. (1988) J. Biol. Chem. 263, 174-181.

Advances in Prostaglandin, Thromboxane, and Leukotriene Research, Vol. 20, edited by B. Samuelsson et al. Raven Press, Ltd., New York © 1990.

Incorportion of Arachidonic Acid into Glycerophospholipids of a Murine Bone Marrow Derived Mast Cell

Laura Bettazzoli, Joseph A. Zirrolli, Charles T. Reidhead, Mona Shahgholi, and Robert C. Murphy

National Jewish Center for Immunology and Respiratory Medicine
Department of Pediatrics
1400 Jackson St.
Denver, Colorado USA 80206

INTRODUCTION

Ten years ago two potent lipid mediators were structurally described: leukotriene C_4, a metabolite of arachidonic acid via the 5-lipoxygenase pathway of oxidative metabolism, and platelet activating factor, a unique alkylether phospholipid. During the intervening decade, a great deal of information has been obtained about the chemistry (1), biochemistry (2), pharmacology (3), and molecular biology (4,5) of these molecules and the proteins involved in biosynthesis (6) and recognition (7). However, a major question still remains as to the source of the biochemical precursors for both of these substances. Furthermore, an interesting question remaining in the field of eicosanoids is whether or not there is a single phospholipid source of arachidonic acid for eicosanoid biosynthesis within various cells. There are numerous reasons why our knowledge has not advanced in these areas, chief among them are 1) the analytical challenges presenting themselves in assessing a unique precursor in the presence of a complex mixture of potential precursors; 2) the biosynthesis of only small quantities of these lipid mediators following a physiologic relevant stimulus from a large mass of precursor; and 3) the complexities of phospholipid turnover and arachidonic acid remodeling within phospholipids. Several years ago we put forth a hypothesis that a common biochemical precursor existed for platelet activating factor and eicosanoids, that being 1-O-hexadecyl-2-arachidonoyl-glycerophosphocholine (8). This substance could be hydrolyzed by phospholipase A_2 generating two intermediates, free arachidonic acid which could be further processed to an active lipid mediator by either cyclooxygenase or 5-lipoxygenase and lyso-platelet activating factor which could be acetylated by acetyl transferase to PAF. These are seen in Figure 1.

Substantial progress has been made in understanding of the unique remodeling of arachidonic acid which takes place with cells, in particular the human polymorphonuclear leukocyte (8). The biochemical pathways illustrated in Figure 1 show partially the complex nature of arachidonic acid remodeling into phospholipid molecular species of phosphatidylcholine. The complicated nature of this remodeling process was not anticipated until most recently. For example, we found that when exogenous arachidonate was added to the human neutrophil, it was rapidly incorporated into 1,2-diacylglycerophospholipids (8) in particular glycerophosphatidylinositol (GPI) and glycerophosphatidylcholine (GPC). In a time dependent process this arachidonate was remodeled within the glycerophosphatidylcholine class into the 1-alkyl subclass of GPC. This appeared to be dependent upon the specificity of arachidonyl transferases for the 1-acyl-2-lyso-glycerophosphatidylcholine (9). Discovery of these multiple steps and time dependent remodeling processes have expanded greatly our understanding of how arachidonate becomes equilibrated within cells.

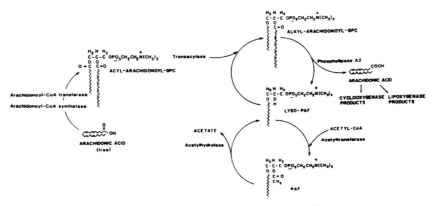

Figure 1 *Incorporation of arachidonic acid into 1-alkyl-2-arachidonoyl-GPC in the human neutrophil and the postulated liberation of free arachidonic acid and lyso-PAF for active lipid mediator biosynthesis (PAF, cyclooxygenase products, and lipoxygenase products) from this single precursor. (With permission, ref. 8)*

In order to elucidate the exact biochemical source cf arachidonic acid which is metabolized to eicosanoids, several strategies were developed over 20 years. However, two schools of thought dominated this area. By far the largest group of investigators employed radiolabeled arachidonic acid to trace its movement into esterified phospholipids, de-esterification and formation of eicosanoid products. Using such an approach in the platelet fcr example, evidence was presented to support the concept that phosphatidylinositol was a major phospholipid class providing arachidonic acid ending up as thromboxane (10). An alternative approach involved the measurement of the mass loss of arachidonate from phospholipid classes and in the platelet most of the mass of arachidonate which goes into thromboxane biosynthesis appeared to come from phosphatidylethanolamine (11). It has been difficult to reconcile these two independent and opposing observations. Both approaches to the arachidonic acid precursor question have different assumptions inherent in interpretation of the data. Therefore, we proposed several years ago to employ both techniques in our studies of the precursor of arachidonate for LTB$_4$ biosynthesis in the human neutrophil. Our approach was to measure specific activities (the ratio between the incorporated radioactive label from tracer arachidonate divided by the mass of the product measured by an independent technique). Specific activity was then used as a parameter to support precursor-product relationships in terms of glycerophospholipid molecular species and eicosanoid.

Studies with the human neutrophil revealed a similar situation to that found with the platelets. A majority of the arachidonic acid esterified to glycerophospholipids was in the glycerophosphatidylethanolamine (GPE) fraction, in particular in the 1-alkenyl-2-arachidonoyl-GPE molecular species. Overall, 18 different molecular species of glycerophospholipids were characterized which had arachidonate esterified at the sn-2 position (12). In experiments with [^{3}H]-arachidonate added as a tracer there was a time dependent remodeling of arachidonate from the 1,2-diacyl species to the 1-alkyl-GPC and -GPE species (8). When human neutrophils were stimulated with A23187, all three major phospholipid classes GPE, GPC, and GPI were hydrolyzed and the mass of arachidonic acid was released in the rank order GPE > GPC > GPI (13). In terms of radioactivity, most of the prelabeled arachidonate was released from GPC and GPI with very little radiolabeled release from GPE. Thus, the data from the stimulated neutrophil was similar to that obtained from the stimulated platelet studies in that the radiolabeled tracer experiment suggested that free arachidonate came from GPC or GPI or both and that the measurement of mass suggested that free arachidonate was liberated primarily from GPE. When specific activities of glycerophospholipid precursors and the specific activities of LTB$_4$ and 20-hydroxy-LTB$_4$ were calculated, it was found that the eicosanoid products had specific activities approximately 20-30 nCi/nmol (14) which was three times higher than any of the GPE subclasses which contained arachidonate. This specific activity of LTB$_4$ was very similar to that for the 1-alkyl-2-arachidonyl-GPC and somewhat lower than the specific activities for the 1-acyl-2-arachidonyl-GPC and the GPI molecular species which contain arachidonate. Thus, some of the arachidonate which was immediately processed by the 5-lipoxygenase enzyme had to come from one of these three lipid classes, but not GPE. Unfortunately, these studies employed a rather strong stimulus, that being the calcium ionophore A23187, which could have recruited alternative sources of arachidonate for the 5-lipoxygenase, perhaps not typically involved when using physiologically relevant stimuli.

The limited life time of the human neutrophil made it difficult to use biochemical techniques that could alter specific activities of phospholipid molecular species. Therefore, we have turned to the bone marrow derived mast cell in culture as a model for the study of arachidonic acid remodeling and a test system for the hypothesis presented in Figure 1 that a single molecular species, 1-alkyl-2-arachidonyl-GPC, is a unique precursor for free arachidonate processed by 5-lipoxygenase and cyclooxygenase. The mast cells employed here could be stimulated with IgE to release PGD$_2$, LTC$_4$, LTB$_4$, and PAF. Initial studies of the incorporation of arachidonic acid into classes and subclasses of this mast cell, release of free arachidonate and production of eicosanoids are presented. Furthermore, the depletion of free arachidonate from the tissue culture media was measured.

METHODS

Murine bone marrow derived mast cells were obtained from Dr. E. Razin (Jerusalem, Israel) which had been transformed by Abelson-MuLV virus to a cell which could be carried in culture (15). These cells were grown in RPMI supplemented with 10% fetal calf serum to a density of 1 x 10^6 cells/mL and fresh media (20 mL) added every two days.

Cells (1 x 10^7/ml) were incubated overnight with monoclonal mouse IgE, anti-DNP antibody (ICN Immunobiologicals) at a concentration of 1 μg/10^6 cells. These IgE sensitized cells were then ready for stimulation with DNP-BSA added in water (stock solution, 50 μg/mL). Before stimulation, the cells were washed with Hank's balanced salt solution (HBSS) then suspended at 10^7/mL. Following warming to 37^0 for 10 min the DNP-BSA was added to a final concentration of 100 ng/10^6 cells. The cell suspension was then agitated for 10 min.

Glycerophospholipids were isolated by the method of Bligh and Dyer (16). The organic extract was subjected to thin layer chromatography on silica gel G developed in $CHCl_3$/MeOH/isopropanol/0.25% KCl/triethylamine (90:27:75:18:54). The silica gel TLC plate had been previously washed in chloroform methanol (1:1) and activated in an oven overnight at 110°. Radioactive content on the TLC plate was measured by a Berthold TLC Linear Analyzer. Mast cell glycerolipids were labeled with [^{3}H]-arachidonate essentially by the methods previously described for the human neutrophil (8). Briefly, [^{3}H]-arachidonate (83 Ci/mM) complexed to HSA (5.0 mg/mL) was added to 1.0 mL cell suspension (5 x 10^6 mast cells), bringing the final concentration of arachidonic to 0.02 μM. Cold arachidonate was added to adjust concentration as indicated. Incubation was maintained at 37° for the times indicated. The reaction was terminated by the addition of cold HBSS containing HSA (0.25 mg/mL). The cells were centrifuged at 300 x g for 15 min and washed one time.

Free arachidonate was measured by the methods of Hadley *et al.* (17) using negative ion chemical ionization mass spectrometry of the pentafluorobenzyl ester. LTC_4 and PGD_2 were measured by enzyme immunoassay as previously described (18).

RESULTS

The distribution of arachidonic acid within the various glycerophospholipids is similar to what has been found for other cells including the human neutrophil. Table I indicates the mass of arachidonic acid in each of the glycerolipids GPS (glycerophosphoserine), GPI, GPC, GPE, and neutral lipids (primarily triglycerides). Furthermore, the distribution of arachidonate within

TABLE I: Mass of esterified arachidonic acid in glycerolipids of virus transformed mass cells determined by quantitative mass spectrometry of hydrolyzed arachidonate (17).

Distribution

Glycero-lipid Class	ng/10^{6}cells[1]	% 1-Acyl	% 1-Akyl	% 1-Alkenyl (plasmalogen)
GPS	2.9 ± 0.54[2]	--	--	--
GPI	25.6 ± 5.0	--	--	--
GPC	30.8 ± 3.5	49.8 ± 2.6	49.8 ± 2.5	2.0[3]
GPE	199 ± 50.1	27.6 ± 5.1	22.6 ± 5.5	51.6 ± 2.0
NL	11.8 ± 5.1	--	--	--

[1] n = 5
[2] ± Standard error of the mean
[3] One cell extract had measurable 1-alkenyl-2-arachidonoyl-GPC

the subclasses of GPC and GPE are also presented. These subclasses represent the 1-acyl, 1-alkyl, and 1-alkenyl-2-arachidonyl species which differ by the attachment of an alkyl chain at sn-1 through an ester, an ether, or a vinyl ether bond. The majority of the arachidonate was primarily found in the ethanolamine class of phospholipids which was six times higher in arachidonate content than the next most abundant lipid class, that being GPC. The distribution of arachidonate into the subclasses of these two abundant species was substantially different in that most of the arachidonate was found in the plasmalogen GPE subclass whereas arachidonate was equally distributed between the 1-acyl and 1-alkyl molecular species of GPC.

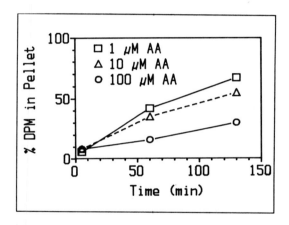

Figure 2 *Time-dependent uptake of exogenous* [³H]-*AA by transformed mast cells as a function of AA concentration.*

When arachidonic acid was added to these virus transformed mast cells, there was a time and concentration dependent uptake of arachidonic acid as shown in Figure 2. This rate of uptake was substantially slower than that measured for the human neutrophil which showed greater than 60% uptake in less than 5 min. The characterization of the esterified arachidonic acid in the cells following different times and exogenous arachidonate concentrations is shown in Table II. At the earliest time points there was a substantial amount of nonesterified, free arachidonic acid which fell to 1 to 2% after 1 hr incubation with all concentrations of arachidonate employed. The esterification of arachidonate appear to be most rapid into the GPC species at all concentrations tested. Even after 1 hr incubation typically greater than 50% of the exogenously added arachidonic acid remained esterified to GPC. Virtually no arachidonate was incorporated into GPS in the time frame of these experiments. The percent of [³H]-arachidonate incorporated into GPI was surprisingly constant in terms of its time course and was maintained around 10%. There was a time dependent increase in the esterification of arachidonate into the GPE classes which were initially low and increased 7-fold after 1 hr incubation at the 1 μM AA concentration, but only a 50% increase after 1 hr at the 100 μM aa concentration. Neutral lipids were

TABLE II: Concentration and time dependent distribution of [³H]-arachidonate in virus transformed murine bone marrow derived mast cells.

% Exogenous [³H]-Arachidonate[1]

Lipid Class	1 μM 5 min	60 min	10 μM 5 min	60 min	100 μM 5 min	60 min
GPS	---	4.4	---	---	---	---
GPI	7.5	7.4	9.6	12	10	9.9
GPC	29.2	57	66	71	60	45
GPE	4.1	28	3.6	9.8	8.6	12
AA	34	1.0	13	2.0	20	2.2
NL	25	2.0	7.2	4.4	0.9	30

[1] Distributions determined by relative area of radioactivity on the TLC separation of lipids. Radioactivity measured by TLC linear analyzer.

significant in terms of [³H]-arachidonate incorporation only at the 100 μM arachidonate concentration where they accounted for approximately 30% of the total arachidonate.

After sensitization of these mast cells with the monoclonal mouse IgE anti-DNP antibody, these cells could be stimulated with DNP-albumin to release free arachidonic acid, PGD$_2$, LTC$_4$, and LTB$_4$ in measurable quantities. When cells were prelabeled with [³H]-arachidonate, all of these products became radiolabeled. The release of β-hexosaminidase could also be measured as an index of stimulation of these mast cells. The time course for the release of LTC$_4$ is shown in Figure 3 where LTC$_4$ synthesis leveled off after 30 min. In a repesentative experiment, the amount of free arachidonate released was 19 ng/10^6 cells; LTC$_4$, 4.6 ng/10^6; and PGD$_2$, 0.77 ng/10^6 cells. The exact amount of LTC$_4$ release (per 10^6 cell) was quite reproducible within a single cell harvest, but somewhat variable as well as other eicosanoids when values were compared between cell batches. For example, using the same antigenic stimulation, PGD$_2$ was found to be produced in concentrations ranging from 0.18 to 0.77 ng/10^6 mast cells over a two month period. The source of this variation was of some concern since the cells were grown under identical conditions in all cases.

One of the parameters which was investigated was the amount of free arachidonic acid in the tissue culture media. Table III shows that fetal calf serum employed contained approximately 13 μM free arachidonate, (4 μg/mL). Since the growth media contained 10% fetal calf serum, this resulted in fresh media containing approximately 400 ng/mL arachidonate in the initial solution in which the cells were suspended. After 48 hr of cell growth in this media this level dropped substantially to approximately 30 ng/mL (0.09 μM) demonstrating utilization of arachidonate by the mast cells. Previous to this, no attempt was made to control the exact time of cell harvesting following exposure to fresh media nonmeasurement of free arachidonic acid present in the media.

Figure 3 *Time course LTC₄ biosynthesis and release from viral transformed mast cells following IgE sensitization and challenge.*

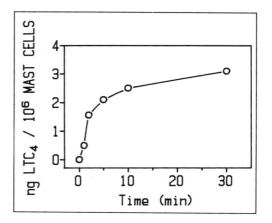

TABLE III: Concentration of unesterified arachidonic acid in tissue culture media[1].

	ng/ml[2]	
Fetal calf serum	3970	(13 μM)
Day 1	412	(1.35 μM)
Day 3[3]	27.5	(0.09 μM)

---

[1] RPMI with 10% fetal calf serum
[2] Averge of 2 determinations
[3] After 48 hours of cells in culture media

DISCUSSION

The Abelson-MuLV virus transformed bone marrow derived mast cell described by Pierce (15) can be carried in culture and has a functional IgE receptor which enable antigenic stimulation of this cell with release of eicosanoids and platelet activating factor. Radiolabeled arachidonic acid is readily incorporated into this cell and four classes of phospholipids become labeled in a time and exogenous arachidonate concentration dependent manner.

The phospholipid classes labeled include glycerophosphatidylcholine, glycerophosphatidylethanolamine, glycerophosphatidylinositol, and to a minor extent glycerophosphatidylserine. The three subclasses of GPC and GPE are also readily labeled. Most of the mass of esterified arachidonic acid is contained within the 1-alkenyl-GPE (plasmalogen) subclass, but this pool is very poorly labeled by exogenous radiolabeled arachidonate. More readily labeled by exogenous arachidonate is the smaller pool of arachidonate in glycerophosphatidylcholine which is equally distributed between 1-acyl and 1-alkyl-GPC. There were substantial variations in the absolute amount of eicosanoids produced following antigenic stimulation of these bone marrow derived mast cells. This was somewhat surprising since care had been taken to standardize protocols for sensitization and challenge of these cells. One uncontroled variable was the length of time these cells had been in culture and exposed to fresh media. The deprivation of free arachidonic acid from cells can have a major impact on PAF biosynthesis (19). Furthermore, there could be substantial reduction in the remodeling of arachidonate into molecular species of glycerophospholipids which are involved in the release of arachidonic acid for eicosanoid biosynthesis.

ACKNOWLEDGMENT

This work was supported, in part, by a grant from the National Institutes of Health (AA03527).

REFERENCES

1. Welton, A.F., G.W. Holland, D.W. Morgan, and M. O'Donnell, *Ann. Reports Med. Chem.* **24**:61 (1989).
2. Lewis, R.A. and K.F. Austen, *J. Clin. Invest.* **73**:889 (1984).
3. Mong, S., J. Miller, H.-L. Wu, and S.T. Crooke, *J. Pharmacol. Exptl. Therap.* **244**:508 (1988).
4. DeWitt, D.L. and W.L. Smith, *Proc. Natl. Acad. Sci. USA*, **85**:1412 (1988).
5. Matsumoto, T., C.D. Funk, O. Radmar, J.-O. Hoog, H. Jornvall, and B. Samuelsson, *Proc. Natl. Acad. Sci. USA*, **85**:26 (1988).
6. Samuelsson, B., M. Goldyne, E. Granstrom, M. Hamberg, S. Hammarstrom, and C. Malmsten, *Ann. Rev. Biochem.* **42**:997 (1978).
7. Braquet, P., T.Y. Shen, L. Touqui, and B.B. Vargaftig, *Pharmacol. Rev.* **32**:97 (1987).
8. Chilton, F.H. and R.C. Murphy, *J. Biol. Chem.* **261**:7771 (1986).
9. Chilton, F.H., J.S. Hadley, and R.C. Murphy, *Biochim. Biophys. Acta* **917**:48 (1987).
10. Prescott, S.M. and P.W. Majerus, *J. Biol. Chem.* **258**:764 (1983).
11. Billah, M.M. and E.G. Lapetina, *J. Biol. Chem.* **257**:5196 (1982).
12. Chilton, F.H. and R.C. Murphy, *Prostaglandin, Leukotriene, Med.* **23**:141 (1986).
13. Chilton, F.H. and T.R. Connell, *J. Biol. Chem.* **263**:5260 (1988).
14. Chilton, F.H. *Biochem. J.* **258**:327 (1989).
15. Pierce, J.H., P.D. DiFiore, S.A. Aaronson, M. Potter, J. Pumphrey, A. Scott, and I.N. Ihle, *Cell* **41**:685 (1985).
16. Bligh, E.G. and W. Dyer, *Can. J. Biochem. Physiol.* **37**:911 (1959).
17. Hadley, J.S., A. Fradin, and R.C. Murphy, *Biomed. Environ. Mass Spectrom.* **15**:175 (1988).
18. Westcott, J.Y., S. Chang, M. Balazy, D.O. Stene, P. Pradelles, M. Maclouf, N.F. Voelkel, and R.C. Murphy, *Prostaglandins* **32**:857 (1986).
19. Ramesha, C.S. and W.C. Pickett, *J. Biol. Chem.* **261**:7592 (1986).

Advances in Prostaglandin, Thromboxane, and Leukotriene Research, Vol. 20, edited by B. Samuelsson et al. Raven Press, Ltd., New York © 1990.

CHARACTERIZATION OF A SECRETABLE PHOSPHOLIPASE A$_2$ FROM HUMAN PLATELETS

Ruth M. Kramer[a], Berit Johansen[b], Catherine Hession[c] and R. Blake Pepinsky[c]

[a] Lilly Research Laboratories, Indianapolis, IN 46285;
[b] Norwegian Institute of Technology, Trondheim, Norway;
[c] Biogen Inc., Cambridge, MA 02142

Introduction

Phospholipases A$_2$ (PLA$_2$s) constitute a diverse family of enzymes that hydrolyze the sn-2 fatty acyl ester bond of phosphoglycerides liberating free fatty acids and lyso-phospholipids (10). Extracellular, secreted PLA$_2$s from snake venoms and pancreas have been sequenced and structurally defined, and the molecular mechanism of enzymatic action has been extensively studied (50, 10). In contrast, until recently, little was known about the molecular structure and properties of non-pancreatic mammalian PLA$_2$s. Knowledge of the structure and mode of action of these PLA$_2$s, however, is a prerequisite for further understanding of their involvement in cellular processes and elucidation of their role in disease.

Mammalian extracellular PLA$_2$s are abundant in pancreatic secretions, but are also present in plasma, lymph and pulmonary alveolar secretions (45). Intracellular PLA$_2$s are found in all tissues and cells (49), where they are located either in the cytosolic compartment associated with the plasma membrane or stored within secretory granules. The granule-associated PLA$_2$s are designed to effectively degrade phospholipids upon exocytosis thereby serving an anti-microbial function (13). In contrast, the cytosolic PLA$_2$s play a key role in the biosynthesis of specifically tailored phospholipids and the degradation of peroxidized phospholipids thus protecting membranes from oxidation damage. Furthermore, such PLA$_2$s are involved in the generation of rate-limiting precursors for various types of lipid mediators (21, 43) that transmit stimulatory signals to other cells or function as intracellular messengers (34, 30). This amplification mechanism is an integral part of the inflammatory response of tissues to injury that normally leads to removal of the inciting agent and repair of injured site.

The control and regulation of enzymatic activity of the granule-associated and cytosolic PLA$_2$s are quite distinct. PLA$_2$s sequestered in granules under conditions that suppress catalytic activity are activated upon secretion into the extracellular space, where conditions for enzyme activity are favourable. The regulation of the activity of cytosolic PLA$_2$s, on the other hand, appears to be subject to many different factors that may act in concert to modulate catalytic activity and direct the enzyme to appropriate target substrates. Thus, changes in intracellular free Ca^{2+}, perturbations of the plasma membrane, protein kinase C and a PLA_2 activating protein have all been implicated in PLA_2 activation (49, 9, 7). More recently, it has been proposed that cytosolic PLA_2s may be directly activated via membrane receptors and guanine nucleotide-binding proteins (2).

Human platelet secretable phospholipase A₂

We have previously characterized a PLA_2 from human platelets that exhibits functional properties typical for a cytosolic PLA_2 (23-25). The enzyme is activated by physiological (submicromolar) concentrations of Ca^{2+}, stimulated by diacylglycerol, hydrolyzes both diacyl-phospholipids and ether-linked PAF precursor phospholipids and is catalytically active at neutral pH. This PLA_2 has a preference for substrate presented in the physical form of sonicated liposomes, has an apparent molecular weight of 60,000 (by gel filtration) and is a rather labile enzyme that is denatured by most detergents, acid and non-physiological salt concentrations. The scarceness of the enzyme in platelets and its lability has hampered purification of the enzyme.

We have observed a second PLA_2 resembling an extracellular enzyme that is secreted by washed platelets upon stimulation with thrombin (Fig. 1.). The secreted PLA_2 was stable in acid (pH < 1) and could only be detected using *E.coli* membranes as substrate. Although the secretable PLA_2 is only a trace protein component of platelets, the great stability in acid was a key property that ultimately allowed us to purify the enzyme to homogeneity (26). The PLA_2 was extracted from lysed platelets at pH 1, dialyzed against acetate buffer (pH 4.5), subjected to cation exchange chromatography, followed by gel filtration and reverse-phase chromatography. Overall, the platelet PLA_2 was

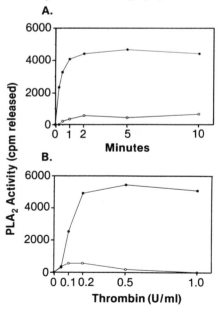

FIG. 1. Time-course (A) and dose-dependence (B) of thrombin induced secretion of PLA_2 from human platelets.

purified over a million-fold with a recovery of 34%. The purified platelet PLA$_2$ had a molecular weight of 14,000 (by SDS-PAGE) and exhibited maximal activity at pH 8-9 in the presence of 10 mM Ca^{2+}. The PLA$_2$ showed a great preference for *E.coli* membrane substrate, hydrolyzed phosphatidylethanolamine more readily than phosphatidylcholine and showed poor activity towards phosphatidylcholine presented in the physical form of liposomes.

The amino-terminal amino acid sequence of the platelet PLA$_2$ was determined to be: NH$_2$-Asn-Leu-Val-Asn-Phe-His-Arg-Met-Ile-Lys-Leu-Thr-Thr-Gly-Lys-Glu-Ala-Ala-Leu. Based on the sequences Asn^4 to Ile^9 and Met^8 to Thr^{13} two overlapping degenerate oligonucleotide probes (17 nucleotides in length; 48- and 144-fold redundant, respectively) were synthesized and used to screen a human genomic phage library by plaque hybridization analysis. One clone hybridized to both probes and contained a genomic DNA insert of 15 kb. This insert comprised a 6.2-kb *Hind*III restriction fragment that hybridized to both probes. The restriction fragment was subcloned and completely sequenced. The restriction map of the 6.2-kb fragment and a portion of the sequence that contains the coding sequences for the PLA$_2$ are shown in Fig. 2. Four exons were identified that encode a 144-amino acid protein. Exon 2 encodes the mature amino-terminal sequence that we obtained by sequencing platelet PLA$_2$. This sequence is preceded by a 20-residue peptide starting with a methionine. The intron-exon structure greatly resembles that of the human pancreatic PLA$_2$ (40).

A.

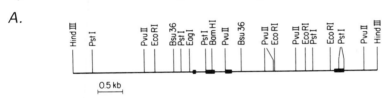

B.

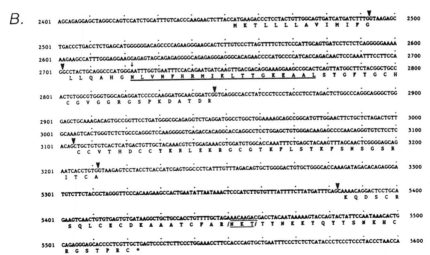

FIG. 2.   PLA$_2$ gene: restriction map (A) and DNA sequence (nucleotides 2401-3300 and 5301-5600) containing translated regions (B); triangles indicate intron-exon boundaries.

Southern blot analysis of human chromosomal DNA digests with a PLA₂ 1.4-kb *Bsu*36 restriction fragment (spanning nucleotides 2055-3414) revealed that a single gene exists for this human PLA₂ (Fig. 3A). A 3.8-kb PLA₂ restriction fragment was transfected into COS-7 cells. Conditioned media from transfected cells contained >100 times more PLA₂ activity than cells transfected with the vector only. Expression of the PLA₂ gene in animal cells confirmed that the gene encodes a functional protein. Furthermore, the fact that transfected cells secrete PLA₂ indicates that the peptide preceding the amino terminus serves as a functional signal sequence. Levels of mRNA in transfected COS-7 cells were monitored by Northern blotting, probing with the PLA₂ 1.4-kb *Bsu*36 restriction fragment. The probe hybridized to a ~1200-base nucleotide in cells transfected with the PLA₂ construct (Fig. 3B) consistent with the predicted size of a PLA₂ transcript.

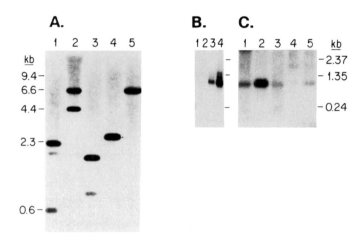

FIG. 3.   Southern analysis (A) of human genomic DNA digested with*Pst*I (1), *Bam*HI (2), *Pvu*II (3), *Eco*RI (4) and *Hind*III (5) and probed with the *Bsu*36 restriction fragment; Northern blotting (B) of RNA from control (1,2) and PLA₂-transfected (3,4) COS-7 cells; Northern analysis (C) of RNA human tonsils (1), placenta (2), kidney (3) and synovial cells from patients with rheumatoid arthritis (4, 5).

Structural features of human platelet secretable phospholipase A₂

Several important structural features of the human PLA₂ are predicted from the amino acid sequence. First, the 20-amino acid extension preceding the amino terminus of the mature protein resembles a signal sequence for translocation from the cytosolic compartment to the central vacuolar system (3). The presence of this element confirms that the platelet PLA₂ is destined for the secretory pathway. Second, the deduced amino acid sequence of the mature protein (Fig. 2) contains highly conserved amino acid residues and sequences characteristic of all PLA₂s sequenced to date (42, 19, 1), including the α-helical amino-terminal segment (residues 1-12), the calcium binding loop (residues 25-37 and 49) and the catalytic site (His[48], Asp[99], Tyr[52] and Tyr[73]). PLA$_2$s have been separated into two distinct structural classes, designated Group I and II (18). As shown in Fig. 4, the human PLA$_2$ sequence exhibits the half-cystine pattern typical of Group II enzymes lacking both Cys[11] and Cys[77], but having Cys[50] and the carboxyl-terminal extension ending with a half-cystine. However, the human PLA$_2$ also possesses a Group I-like feature within the structural segment called the "surface loop" (residue 54-66), since it is missing only six residues out of the total thirteen residues present in pancreatic PLA$_2$s (12). Overall, the homology with representative Group I and Group II PLA$_2$s (e. g. PLA$_2$ from bovine pancreas and *C.atrox* venom) is 37% and 44%, respectively. The amino acid sequence of rat platelet PLA$_2$ has been reported (17). Alignment of the protein sequence of the human and rat platelet PLA$_2$ (Fig. 4) reveals many identical structural segments and an overall sequence homology of 69%. Furthermore, some highly conserved residues are changed in both platelet PLA$_2$s, e.g. Tyr[28] and Tyr[75] are replaced by His[28] and Phe[75], respectively. Recently, full length amino acid sequence of a PLA$_2$ present in human rheumatoid arthritic fluid has been reported (41, 26). Interestingly, this enzyme is identical to the human platelet enzyme.

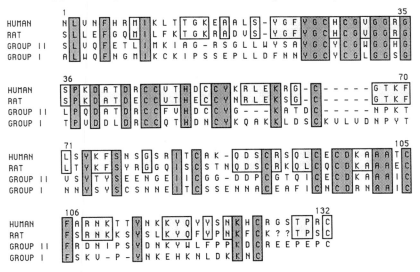

Fig. 4.   Alignment of amino acid sequences of PLA$_2$ from human platelet, rat platelet, *C.atrox* venom (Group II) and bovine pancreas (Group I). Identical residues are boxed (dark shading: homology between all PLA$_2$s; light shading: sequence identity between human and rat platelet PLA$_2$).

Phospholipases A$_2$ and disease

There is significant evidence to indicate that PLA$_2$s are involved in the pathogenesis of many diseases. Thus, local and circulating levels of PLA$_2$ enzyme are elevated during infections, inflammatory diseases, tissue injury and brain dysfunction (45, 6, 14) and correlate with the severity, magnitude and duration of theses disorders (15, 45-47, 37). Excessive PLA$_2$ activity may promote chronic inflammation, allergic reactions, tissue injury and pathophysiological complications. These effects may be the result of accumulating PLA_2 products (lysophospholipids and free fatty acids) and destruction of key structural phospholipid components, but undoubtedly are potentiated by secondary metabolites, such as eicosanoids and platelet-activating factor. PLA_2 products or lipid mediators derived thereof have been implicated in numerous activities that are an integral part in effector cell activation, chemotaxis, adhesion, degranulation, phago-cytosis and aggregation (34). The (patho)physiological sequelae of these cellular events include changes in smooth muscle tone, vascular permeability and blood flow and result in influx of inflammatory cells, tissue damage, fever and pain (30, 8).

PLA_2s secreted excessively at local sites may be responsible for tissue damage common to rheumatic disorders, alveolar epithelial injury of lung diseases and reperfusion damage (45, 6). Moreover, massive release of such PLA_2s into the circulation and air-ways may provide for the disturbed functions of the renal, circulatory and respiratory organ systems in acute pancreatitis, adult respiratory distress syndrom and septic shock. The source of locally emerging and systemically circulating PLA_2s is unknown. Various cells, including macrophages (44), neutrophils (29), platelets (20, 26), chondro-cytes (5), synoviocytes (19), renal mesanglial cells (35) and smooth muscle cells (36) were found to release PLA_2 upon stimulation. Moreover, interleukin 1, a polypeptide that is produced after infection, injury or antigenic challenge (11), was reported to induce cellular biosynthesis of PLA_2 (5). Human secreted PLA_2 mRNA has been detected in human tonsils, kidney and placenta, as well as in cells derived from human rheuma-toid arthritic synovial fluid (Fig. 3C), inflamed synovial tissue and peritoneal exudate (41). Such mRNA was, however, not detectable in pancreas, spleen and liver (41). Although the presence of PLA_2 transcripts in isolated polymorphonuclear leucocytes, monocytes and macrophages remains to be demonstrated, it appears that extracellular PLA_2s may originate not only from platelets and cells of the myelomonocytic phagocyte system, but also from cells constituting inflamed or damaged tissues.

Direct evidence for the involvement of PLA_2 in the pathogenesis of disease has been obtained in studies using in vitro or animal models of disease, where administration of purified PLA_2s was found to cause disease-like symptoms (45). Exogenous PLA_2 was found to induce release of eicosanoids from leukocytes (28) and potentiate stimulation of neutrophils by the chemotactic peptide fMLF (27). More recently, PLA_2 isolated from septic shock plasma was reported to promote systemic hypotension upon reinfusion (47). Intra-articular injection of purified PLA_2 elicited acute inflammatory and destructive changes of joints (48). PLA_2 was also found to induce nonspecific airway hyper-reactivity that is a hallmark of asthma (4). Further, PLA_2 was reported to readily degrade lung surfactant, change the barrier properties of the alveolar epithelium and promote functional and morphological changes indicative of severe epithelial cell injury (33). Similarly, exogenous PLA_2 produced renal tubular cell injury that was poten-tiated under hypoxic conditions (32).

Taken together these findings support the contention that secreted PLA_2s are inti-mately involved in the pathogenesis of many diseases, including pulmonary dysfunc-tion, reperfusion injury, gastrointesinal disorders, connective tissue and skin diseases, disordered brain function and septic shock. Control of excessive PLA_2 secretion, activa-tion and induction as well as inhibition of exorbitant enzymatic activity may therefore provide adjunctive therapy in the prevention or treatment of these disorders.

Conclusions

PLA_2 present in human platelets closely resembles PLA_2s from the venoms of snake and exhibits structural and functional properties of a secreted enzyme. Undoubtedly, intracellular, cytosolic platelet PLA_2s that are activated by submicromolar Ca^{2+} and prefer phosphatidylcholine substrates (31, 25) are distinct enzymes and their structural properties remain to be elucidated.

It is well known that snake venom PLA_2s, although exhibiting a high degree of structural homology, differ greatly in their pharmacological properties. The pharmacological potency is most pronounced for basic PLA_2s. There is evidence to indicate that these pharmacological properties may not be solely due to hydrolytic activity, but also depend on structural features of the PLA_2 protein (39). The human PLA_2 is most homologous to basic snake venom PLA_2s and the full spectrum of its biological activities remains to be determined. The availability of sufficient quantities of recombinant PLA_2 for crystallographic analysis will play a key role in the discovery and design of potential drugs. Furthermore, molecular PLA_2 probes will enable the study of regulation of PLA_2 at the transcriptional level. Such investigations may provide new insights into the involvement of secreted PLA_2s in the pathophysiology of chronic diseases and reveal new points of pharmacological intervention.

References

1. Achari, A., Scott, D., Barlow, P., Vidal, J.C., Otwinowski, Z., Brunie, S. and Sigler, P. (1987) Cold Spring Harbour Symp. Quant. Biol. 52, 441-452
2. Axelrod, J., Burch, R.M. and Jelsema, C.L. (1988) Trends Neurochem. Sci. 11,117-123
3. Blobel, G. (1988) Proc.Natl.Acad.Sci. 77, 1496-1500
4. Chand, N., Diamantis, W., Mahoney, T.P. and Sofia, R.D. (1988) Br.J.Pharmacol. 94, 1057-1062
5. Chang, J., Gilman, S.C. and Lewis, A.J. (1986) J.Immunol. 136, 1283-1287
6. Chang, J., Musser, J.H. and McGregor, H. (1987) Biochem.Pharmacol. 36, 2429-2436
7. Clark, M.A., Conway, T.M., Shorr, R.G.L. and Crooke, S. (1987) J.Biol.Chem. 262, 4402-4406
8. Davies, P., Bailey, P.J. and Goldenberg, M.M. (1984) Ann.Rev. Immunol. 2, 335-357
9. Dawson, R.M.C., Hemington, N.L. and Irvine, R.F. (1983) Biochem.Biophys. Res.Commun. 117, 196-201
10. Dennis, E.A. (1983) in The Enzymes (ed. Boyer, P.) Vol 16, pp. 307-353, Academic Press, New York
11. Dinarello, C. (1988) Faseb J. 2, 108-115
12. Dufton, M.J., Eaker, D. and Hider, R.C. (1983) Eur.J.Biochem. 137, 537-544
13. Elsbach, P. (1980) Rev.Infect.Dis. 2, 106-128
14. Farooqui, A.A., Taylor, W.A. and Horrocks, L.A. (1987) Neurochem. Pathol. 7, 99-128
15. Gattaz, W.F., Kollisch, M., Thuren, T., Virtanen, J.A. and Kinnunen, P.K.J. (1987) Biol.Psychiatry 22, 421-426
16. Gilman, S.C., Chang, J., Zeigler, P.R., Uhl, J. and Mochan, E. (1988) Arthritis Rheum. 31, 126-130
17. Hayakawa, M., Kudo, I., Tomita, M., Nojima, S. and Inoue K. (1988) J.Biochem. 104, 767-772
18. Heinrikson, R.L., Krueger, E.T. and Keim, P.S. (1977) J.Biol.Chem. 252, 4913-4921
19. Heinrikson, R.L. (1982) in Proteins in Biology and Medicine (Bradshaw, R.A.,

Hill, R.L., Tang, J., Chiah-chuan, L., Tien-chin, T. and Chen-lu, T. eds.) pp. 131-152, Academic Press, New York

20. Horigome, K., Hayakawa, M., Inoue, K. and Nojima, S. (1987) J.Biochem 204, 53-61
21. Irvine, R.F. (1982) Biochem.J. 204, 3-16
22. Kini, R.M. and Evans, H.J. (1987) J.Biol.Chem. 262, 14402-14407
23. Kramer, R.M., Checani, G.C., Deykin, A., Pritzker, C.R. and Deykin, D. (1986) Biochim.Biophys.Acta 878, 394-403
24. Kramer, R.M., Checani, G.C. and Deykin, D. (1987) Biochem. J. 248, 779-783
25. Kramer, R.M., Jakubowski, J.A. and Deykin, D. (1988) Biochim. Biophys.Acta 959, 269-279
26. Kramer, R.M., Hession, C., Johansen, B., Hayes, G., McGray, P., Chow, E.P., Tizard, R. and Pepinsky, R.B. (1989) J.Biol.Chem. 264, 5768-5775
27. Lackie, J.M. and Lawrence, A.J. (1987) Biochem.Pharmacol. 36, 1941-1945
28. Lam, B.K., Lee, C.Y. and Wong, P. Y-K (1988) Ann.N.Y. Acad.Sci. 524, 27-34
29. Lanni, C. and Becker, E.L. (1983) Am.J.Pathol. 113, 90-94
30. Larsen, G.L. and Henson, P.M. (1983) Ann.Rev.Immunol. 1, 335-359
31. Loeb, L. and Gross, R. (1986) J.Biol.Chem. 261, 10467-10470
32. Nguyen, V.D., Cieslinski, D.A. and Humes H.D. (1988) J.Clin.Invest. 82, 1098-1105
33. Niewoehner, D.E., Rice K., Duane, P., Sinha, A.A., Gebhard R. & Wangensteen, D. (1989) J.Appl.Physiol. 66, 261-267
34. O'Flaherty, J.T. (1982) Lab.Invest. 47, 314-329
35. Pfeilschifter, J., Pignat, W., Vosbeck, K. and Marki, F. (1989) Biochem. Biophys.Res.Commun. 159, 385-394
36. Pfeilschifter, J., Pignat, W., Marki, F. and Wiesenberg, I. (1989) Eur.J.Biochem. 181, 237-242
37. Pruzanski, W., Keystone, E.C., Sternby, B. ,Bombardier, C., Snow, K.M. and Vadas, P. (1988) J.Rheumatol. 15, 1351-1355
38. Renetseder, R., Brunie, S., Dijkstra, B.W., Drenth, J. and Sigler, P.B. (1985) J.Biol.Chem. 260, 11627-11634
39. Rosenberg, P. (1986) in Natural Toxins (Harris, J.R., ed.) pp.129-174, Oxford University Press, Oxford
40. Seilhamer, J.J., Randall, T.L., Yamanaka, M. and Johnson, L.K. (1986) DNA 5, 519-527
41. Seilhamer, J.J., Pruzanski, W., Vadas, P., Plant, S., Miller, J.A., Kloss, J. and Johnson, L.K. (1989) J.Biol.Chem. 264, 5335-5338
42. Slotboom, A.J., Verheij, H.M. and de Haas, G.H. (1982) in New Comprehensive Biochemistry (Neuberger, A. and van Deenen, L.L.M., eds) Vol 4, pp. 359-434, Elsevier Science Publishers B. V., Amsterdam
43. Snyder, F. (1985) Med.Res.Rev. 5, 107-140
44. Traynor, J.R. and Authi, K.S. (1981) Biochim.Biophys.Acta 665, 571-577
45. Vadas P. and Pruzanski, W. (1986) Lab.Invest. 4, 391-404
46. Vadas, P. , Pruzanski, W., Stefanski, E., Sternby, B., Mustard, R., Bohnen, J., Frazer, I., Farewell, V. and Bombardier, C. (1988) Crit.Care Med. 16, 1-7
47. Vadas, P., Pruzanski, W. and Stefanski, E. (1988) Agents and Actions 24, 320-325
48. Vadas, P., Pruzanski, W., Kim, J. and Fornasier, V. (1989) Am.J.Pathol. 134, 807-811
49. Van den Bosch, H. (1980) Biochim.Biophys.Acta 604, 191-246
50. Verheij, H.M., Slotboom, A.J. and de Haas, G.H. (1981) Rev. Physiol.Biochem. Pharmacol. 91, 91-203

Advances in Prostaglandin, Thromboxane, and Leukotriene Research, Vol. 20,
edited by B. Samuelsson et al.
Raven Press, Ltd., New York © 1990.

Novel Eicosanoids Generated by Cytochrome P450: Effects on Platelet Aggregation and Protein Phosphorylation

K. Malcolm[1], J.R. Falck[2] and F.A. Fitzpatrick[1]

[1]University of Colorado Health Sciences Center
Department of Pharmacology C236
4200 E. Ninth Avenue
Denver, Colorado USA 80262

[2]Department of Molecular Genetics
University of Texas Health Science Center
Dallas, Texas USA 75235

INTRODUCTION

The eicosanoid family includes : i) prostaglandins and thromboxanes derived from the cyclooxygenase enzyme   ii) leukotrienes   derived from the 5-lipoxygenase enzyme (1) iii) other mono -, di-, or trihydroxy eicosatetraenoic acid metabolites derived from regiospecific lipoxygenase enzymes (2)   iv) epoxyeicosatrienoic acids (EETs) or hydroxy-eicosatetraenoic acids (HETEs) derived from cytochrome P-450 mixed function monoxygenase (3). Compared to classical eicosanoids, the latter group of 'epoxygenase' eicosanoids has distinctive biosynthetic origins and prominent effects on stimulus-response coupling in cardiac, renal, and secretory cells (4-10). In some cases,typified by the renal system, the relationships between their occurrence, activity, and mechanism suggests that the EETs may have a physiological role (11). In other systems their physiological roles are controversial, but their pharmacological traits are interesting.

Effects on Cyclooxygenase

We began to investigate the EETs because of uncertainties about their mechanism of action. Inhibition of Na^+/K^+ ATPase accounts for the activity of the EETs in renal and ocular systems, but not in other systems (8). Based on a precedent by Oliw (12) who demonstrated that 5,6-cis-EET was a substrate for the cyclooxygenase we proposed that other EETs acted, in part, by competitive inhibition of this enzyme.We confirmed that both 14,15-cis-EET and 8,9-cis-EET inhibited isolated cyclooxygenase enzyme in a dose dependent manner at concentrations from 1 to 50 μM.   The 11,12-cis-EET analog was ineffective at concentrations below 100 μM. We extended our investigation to include four stereoisomers of 14,15-EET. Among these, only the (14R,15S) stereoisomer was active. (14S,15R)-cis-EET, (14S,15S)-trans-EET, (14R,15R)-trans-EET and the erythro and threo vicinal 14,15-diols were inactive (13).   Three points were noteworthy: i) the inhibition of cyclooxygenase was stereospecific   ii) the effect of (14R,15S)-cis-EET conformed to a pattern establishing the dextrorotary isomer as the more potent member of an enantiomeric pair, and iii) epoxidation of arachidonic acid by cytochrome P-450 *in vitro* proceeds stereoselectively with predominant formation of the active species (14R,15S)-cis-EET (14).

Effects on Human Platelets

Next, we conducted experiments to characterize the effects of EETs on cellular cyclooxygenase activity, using human platelets as a model system. Platelets are useful in this regard because their principal cyclooxygenase metabolite, thromboxane A_2 (TxA$_2$), is conveniently determined by immunoassay for its hydration product, TxB$_2$ and the results can be correlated with the corresponding platelet aggregation. These experiments showed that potency and stereospecific effects were maintained within platelets, *in vitro*: only (14R,15S)-cis-EET inhibited the cellular cyclooxygenase. However, all EET isomers, without evident stereospecificity, inhibited platelet aggregation induced by exogenous arachidonic acid. Inhibition of TxB$_2$ formation was dissociated from inhibition of aggregation. Ordinarily, these two parameters correspond.

Because of this unusual effect on human platelets we continued to investigate the scope and mechanism of the platelet antiaggregatory activity of the EETs. We focused on 14,15-cis-EET because it may occur in endothelial cells and platelets (15,16). We also examined its episulfide and aza analogs, and its 14,15-trans isomer because these do not inhibit the cyclooxygenase enzyme.

EXPERIMENTAL

Human platelet rich plasma (45 ml) was mixed with 93 mM sodium citrate/7 mM citric acid/0.14 mM dextrose anticoagulant (5 ml) and centrifuged at 200 x g for 12 minutes. The platelet pellet was resuspended in 20 ml of Ca^{++} free Hank's balanced salt solution and 2 ml of plasma. This mixture was incubated with 1 mCi of [^{32}P] orthophosphoric acid for 1 hr at 37°C. Excess [^{32}P] phosphate was removed by washing the platelets once with Ca^{++} free Hanks. The platelets were finally resuspended in buffer containing 1.4 mM Ca^{++} and 0.7 mM Mg^{++}. When phosphoprotein formation was quantitated, phosphate free Hank's was used.

Suspensions of washed platelets labeled with [^{32}P]-phosphate were incubated for 2 min at 37°C with 0-100 nanomoles of 14,15-cis-EET or an analog. Aggregation, and corresponding biochemical events such as protein phosphorylation, were initiated by adding thrombin (0.1 units/ml), divalent Ca^{++} ionophore A23187 (1 μM) or PMA (20 ng/ml). Aggregation was monitored photometrically. Samples (0.2 ml) were withdrawn and quenched in a 3x concentrate of Laemmli sample buffer. Platelet proteins were separated by electrophoresis on a 10% SDS-PAGE gel (17). Proteins were visualized by staining with Comassie blue. Protein phosphorylation was visualized by autoradiography on Kodak ARO x-ray film. In certain experiments, the extent of phosphoprotein formation was measured by cutting a band from the dried gel and measuring the radioactivity by liquid scintillation spectrometry.

RESULTS

Table I lists the potency of 14,15-cis-EET; 14,15-episulfide-cis-ET; 14,15-aza-ET, and 14,15-trans-EET as inhibitors of platelet aggregation. 14,15-cis-EET and its episulfide isomer inhibit aggregation induced by arachidonic acid, the thromboxane A_2 mimetic U46619, the divalent calcium ionophore A23187, and collagen. The IC$_{50}$ value is below 10 μM in these instances. The aza-

TABLE I. IC_{50} values for inhibition of platelet aggregation by epoxyeicosatrienoic acid analogs.

Agonist	(±)14,15-cis-EET	(±)14,15-cis-thia-Et	(±)14,15-cis-AzA-ET	(±)14,15-trans-ET
AA-3 μM	3.9 ± 1.0	6.0 ± 1.8	>50 μM	5.8 ± 1.3
U-46619 (1 μM)	6.7 ± 2.7	3.4 ± 1.1	15 μM	16 ± 7.2
A-23187 (2 μM)	6.3 ± 1.2	7.2 ± 2.6		34.3 ± 11.6
Thrombin* (0.1 U/ml)	100 μM n/i	100 μM n/i	100 μM n/i	100 μM n/i
Collagen (2 μg/ml)	7.9 ± 2.6	12 ± 3.2	>30	8 ± 3 μM
PMA+ (20 ng/ml)	100 μM n/i	50 μM n/i	50 μM n/i	100 μM n/i

Values represent mean $\pm$ S.E.M. IC_{50} in μM. IC_{50} equals concentration that inhibits the initial rate or maximal response by half of its maximal value.

The number of experiments involving separate blood donors was n>3.

*n/i refers to no change in the initial rate or the magnitude of the response.

+n/i refers to no change in the initial rate or the magnitude of the response. The initiation of aggregation was delayed by 1 minute at these concentrations.

analog and the 14,15-trans EET analog were less potent inhibitors. None of the 14,15-EET analogs, at concentrations up to 100 μM, inhibited aggregation induced by thrombin or phorbol myristyl acetate, a direct activator of protein kinase C. These data indicate that 14,15-cis-EET and its episulfide analog do not act by established mechanisms such as cyclooxygenase inhibition; antagonism of the PGH_2/TxA_2 receptor; or elevation of intracellular cyclic adenosine monophosphate. For example, a cyclooxygenase inhibitor, typified by aspirin, will inhibit arachidonic acid and collagen induced aggregation, but not U46619 or A23187 induced aggregation. In contrast, 14,15-cis EET and the episulfide analog inhibit all four agonists. Furthermore, the episulfide analog of 14,15-cis EET does not inhibit the isolated cyclooxygenase enzyme, nor does it inhibit thromboxane B_2 formation by platelets stimulated with exogenous arachidonic acid (1 μg/ml) . Platelets produced 203 ± 25 ng TxB_2/ml in the presence of 50 μM 14,15-cis-episulfide ET. This was statistically indistinguishable from the control value of 213 ± 15 ng/ml.

The EETs examined do not act by receptor antagonism of the PGH_2 receptor or by elevation of intracellular cyclic AMP. This conclusion may be derived from the data in Table I. PGH_2/TxA_2 receptor antagonists, typified by LY 655,240 or BM 13.177 will inhibit U46619, arachidonic acid, and collagen induced aggregation, but not A23187 induced aggregation. In contrast, 14,15-cis-EET and the episulfide analog inhibited all four agonists. Furthermore, receptor level antagonists do not inhibit TxB_2 formation derived from endogenous arachidonic acid. In contrast, for platelets stimulated by collagen, TxB_2 levels declined from control values of 189 ± 11 ng/ml to 107 ± 1; 90 ± 13; and 64 ± 10 ng TxB_2/ml in the presence of 7.5 μM, 15 μM, and 30 μM 14,15-cis-episulfide-EET, respectively. Agents that will elevate platelet cyclic AMP inhibit both thrombin and A23187 induced aggregation. In contrast, the EETs displayed a differential effect on these agonists.

To probe their mechanism of action we examined the effect of EETs on aggregation and phosphoprotein formation by platelets stimulated with A23187, thrombin, U46619, and PMA, an agonist which activates protein kinase C directly (18). At concentrations of 50 -100 μM neither 14,15-cis-EET nor the corresponding sulfur and nitrogen analogs inhibited platelet aggregation induced by thrombin (0.1 unit/ml). Phosphorylation of a 40 kilodalton substrate (19) and other phosphoproteins was indistinguishable between control and EET treated samples [Figure 1]. Unlike the case with thrombin, 14,15-cis-EET and its episulfide EET analog inhibited aggregation induced by the

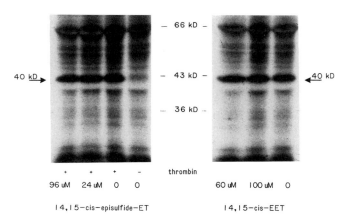

Figure 1. *Effect of 14,15 EET analogs on thrombin induced platelet aggregation and phosphoprotein formation. The left panel shows results with 14,15-cis-episulfide-ET. The right panel shows results with 14,15-cis-EET. Platelets were incubated for 2 min with the concentrations indicated, then stimulated with 0.1 units thrombin/ml. There was no detectable inhibition of aggregation or phosphoprotein formation with concentrations approaching 100 μM.*

divalent Ca^{++} ionophore A23187. There was a corresponding, concentration dependent reduction in the formation of a 40 kilodalton phosphoprotein associated with platelet activation by A23187 [Figure 2]. Rittenhouse (20) has shown that the activation of human platelet phospholipase C by A23187 is totally dependent on TxA_2 and ADP. Therefore, we examined the effect of the EETs on platelets stimulated with U46619, a TxA_2 mimetic. 14,15-cis-

EET and 14,15-cis-episulfide-ET inhibited aggregation and phosphoprotein formation in a concentration dependent manner when platelets were stimulated with U46619 [Figure 3].

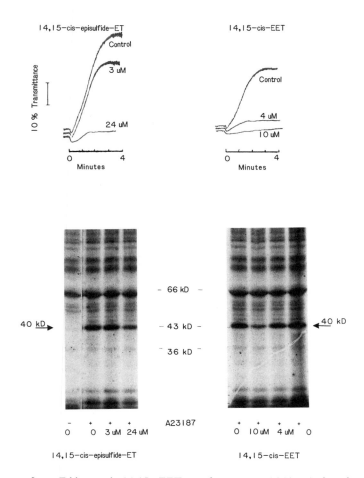

Figure 2. *Effect of 14,15 EET analogs on A23187 induced platelet aggregation and phosphoprotein formation. The left panel shows results with 14,15-cis-episulfide-ET. The right panel shows results with 14,15-cis-EET. Platelets were incubated for 2 min with the concentrations indicated, then stimulated with 3 μM A23187. There was detectable inhibition of phosphoprotein formation with 24 μM 14,15-cis-episulfide-ET and 10 μM 14,15-cis-EET. Aggregation was completely inhibited at these concentrations.*

The EET analogs (50-100 μM) did not alter the initial rate or the magnitude of the aggregation response for platelets stimulated with PMA. However, the onset of aggregation was delayed by approximately one minute. This delay was not attributable to inhibition of protein kinase C activation. Neither 14,15-

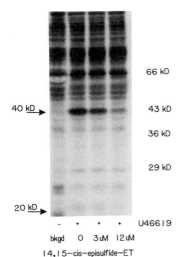

Figure 3. *Effect of 14,15-cis-episulfide-ET analog on U46619 induced platelet aggregation and phosphoprotein formation. There was a dose dependent suppression of both aggregation and 40 kilodalton protein phosphorylation. Results were similar with 14,15-cis-EET and 14,15-trans-EET.*

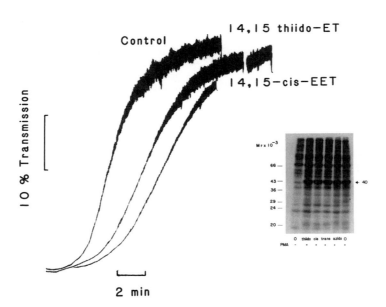

Figure 4. *Effect of 14,15 EET analogs on PMA induced platelet aggregation and phosphoprotein formation. 85 μM 14,15-cis-episulfide-ET or 100 μM 14,15-cis-EET did not alter the initial rate or maximum aggregatory response when platelets were stimulated with 20 ng PMA/ml. The delay in the aggregation response was not attributable to inhibition of protein kinase C (insert). Thirty seconds after stimulation the phosphorylation of a 40 kilodalton substrate was unaltered by any EET analog examined at doses from 50-100 μM.*

cis-EET nor its corresponding sulfur or nitrogen analogs inhibited platelet phosphorylation of a 40 kilodalton substrate, or other phosphoproteins 30 seconds after stimulation with 20 ng/ml PMA [Figure 4].

DISCUSSION

Yamanishi *et al.* have examined the contribution of cellular Ca^{++} metabolism to platelet activation following stimulation by thrombin or PMA (21). Thrombin activates protein kinase C and mobilizes Ca^{++} from the dense tubular system. PMA activates protein kinase C without appreciable mobilization of Ca^{++}. If the EETs inhibited protein kinase C activation one would expect an inhibition of aggregation induced by either thrombin or PMA, and one would expect diminished phosphorylation of the 40 kilodalton substrate for protein kinase C. This did not happen. Consequently, inhibition of protein kinase C does not account for the antiaggregatory properties of the EETs.

Several EET analogs inhibited aggregation and protein phosphorylation by the Ca^{++} ionophore A23187, suggesting that their action involves a modulation of platelet cytosolic Ca^{++} levels. Two questions are pertinent: i) Can this account for their differential activity against A23187 and thrombin? ii) Is it consistent with all available data? Both A23187 and thrombin require Ca^{++} for shape change and aggregation (22,23). However, intracellular Ca^{++} may be mobilized differently by these agonists. For instance, thrombin increases Ca^{++} by ATP dependent processes (24) and activation of phospholipase C (20). A23187 can increase Ca^{++} independently of ATP or phospholipase C (24). The relative importance of extracellular and intracellular Ca^{++} also differs between these two agents. A23187 facilitates uptake of extracellular Ca^{++} more than thrombin does (25). Consequently, Ca^{++} levels rise in many cellular compartments for platelets stimulated with A23187. With thrombin, intracellular compartments, typified by the dense tubular system are more prominent (25). Thus, an effect of EETs on uptake rather than redistribution would be compatible with the results of the aggregation experiments. It is likely that the inhibition of A23187 dependent phosphorylation of a 40 kilodalton protein is a consequence of inhibition of platelet aggregation, rather than its cause. The blockade of phosphorylation occurs indirectly, by inhibiting phosphorylation due to Ca^{++} dependent release of ADP or TxA_2. Had the EETs inhibited phosphorylation as a basis of their antiaggregatory mechanism one might have expected a uniform effect against A23187, thrombin, and PMA.

The effect of the EETs on influx of extracellular Ca^{++}, rather than redistribution from intracellular sources, is consistent with other data. For example, their action is reversible: washing with albumin sequesters the EETs and restores the aggregation response. If the EETs acted at the dense tubular system or other intracellular sites it is unlikely that their effects could be readily reversed. We draw attention to the fact that the 14,15-cis-episulfide ET and certain other EETs do not inhibit the cyclooxygenase. However they reduce TxB_2 formation derived from mobilization of endogenous arachidonic acid by collagen. The latter effect would also be consistent with diminishing the Ca^{++} levels which regulate phospholipase A_2 activity. Using the Ca^{++} indicator INDO-1 we have recently obtained direct evidence that 14,15-cis-episulfide ET suppresses the increase in cytosolic Ca^{++} levels following stimulation of platelets by ionophore A23187 (data not shown).

ACKNOWLEDGMENTS

Grants RO1 GM41026 and BRSG-05357 awarded by the General Medical Science Division of the NIH supported F.A. Fitzpatrick; grant RO1 GM 31278 supported the work by J.R. Falck.

REFERENCES

1. Samuelsson, B. (1983): *Science*, 220:568-575.
2. Samuelsson, B., Dahlen, S.E., Lindgren, J.A., Rouzer, C., and Serhan, C. (1987): *Science*, 237:1171-1176.
3. Fitzpatrick, F.A. and Murphy, R.C. (1989); *Pharmacological Reviews*, 40:229-241.
4. Capdevila, J., Chacos, N., Falck, J.R., Manna, S., Negro-Vilar, A., and Ojeda, S. (1983); *Endocrinology*, 113:421-423.
5. Carroll, M., Schwartzman, M., Capdevila, J., Falck, J.R., and McGiff, J. (1987); *Eur. J. Pharmacol.*, 138:281-283.
6. Kutsky, P., Falck, J.R., Weiss, G., Manna, S., Chacos, N., and Capdevila, J. (1983); *Prostaglandins*, 26:13-21.
7. Murphy, R.C., Falck, J.R., Lumin, S., Yadigiri, P., Zirrolli, J., Balazy, M., Masferrer, J., Abraham, N., and Schwartzman, M. (1988); *J. Biol. Chem.*, 263:17197-17202.
8. Schwartzman, M., Ferrer, N., Carroll, M., Songu-Mize, E., and McGiff, J. (1985); *Nature*, 317: 620-622.
9. Snyder, G., Lattanzio, L., Yadagiri, P., Falck, J.R., and Capdevila, J. (1986); *Biochem. Biophys. Res. Commun.*, 139:1188-1194.
10. Sacerdoti, D., Abraham, N., McGiff, J., and Schwartzman, M. (1988); *Biochemical Pharmacology*, 37:521-527.
11. McGiff, J. and Laniado-Schwartzman, M. (1988); *Clin. Physiol. Biochem.*, 6:179-187.
12. Oliw, E. (1984); *FEBS Lett.*, 172:279-283.
13. Fitzpatrick, F., Ennis, M., Baze, M., Wynalda, M., McGee, J., and Liggett, W. (1986); *J. Biol. Chem.*, 261:15334-15338.
14. Falck, J.R., Manna, S., Jacobson, H., Estabrook, R., Chacos, N., and Capdevila, J. (1984); *J. Am. Chem. Soc.* , 106:3334-3336.
15. Ballou, L., Lam, B., Wong, P.K., and Cheung, W.Y. (1987); *Proc. Natl. Acad. Sci. USA*, 84:6990-6994.
16. Revtyak, G., Johnson, A., and Campbell, W. (1988); *Am. J. Physiol.*, 254:C8-C16.
17. Laemmli, U.K. (1970); *Nature*, 227:680-685.
18. Nishizuka, Y. (1984) *Nature*, 308:693-698.
19. Lyons, R., Stanford, N., and Majerus, P. (1975); *J. Clin. Invest.*, 56:924-936.
20. Rittenhouse, S. (1984); *Biochem J.*, 222:103-110.
21. Yamanishi, J., Takai, Y., Kaibuchi, K., Sano, K., Castagna, M., and Nishizuka, Y. (1983); *Biochem. Biophys. Res. Commun.*, 112:778-785.
22. Le Breton, G., Dinerstein, R., Roth, L., and Feinberg, H. (1976); *Biochem. Biophys. Res. Commun.*, 71:362-370.
23. Charo, I., Feinman, R., and Detweiler, T.C. (1976); *Biochem. Biophys. Res. Commun.*, 72:1462-1467.
24. Rittenhouse-Simmons, S., and Deykin, D. (1977); *J. Clin. Invest.*, 60:495-498.
25. Massini, P., and Luscher, E. (1974); *Biochim. Biophys. Acta* , 372:109-121.

Advances in Prostaglandin, Thromboxane,
and Leukotriene Research, Vol. 20,
edited by B. Samuelsson et al.
Raven Press, Ltd., New York © 1990.

A CONCEPT FOR THE MECHANISM OF PROSTACYCLIN AND THROMBOXANE A2 BIOSYNTHESIS

Volker Ullrich and Markus Hecker

Faculty of Biology, University of Konstanz, P.O. Box 5560, D-7750 Konstanz,
Federal Republic of Germany

Prostaglandins (PG) are derived from their parent compound PGH2 by isomerization reactions which are driven by the high reactivity of the endoperoxide group. Scission of this bond results in formation of PGD2 and PGE2 by intramolecular dismutation reactions, whereas the isomerizations to prostacyclin (PGI2) and thromboxane A2 (TXA2) appear to be rather complicated due to formation of heterocyclic ring systems. Shortly after the discovery of PGI2 a polar reaction mechanism based on the addition of the oxygen atom at C-9 to the Δ^5-double bond was postulated (1,3). Others favored a radical mechanism catalyzed by a Fe(II)/Fe(III) cycle (18) which found experimental proof in a subsequent report showing that Fe(II)-catalyzed decomposition of a model endoperoxide led to formation of the corresponding PGI2 analog (14).

For TXA2 formation any valid mechanism must not only explain the cyclization but also the concomitant fragmentation into 12-hydroxy-5,8,10-heptadecatrienoic acid (HHT) and malondialdehyde (MDA). A polar mechanism (2) but also an electron transfer model (18) which fit these criteria have been proposed. However, as for PGI2 formation, only the Fe(II)-catalyzed conversion yielded small amounts of a TXB2 analog (16). In our own experiments with ferrous salts, however, we could not confirm the formation of significant amounts of PGI2 or TXA2 from PGH2, whereas ferric ions and especially hemin were clearly active (10).

Thus, model systems favor a radical mechanism over a polar electrophilic reaction. The necessary radical intermediates, however, may exist only within the "cage" of the active site of prostacyclin and thromboxane synthase since, otherwise, a chain reaction with destructive effects on the protein and the surrounding membrane phospholipids would be a consequence. Such a "cage-radical mechanism" originating from an [Fe-O•] intermediate has been postulated for biological hydroxylation reactions catalyzed by cytochrome P450 (19). A meanwhile commonly accepted reaction scheme involves such an active oxygen species which can be generated also by organic hydroperoxides (Scheme 1).

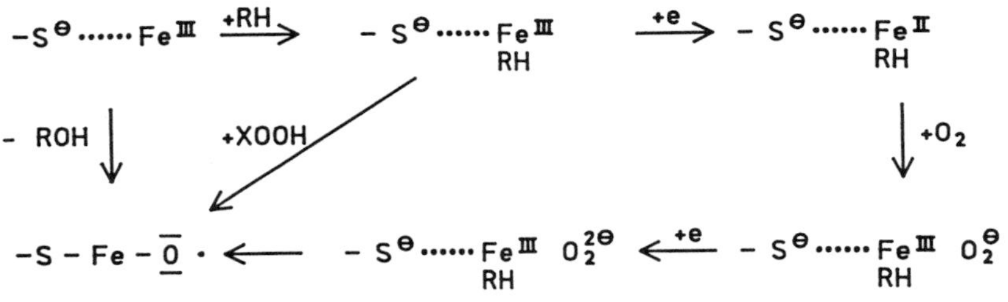

$$-S^{\ominus}\cdots Fe^{III} \xrightarrow{+RH} \quad -S^{\ominus}\cdots Fe^{III} \underset{RH}{} \xrightarrow{+e} \quad -S^{\ominus}\cdots Fe^{II} \underset{RH}{}$$

$$\Big\downarrow -ROH \qquad +XOOH \qquad\qquad\qquad \Big\downarrow +O_2$$

$$-S-Fe-\underline{\overline{0}}\cdot \longleftarrow \quad -S^{\ominus}\cdots Fe^{III}\,O_2^{2\ominus} \underset{RH}{} \xleftarrow{+e} \quad -S^{\ominus}\cdots Fe^{III}\,O_2^{\ominus} \underset{RH}{}$$

SCHEME 1

PROSTACYCLIN SYNTHASE

When comparing the chemistry of cytochrome P450 with the rearrangement of the endoperoxide by prostacyclin or thromboxane synthase, one finds analogies in the activation of peroxides which have led us to suggest that both enzymes catalyze a cytochrome P450-like mechanism. Since none of the two enzymes were isolated or characterized at that time, we developed a solubilization and fractionation procedure for porcine aortic microsomes and found indications that prostacyclin synthase is a cytochrome P450-type hemoprotein (20). The subsequent isolation of the homogeneous enzyme from porcine aorta established this finding (4). In contrast to cytochrome P450-dependent monooxygenases, prostacyclin synthase could not be reduced enzymatically in the presence of carbon monoxide (CO) to give the characteristic band at 450 nm, only chemical reduction with dithionite was effective. CO was not able to inhibit PGI$_2$ formation from PGH$_2$ in agreement with our proposal that only the ferric enzyme is active in catalysis (21). With respect to its substrate specificity we could confirm earlier findings (11) that the D^5-double bond is essential for PGI$_2$ formation (10). The trans-stereochemistry at the cyclopentane ring also seems to be important, since 8-iso-PGH$_2$, likewise PHG$_1$, interestingly yielded only the corresponding C$_{17}$ hydroxy acid and MDA. The formation of these C$_{17}$ hydroxy acids can be conveniently followed photometrically (7) and therefore we could determine the molecular activity of bovine aortic prostacyclin synthase with PGH$_1$ to be 2701 x min^{-1}. This value is about 10-fold higher than the molecular activity for PGH$_2$, indicating that PGI$_2$ formation involves a slow rate-limiting step which is not required for the fragmentation process.

Inhibitor studies with tranylcypromine and minoxidil (8) revealed binding of a nitrogen ligand to the ferric iron, suggesting that the sixth ligand position is required for catalysis. In the presence of the stable PGH$_2$ analogs 9,11-epoxymethano-PGF$_{2\alpha}$ (U44069) and 11,9-epoxymethano-PGF$_{2\alpha}$ (U46619) characteristic and stable difference spectra were observed (Fig. 1). With the methylene group at C-11, U44069 caused formation of a small peak at 390 nm and a trough at 421 nm which closely resembles the substrate binding spectra of cytochrome P450-dependent monooxygenases (15). In contrast, U46619 led to a redshift of the peak in the difference spectrum known for oxygen ligands at the ferric heme (17). We shall come back to the interpretation of this spectral data after a look at the properties of thromboxane synthase.

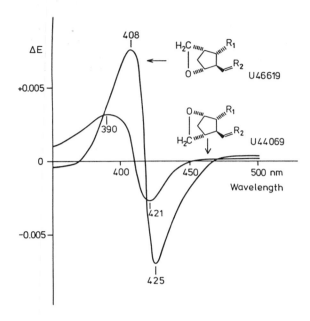

FIG. 1. OPTICAL DIFFERENCE SPECTRA OF
SOLUBILIZED PROSTACYCLIN SYNTHASE
WITH U44069 AND U46619. Solubilized bovine
aortic prostacyclin synthase (1.19 nmol/ml; 0.5
ml) was incubated with 0.286 mmol/l of U44069
or U46619 (dissolved in ethanol; 0.2 %, v/v),
respectively. After 1 min at 10°C a difference
spectrum was recorded versus ethanol (0.2 %,
v/v) added to the reference cuvette.

THROMBOXANE SYNTHASE

The chemically related isomerizations of PGH_2 to PGI_2 and TXA_2
suggested to us an analogous cytochrome P450 structure for thromboxane
synthase. Human platelets contain a cytochrome P450 protein which we could
isolate as a homogeneous protein exhibiting high TXA_2-synthesizing activity
(5). With a molecular weight of 58.8 kD the enzyme contains one heme per
polypeptide chain and was found spectrally to be indistinguishable from
prostacyclin synthase. With PGH_2 as a substrate TXA_2, HHT and MDA were
formed in equimolar amounts with a molecular activity of 3198 x min^{-1} (7,10).
Under no experimental conditions could this 1:1:1 ratio be changed. With
PGH_1 only 12-hydroxy-8,10-heptadecadienoic acid (HHD) and MDA
appeared as products with a similar turnover of 3563 x min^{-1}. It seems likely
therefore that the cyclization reaction to TXA_2 is not a rate-limiting step. It is
interesting to note, however, that product formation with all substrates tested
proceeds with the same molecular activity of about 2000-3000 x min^{-1}. This

turnover number is in the same range as HHD and MDA formation from PGH$_1$ by prostacyclin synthase, indicating that cleavage of the endoperoxide may be the slowest reaction step in TXA$_2$ biosynthesis. Rather illuminating and a clue to the mechanism was the spectral investigation of the binding of the two PGH$_2$ analogs. Just opposite to prostacyclin synthase the methylene group in position 9 led to a peak at 391 nm, whereas the ligand-type difference spectrum appeared with the other isomer (Fig. 2).

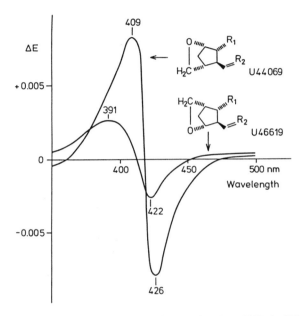

FIG. 2. OPTICAL DIFFERENCE SPECTRA OF SOLUBILIZED THROMBOXANE SYNTHASE WITH U44069 AND U46619. Solubilized human platelet thromboxane synthase (0.363 nmol/ml; 0.5 ml) was incubated with 0.286 mmol/l of U44069 or U46619 (dissolved in ethanol; 0.2 %, v/v), respectively. After 1 min at 10°C a difference spectrum was recorded versus ethanol (0.2 %, v/v) added to the reference cuvette.

Together with QSAR studies of various imidazole and pyridine-based thromboxane synthase inhibitors (6) there is no doubt that PGH$_2$ in thromboxane synthase is oriented with the 9-oxygen atom of the endoperoxide bridge towards the heme iron. In contrast, the heme of prostacyclin synthase must bind PGH$_2$ with the 11-oxygen atom. Any model for the mechanism of both enzymes must take this into account as well as the involvement of a ferric heme-thiolate catalytic site.

A CONCEPT FOR THE MECHANISM OF PGI$_2$ AND TXA$_2$ BIOSYNTHESIS

The highly potent thromboxane synthase inhibitors are inactive for prostacyclin synthase, whereas, vice versa, tranylcypromine and minoxidil do not interact with thromboxane synthase. Only the PGH$_2$ analogs are effective for both enzymes. Since it appears to be essential for both enzymes to fix the PGH$_2$ molecule at the endoperoxide bridge, however differently at the two oxygen atoms, it becomes obvious that the stereochemical orientation of the substrate should be very different. It may be anticipated that after formation of the enzyme-substrate complex the subsequent event of endoperoxide cleavage is the same for both enzymes. However, a homolytic as well as a heterolytic scission can be formulated. In order to generate an electrophilic oxygen atom at C-9 for PGI$_2$ synthesis, a homolytic reaction would yield an oxygen radical, whereas the heterolytic reaction forms an alkoxy cation. If the latter reaction would occur, the ferric iron must be an extremely strong Lewis acid which, in view of the trans thiolate ligand, is difficult to imagine. In contrast, cytochrome P450 seems to stabilize electron deficient ligands which makes the alkoxy cation at C-9 an unlikely candidate.

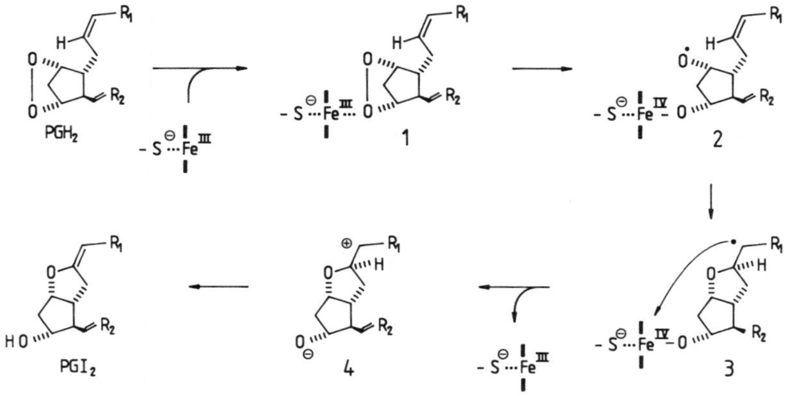

SCHEME 2
(R$_1$=(CH$_2$)$_3$-CO$_2$H; R$_2$=CH-CHOH-(CH$_2$)$_4$-CH$_3$)

Therefore, favoring homolytic splitting, the driving force for this bond scission must be derived from a stabilization of the resulting 11-alkoxy radical by the Fe(III)-thiolate center. This may occur either by spin coupling or bond formation. The remaining free alkoxy radical at C-9 is closely located at the D^5-double bond and could readily react by addition to the π-system under formation of a carbon radical at C-5. This radical intermediate then must become oxidized in order to eliminate a proton at C-6 necessary for PGI$_2$ to be released (Scheme 2).

This mechanism can explain all findings and is consistent with our chemical knowledge. Substrates which lack the Δ^5-double bond undergo fragmentation to the corresponding C$_{17}$ hydroxy acid and MDA which is a well-known consequence of radical lipid peroxidation reactions (13). Fragmentation also must occur if, like in 8-iso-PGH_2, the double bond is sterically not able to react with the 9-alkoxy radical. Since this fragmenation proceeds about 10-times faster than PGI_2 formation, the rate-limiting step must occur after cleavage of the endoperoxide bond.

The same initial event of homolytic endoperoxide scission must be postulated for thromboxane synthase, but now stabilization of the alkoxy radical occurs at C-9 (Scheme 3).The well-known fact that the Δ^{13}-double bond is essential for TXA_2 synthesis (11) makes it likely that a stabilization of a carbon radical at C-12 by mesomeric effects is the crucial prerequisite for ring opening between C-11 and C-12. An inevitable step to reach the necessary polar cyclization process is oxidation of this radical to a carbocation. However, if the electron transfer to the heme-thiyl moiety does not follow immediately, fragmentation into HHT and MDA would be the most likely consequence. This pathway, therefore, is easy to understand as part of the synthase reaction but, by our present knowledge, cannot readily explain why a strict 1:1 ratio between TXA_2 formation and fragmentation into HHT and MDA results. Thus, it is still uncertain whether this ratio is the best the enzyme can achieve for chemical reasons, or whether HHT and/or MDA are deliberately formed as additional second messengers. Some properties of HHT and its oxidation product 12-keto-5,8,10-heptadecatrienoic acid favor the latter hypothesis (9,12).

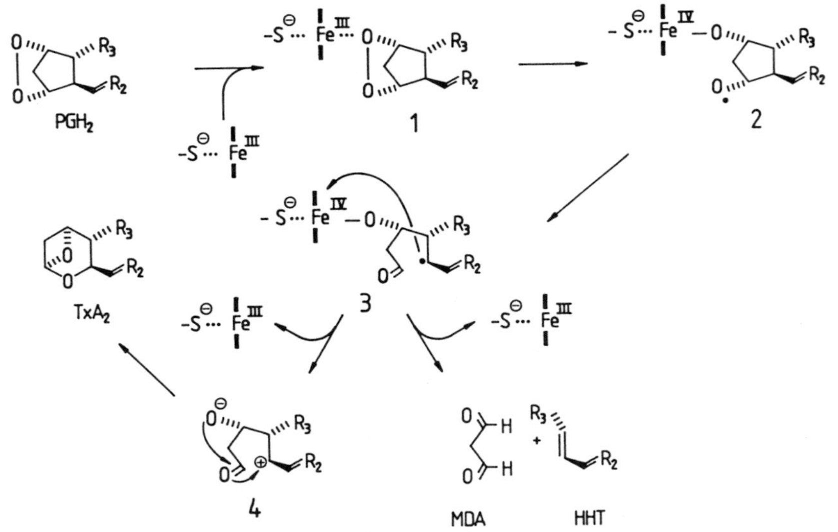

SCHEME 3
(R_2=CH-CHOH-$(CH_2)_4$-CH_3, R_3=CH_2-CH=CH-$(CH_2)_3$-CO_2H)

Where then are the mechanistic homologies of cytochrome P450-catalyzed monooxygenations and the two P450-catalyzed isomerisation reactions? Two aspects seem to be common for all mechanism: i) stabilization of an oxygen radical species and ii) rapid oxidation of a carbon-centered radical. Especially for the second function the resonance structures with the thiyl radicals point to a particular role of the thiolate ligand in this redox reaction. Thus, nature makes use of the low activation energies of radical reactions but by rapid oxidation of carbon radical intermediates prevents chain reactions with their inherent unspecificity and even toxicity.

REFERENCES

1. Corey, E.J., Keckl, G.E., and Sekely, I. (1977): *J. Am. Chem. Soc.* 99:2207.
2. Diczfalusy, U., Falardeau, P., and Hammarström, S. (1977): *FEBS Lett.* 84:271.
3. Fried, J., and Barton, J. (1977): *Proc. Natl. Acad. Sci. USA* 74:2199.
4. Graf, H., and Ullrich, V. (1982): In: *Cytochrome P450 - Biochemistry, Biophysics and Environmental Implications*, edited by E. Hietanen, M. Laitinen, and O. Häninen, pp. 103. Elsevier, Amsterdam.
5. Haurand, M., and Ullrich, V. (1985): *J. Biol. Chem.* 260:15059-15067.
6. Hecker, M., Haurand, M., Ullrich, V., and Terao, S. (1986): *Eur. J. Biochem.* 157:217-223.
7. Hecker, M., Haurand, M., Ullrich, V., Diczfalusy, U., and Hammarström, S. (1987): *Arch. Biochem. Biophys.* 254:124-135.
8. Hecker, M., and Ullrich, V. (1988): *Biochem. Pharmacol.* 37:3363-3365.
9. Hecker, M., and Ullrich, V. (1988): *Eicosanoids* 1:19-25.
10. Hecker, M., and Ullrich, V. (1989): *J. Biol. Chem.* 264:141-150.
11. Johnson, R.A. (1985): *Adv. Prostaglandin Thromboxane Leukotriene Res.* 14:131-154.
12. Liu, Y., Yoden, K., Shen, R.-F., and Tai, H.-H. (1985): *Biochem. Biophys. Res. Commun.* 129:268-274.
13. Porter, N.A. (1980): In: *Free Radicals in Biology*, edited by W.A. Pryor, Vol. 4, pp. 261-294. Academic Press, New York.
14. Porter, N.A., and Mebane, R.C. (1982): *Tetrahedron Lett.* 23:2289-2292.
15. Schenkman, J.B., Remmer, H., and Estabrook, R.W. (1967): *Mol. Pharmacol.* 3:113-123.
16. Takahashi, K., and Kishi, M. (1987): *J. Chem. Soc. Chem. Commun.*:722-724.
17. Tang, S.C., Koch, S., Papaetthymiou, G.C., Foner, S., Frankel, R., Ibers, J.A., and Holm, R.H. (1976): *J. Am. Chem. Soc.* 98:2414.
18. Turner, J.A., and Herz, W. (1977): *Experientia (Basel)* 33:1133-1134.
19. Ullrich, V. (1969): *Hoppe-Seyler's Z. Physiol. Chem.* 350:357-365.
20. Ullrich, V., Castle, L., and Weber, P. (1981): *Biochem. Pharmacol.* 30:2033-2036.
21. Ullrich, V., and Graf, H. (1984): *Trends Pharmacol. Sci.* 5:352-355.

Advances in Prostaglandin, Thromboxane, and Leukotriene Research, Vol. 20, edited by B. Samuelsson et al. Raven Press, Ltd., New York © 1990.

I-BOP, THE MOST POTENT RADIOLABELLED AGONIST FOR THE TXA$_2$/PGH$_2$ RECEPTOR

T.A. Morinelli, D.E. Mais, J.E. Oatis, P.R. Mayeux, A.K. Okwu, A. Masuda, D.R. Knapp and P.V. Halushka

Departments of Cell and Molecular Pharmacology and Experimental Therapeutics and Medicine Medical University of South Carolina 171 Ashley Avenue Charleston, SC 29425

The labile arachidonic acid metabolites prostaglandin H$_2$ (PGH$_2$) and thromboxane A$_2$ (TXA$_2$) cause constriction of vascular smooth muscle and aggregation of platelets (3,7,20-22). These common pharmacologic properties, are thought to be mediated via a common receptor (TXA$_2$/PGH$_2$ receptor). Since both PGH$_2$ and TXA$_2$ have limited stability, much of the study of the physiological and pathophysiological roles of these lipids have relied upon the availability of stable mimetics, such as U46619 and U44069 (2). Recently, EP171, a 7-oxabicycloheptane derivative has been described as the most potent agonist with EC$_{50}$ values in washed human platelets of approximately 5 to 10 nM and 0.35 nM for contraction of canine saphenous veins (9).

High affinity radiolabelled ligands have been extensively used to characterize putative receptors. Several TXA$_2$/PGH$_2$ receptor antagonists have been radiolabelled with either ^{3}H or ^{125}I and used to characterize platelet and vascular TXA$_2$/PGH$_2$ receptors (6). However, to date there have been only two stable agonists that have been used in radioligand binding studies [3H]-U46619 and [3H]-U44069. A study employing [3H]-U44069 estimated three classes of TXA$_2$/PGH$_2$ receptors on human platelets. The highest affinity site had a K$_d$ of 75 nM and a B$_{max}$ of 1700 sites/platelet (1) while the other two classes were not saturable. [3H]-U46619 has also been employed to characterize TXA$_2$/PGH$_2$ receptors on human platelets. The affinity of [3H]-U46619 for TXA$_2$/PGH$_2$ receptors was quite variable and has been reported to range from 20 to 131 nM with 550 to 2000 sites per platelet (8,10,11,17). Specific binding of [3H]-U46619 was also very low, being 40 to 50 percent.

Although these ligands have been used in the characterization of the TXA_2/PGH_2 receptor, their usefulness has been limited by virtue of their low specific activity and low specific binding. In an attempt to overcome these problems, we synthesized a stable high affinity [^{125}I] radiolabelled TXA_2/PGH_2 receptor agonist, [1S-(1α,2ß(5Z),3α (1E,3S*),4α)]-7-[3-(3-hydroxy-4-(4'-iodophenoxy)-1-butenyl)-7-oxabicyclo-[2.2.1]heptan-2-yl]-5-heptenoic acid (I-BOP).

METHODS

Materials

The synthesis of optically active [1S-(1α,2ß(5Z),3α(1E,3S*),4α)]-7-[3-(3-hydroxy-4-(4'-iodophenoxy)-1-butenyl)-7-oxabicyclo-[2.2.1]heptan-2-yl]-5-heptenoic acid (I-BOP) (figure 1) was performed as described (18).

The following were gifts: SQ29550, the optically active precursor to I-BOP and [^{125}I]-BOP, SQ29548 and 9,11 azo PGH_2, Squibb Institute for Medical Research; ONO11,113 (9,11-epithio-11,12 methano-TXA_2), ONO Pharmaceutical Company; U46619, the Upjohn Company; and the stereoisomeric pair of TXA_2/PGH_2 receptor antagonists L657925 and L657926, Merck Frosst Canada Inc. Fura-2 pentacetoxymethyl ester was purchased from Behring diagnostics (LaJolla, Ca).

Platelet aggregation and shape change were performed as previously described (12-14). Intracellular free calcium was measured using Fura-2 flourescence as previously described (4,18). Saphenous vein contractions were measured as previously described (18).

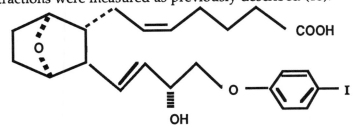

FIG. 1. Structure of I-BOP

Binding of [^{125}I]-BOP to Washed Human Platelets

Incubations (200 µl) containing 1×10^7 platelets were performed in silanized (12 X 75 mm) glass tubes at 37°C for 30 min. The incubation media consisted of the Tris/NaCl buffer and ≈ 0.02 to 0.2 nM (≈ 0.1 to 1×10^5 cpm) [^{125}I]-BOP per tube. For equilibrium binding and competition binding experiments, concentrations of agonists or antagonists ranging from 10^{-11} to 10^{-4}M were also included. The reaction was terminated by the addition of 4 ml of ice-cold 50 mM

Tris/100 mM NaCl buffer at pH 7.4, followed by rapid filtration through Whatman GF/C glass fiber filters (Whatman, Inc., Clifton, NJ). The filters were washed three more times with 4 ml of the ice cold buffer. The filtration procedure was complete within 10 secs. Non-specific binding was defined as that amount of radioactivity bound in the presence of 10 μM L657925, a TXA$_2$/PGH$_2$ receptor antagonist (15). Specific binding was 90 ± 0.9% (n=19) of the total binding.

Statistics

Data from equilibrium binding experiments were analyzed according to Scatchard (23) using the LIGAND computer program (19). EC$_{50}$ and IC$_{50}$ values were determined from a log- logit transformation of the individual concentration-response curves. The EC$_{50}$ is defined as the agonist concentration producing a half-maximal response. The IC$_{50}$ is defined as the concentration of competing agent that produces a 50% inhibition of specifically bound [^{125}I]-BOP.

RESULTS

Platelet Function and Saphenous Vein Contraction

I-BOP produced concentration dependent aggregation of isolated human platelets with an EC$_{50}$ value of 10.8 ± 3 nM (n=9). The EC$_{50}$ value for U46619 was 121 ± 18 nM (n=7). I-BOP induced aggregation was inhibited by the TXA$_2$/PGH$_2$ receptor antagonist, L657925 (15) confirming that I-BOP was stimulating platelets through the TXA$_2$/PGH$_2$ receptor. I-BOP also produced a concentration-dependent shape change of isolated platelets with an EC$_{50}$ value of 0.21 ± 0.05 nM (n=4).

The EC$_{50}$ value for I-BOP stimulated increase in intracellular free calcium concentration was 4.1 ± 1.1 nM (n=4). U46619, for comparison, produced the same effect with an EC$_{50}$ value of 148 nM (n=2). The TXA$_2$/PGH$_2$ receptor antagonist, L657925, at a concentration of 7.5 nM inhibited the increase in fluorescence caused by 1 nM I-BOP by more than 50%, indicating that calcium mobilization induced by I-BOP is mediated by the TXA$_2$/PGH$_2$ receptor.

I-BOP produced a concentration-dependent contraction of canine saphenous veins with an EC$_{50}$ value of 0.038 ± 0.007 nM (n=8).

Radioligand Binding Studies

The association rate constant (k$_1$) for the ligand-binding site complex was determined from the time course for binding of [^{125}I]-BOP. Binding reached equilibrium within 20 minutes at room temperature (figure 2). The observed rate constant (k$_{obs}$) was 0.199 ±

0.053 min^{-1}. Dissociation of the receptor-ligand complex demonstrated an exponential decrease (figure 2) with a k$_{-1}$ of 0.096 ± 0.02 min^{-1}. The association rate constant, k$_1$, was determined from the formula: k$_1$=(k$_{obs}$-k$_{-1}$)/[L], where [L] = the total ligand concentration and was 0.119 ± 0.03. The kinetically determined dissociation constant, K$_d$, was 1.02 ± 0.33 nM, (n=4) (K$_d$ = k$_{-1}$/k$_1$).

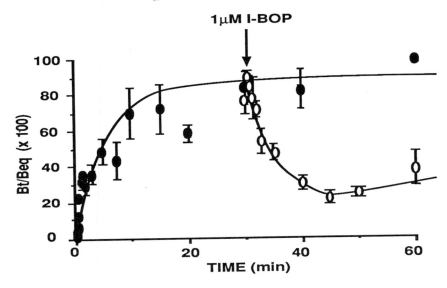

FIG. 2. Kinetic analysis of [^{125}I]-BOP binding to washed human platelets. At each time point during the association, both total binding and non-specific (binding in the presence of 1 μM ^{127}I-BOP) was measured. Specific binding is shown as a percentage of that seen at equilibrium (Bt/Beq) and is shown as a function of time. Dissociation was initiated by the addition of 1 μM I-BOP and terminated at various time points, as described in Methods. Values shown for both association and dissociation are the mean ± standard error of the mean at each time point from four similar experiments. Reprinted from Morinelli et al. (1989) with permission.

Equilibrium binding experiments indicated that binding of [^{125}I]-BOP to the platelet TXA$_2$/PGH$_2$ receptor was saturable. Scatchard analysis of the binding isotherms revealed a K$_d$ value for I-BOP of 2.2 ± 0.3 nM, with a B$_{max}$ = 0.028 ± 0.002 X 10^{-12} moles/10^{7}platelets (1699 ± 162 sites per platelet n=9) (Figure 3).

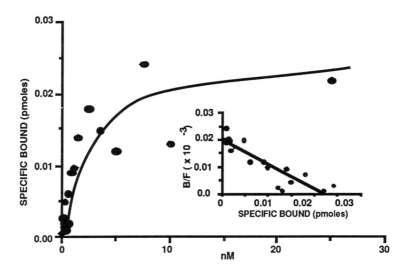

FIG. 3. Representative equilibrium binding analysis of [125I]-BOP to isolated human platelets. Insert shows Scatchard analysis of saturation binding data. Bound/free (pmoles/10^7 plts/pM) is shown as a function of specifically bound pmoles. The K_d was 1.04 nM with B_{max} = 0.022 X 10^{-12} moles/10^7 platelets and 1352 sites/platelet. Representative of nine experiments. Reprinted from Morinelli et al. (1989) with permission.

To determine if [125I]-BOP was interacting with TXA_2/PGH_2 receptors, competition binding studies were performed using a series of TXA_2/PGH_2 receptor agonists; ONO11,113, 9,11azo-PGH_2 and U46619 and TXA_2/PGH_2 receptor antagonists, SQ29548, and the stereoisomeric pair L657925 and L657926. Table 1 shows the IC_{50} values for each of the compounds tested. The rank order for the agonists to displace [125I]-BOP from the receptor was I-BOP> ONO11113> 9,11azo-PGH_2≥U46619 while for the antagonists it was SQ29548>L657925>L657926. For both the agonists and antagonists their rank order correlated with their pharmacological rank order potencies for interacting with the platelet TXA_2/PGH_2 receptor (5). The stereoselective displacement seen for L657925 and L657926, agrees with previous findings for these isomeric pairs and their affinities for the platelet TXA_2/ PGH_2 receptor (15). PGE_1, PGD_2 and TXB_2 at concentrations of 10 µM displaced [125I]-BOP by 11, 51 and 22%, respectively (data not shown).

TABLE 1. <u>Potencies of a series of TXA_2 /PGH_2 agonists and antagonists for competing with [^{125}I]-BOP binding to human platelets.</u>

	IC_{50}[nM]	EC_{50}[nM][a]
Agonists		
ONO11,113	17 ± 1.8 (3)	18 ± 2[a]
9,11azo-PGH_2	41 ± 2.2 (4)	61 ± 5[a]
U46619	62 ± 13 (6)	64 ± 6[a]
Antagonists		K_d [nM]
SQ29548	4.7 ± 0.5 (3)	2.3 ± 0.2[a]
L657925	15 ± 4 (7)	1.8 ± 0.9[b]
L657926	424 ± 90 (7)	186 ± 71[b]

[a]Halushka et al., 1988; [b]Mais et al., 1989.

The IC_{50} values are compared to the EC_{50} and K_d values obtained in previous studies. The K_d values were determined pharmacologically.

DISCUSSION

I-BOP is the first ^{125}I-labelled agonist for TXA_2/PGH_2 receptors. In platelets, I-BOP increased cytoplasmic free calcium concentrations, induced shape change and aggregation. It also contracted canine saphenous veins in a concentration-dependent manner. It mimicked the actions of the naturally occuring agonists TXA_2 and PGH_2 and was more potent in stimulating platelet aggregation than either PGH_2 or TXA_2 (16) or U46619. These effects of I-BOP were produced via stimulation of the platelet TXA_2/PGH_2 receptor, since L657925 a TXA_2/PGH_2 receptor antagonist, inhibited its effects.

The radioligand binding studies performed in Tris-Saline buffer indicated that I-BOP interacted with a single class of high affinity receptors on the platelet. In Hepes-Saline buffer, the affinity of I-BOP for the receptor appears to be somewhat higher and there are two classes of apparent binding sites (unpublished observations). The competition binding studies using analogs of TXA_2 and PGH_2 indicated that I-BOP bound to the TXA_2/PGH_2 receptor in a specific manner. The rank order potency for the analogs to displace [^{125}I]-BOP from its receptor is comparable to their reported pharmacologic potencies to either induce or inhibit TXA_2/PGH_2 mimetic activation of platelets (ONO11,113>9,11azoPGH_2≥U46619, for agonists; SQ29548> L657925>L657926 for antagonists) (5). The IC_{50} values for the antagonists in the binding assay are greater than the published K_d values determined in a pharmacologic assay. In the previous study, the K_d values for the antagonists were determined from Schild analysis of inhibition of U46619 stimulated aggregation, unlike the present study, which determined IC_{50} values from the competition with [^{125}I]-BOP. Also the rank order for SQ29548 and L657925 were different in the binding assay compared to the pharmacologic assay. The reason for these discrepancies is unknown. With further studies of [^{125}I]-BOP binding an explanation may be found.

Additional evidence that [^{125}I]-BOP is binding to the platelet TXA$_2$/PGH$_2$ receptor is provided by the competition studies employing the stereoisomeric pair of TXA$_2$/PGH$_2$ receptor antagonists, L657925 and L657926. L657925 was approximately 30 times more potent than L657926 at competing for binding with [^{125}I]-BOP to the platelet. The relative potencies of these two compounds, in this study, is similar to that previously determined (15).

Previous studies employing the tritiated agonists [^{3}H]-U46619 and [^{3}H]-U44069 in washed human platelets have found similar receptor densities to the values reported in this study (550-2200 sites/platelet, 1,8,10,11,17). The affinity of the agonists for the receptor, however, were much lower in those studies, ranging from 20 nM (11) to 131 nM (8). The discrepancies in the reported affinity for these ligands may be due in part to their poor specific binding. The tritiated agonists [^{3}H]-U44069 and [^{3}H]- U46619, were reported to have forty to fifty percent displaceable binding. I-BOP has a much higher specific binding (90%) allowing for a more accurate estimation of both receptor affinity and density, compared to [^{3}H]-U46619 and [^{3}H]-U44069. Thus, it provides a significant advance over these previous radiolabelled agonists. Ushikubi et al. (24) recently reported two new radiolabelled ligands [^{3}H]-S-145 and [^{125}I]-S-145-OH. S-145 is an antagonist with specific binding similar to I-BOP, but I-BOP has a higher affinity in platelets at pH 7.4. At pH 6, the optimum pH for I-BOP binding to washed human platelets, its K$_d$ is approximately 0.5 nM (unpublished observations).

Besides the high affinity and specific binding for I-BOP, the other advantage of this new agonist is its high specific activity ($\approx$2000 Ci/mmole). The higher specific activity allows for the assay of smaller amounts of receptor compared to using ^{3}H. This is particularly advantageous during purification procedures or when the receptor density is very low. I-BOP has already proven to be of great utility. High affinity I-BOP binding sites have already been identified in other tissues and cultured cells (Table 2).

TABLE 2.   Tissue and cells that have a TXA$_2$/PGH$_2$ receptor detected through the use of radioligand binding studies with [^{125}I]-BOP.[a]

Human vascular smooth muscle cells	Washed rat platelets
Equine peripheral blood mononuclear cells	Rat aortic membranes
Cultured rat aortic smooth muscle cells	Rat renal glomeruli
Guinea pig lung membranes	Rabbit aortic membranes

[a]unpublished observations

In summary, I-BOP should prove to be an extremely useful radioligand for future studies involving the characterization, as well as the regulation, of TXA$_2$/PGH$_2$ receptors on various tissues.

REFERENCES

1. Armstrong, R.A., Jones, R.L., and Wilson, N.H. (1983): *Br. J. Pharmacol.* 79:953-964.
2. Bundy, G. (1975): *Tetrahedron Letters* 24: 1957-1960.
3. Claesson, H.E., and Malmsten, C. (1977): *Eur. J. Biochem.* 76: 277 284.
4. Grynkiewicz, G., Poenie, M., and Tsien, R.Y. (1985): *J. Biol.Chem.* 260:3440-3450.
5. Halushka, P.V., Kochel, P.J., and Mais, D.E. (1987): *Br. J.Pharmacol.* 91:223-227.
6. Halushka, P.V., Mais, D.E., Mayeux, P.R., and Morinelli, T.A. (1989): *Ann Rev. Pharm. Tox.* 29:213-239.
7. Hamberg, M., Svensson, J., and Samuelsson, B. (1975): *Proc.Natl. Acad. SciU.S.A.* 72:2994-2998.
8. Johnson, G.J., Dunlop, P.C., Leis, L.A., and From, A.H.L. (1988): *Circ. Res.* 62:494-505.
9. Jones, R.L., MacIntyre, Pollack, W.K., Shaw, A.M., and Wilson, N.H. (1985): *Br. J. Pharmacol.* 84:148P.
10. Kattelman, E.J., Venton, D.L., and LeBreton, G.C. (1986): *Thromb. Res.* 41:471-481.
11. Liel, N., Mais, D.E., and Halushka, P.V. (1987): *Prostaglandins* 33:789-797.
12. Mais, D.E., Burch, R.M., Saussy, D.L., Kochel, P.J. ,and Halushka, P.V. (1985): *J. Pharmacol. Exp. Ther.* 235: 729-734.
13. Mais, D.E., Saussy, D.L., Chaikhouni, A., Kochel, P.J., Knapp, D.R., Hamanaka,N., and Halushka, P.V. (1985):*J. Pharmacol. Exp. Ther.* 233:418-424.
14. Mais, D.E., DeHoll, D., Sightler, H., and Halushka, P.V. (1988): *European J. Pharmacol.* 148:309-315.
15. Mais, D.E. Yoakim, C., Guindon, Y., Gillard, J., Rokach, J., and Halushka, P.V. (1989): *Biochem. Biophys. Acta:* 1012:184-190.
16. Mayeux, P.R., Morton, H.E., Gillard, J., Lord, A., Morinelli, T.A. Boehm, A., Mais, D.E., and Halushka, P.V. (1988): *Biochem. Biophys. Res. Commun..* 157:733-739.
17. Morinelli, T.A., Niewiarowski, S., Daniel, J.L., and Smith, J.B. (1987): *Am. J. Physiol.* 253:H1035-H1043.
18. Morinelli, T.A., Oatis, J.E., Okwu, A.K., Mais,D.E., Mayeux, P.R., Masuda, A.,Knapp, D.R., and Halushka, P.V. (1989):*J. Pharmacol. Exp. Ther.*: in press.
19. Munson, P.J. and Rodbard, D. (1980): *Anal. Biochem.* 107: 220-239.
20. Needleman, P.M., Minkes, M., and Raz, A.: *Science* 193:163-165.
21. Needleman, P., Moncada, S., Bunting, S., Vane, J., Hamberg, M., and Samuelsson, B. (1976): *Nature* 261:558-560.
22. Ogletree, M.L. (1987): *Fed. Proc.* 46:133-138.
23. Scatchard, G. (1949): *N.Y. Acad. Sci.* 51:660-672.
24. Ushikubi, F., Nakajima, M., Yamamoto, M., Ohtsu, K., Kimura, Y., Okuma, M.,Uchino, I., Fujiwara,M., and Narumiya, S. (1989): *Eicosanoids* 2:21-27.

Advances in Prostaglandin, Thromboxane,
and Leukotriene Research, Vol. 20,
edited by B. Samuelsson et al.
Raven Press, Ltd., New York © 1990.

CLASSIFICATION OF PROSTANOID RECEPTORS

PHILLIP J. GARDINER

BAYER U.K. RESEARCH DEPT.
PHARMACEUTICAL BUSINESS GROUP
STOKE COURT, STOKE POGES, SL2 4LY ENGLAND

Although the structures of the prostanoids were identified some twenty years ago there has been limited progress in the development of new therapeutics in this field. This seems surprising if one considers the large number of areas in which the prostanoids have been proposed to have pathophysiological roles i.e., asthma, thrombosis, inflammation etc. A wide spectrum of biological actions coupled with the ability to induce opposing actions in the same tissue/system [e.g., PGE_2 can contract and/or relax airway smooth muscle (1)] has led to immense problems in the identification of selective prostanoid agonists or antagonists. As in the past with adrenergic and histamine receptors, the classification of prostanoid receptors seems the most likely solution to such problems.

METHODS OF CLASSIFICATION

At present three methods have been used to provide a preliminary classification of prostanoid receptors. They comprise of : - (a) A comparison of rank orders of potency using natural agonists. Numerous factors such as diffusion, metabolism, uptake etc. can lead to large differences in such rank orders, consequently it can only be used to establish a working hypothesis until further pharmacological tools are available (2). (b) A comparison of the potency, (pK_B, negative log of the dissociation constant) of a competitive antagonist on a range of tissues. This method is less prone to the problems in (a) and is generally of more value in setting up a classification. (c) Identification and characterisation of ligand-binding sites using radiolabelled agonists or antagonists. Ligand binding studies will not be dealt with here although it has been suggested that the limited studies that do exist with the prostanoids corroborate the functional studies (3). Halushka et al (4) have recently prepared a comprehensive review of such binding studies.

PRELIMINARY CLASSIFICATION OF PROSTANOID RECEPTORS

A systematic search of a wide range of tissues identified groups of tissues in which one prostanoid was significantly more potent than all of the others (3). The four following rank orders of agonist potency were established using this technique and each was proposed as representing a distinct receptor type.

$$PGE_2 > PGI_2 > PGF_{2\alpha} > PGD_2 > U46619$$
$$PGF_{2\alpha,} > PGD_2 > PGE_2 > PGI_2 > U46619$$
$$U46619 \gg PGD_2 > PGF_{2\alpha} = PGI_2 > PGE_2$$
$$PGI_2 \gg PGD_2 \gg PGE_2 = PGF_{2\alpha} \gg U46619 = 0$$

Initially it seemed that no distinct PGD_2 receptor type existed. However, a comparison of the anti-aggregatory potencies of PGI_2 and PGD_2 in a range of species coupled with cross desensitisation studies with these agonists led to the suggestion that a distinct PGD_2 receptor exists (5,6). The rank order of agonist potency for this receptor has not as yet been determined.

An alternative approach using a limited number of tissues classified prostanoid receptors according to their functional activity (1,7). This led to the proposal that two distinct receptor types exist, one representing contractile/stimulant activity χ and the other relaxant/inhibitory activity, ψ. The different rank orders of agonist potency which occur within each receptor type were proposed as subtypes with three occurring for the contractile/stimulant receptor and two for the relaxant/inhibitory receptor.

A major problem in assessing whether one or more of the prostanoid receptor types is present on a tissue, or involved in a disease process, is the ability of each prostanoid to interact with all of the other receptor (sub) types. Consequently although one prostanoid might be active in a test system this does not indicate that its receptor type is present.

SELECTIVE RECEPTOR AGONISTS AND ANTAGONISTS

Confirmation of the existence of distinct prostanoid types and/or subtypes was then sought by the identification of selective agonists and antagonists for each type (Fig. 1). These compounds are also highly valuable in determining whether one or more of the receptor (sub)types has a major role in a range of diseases.

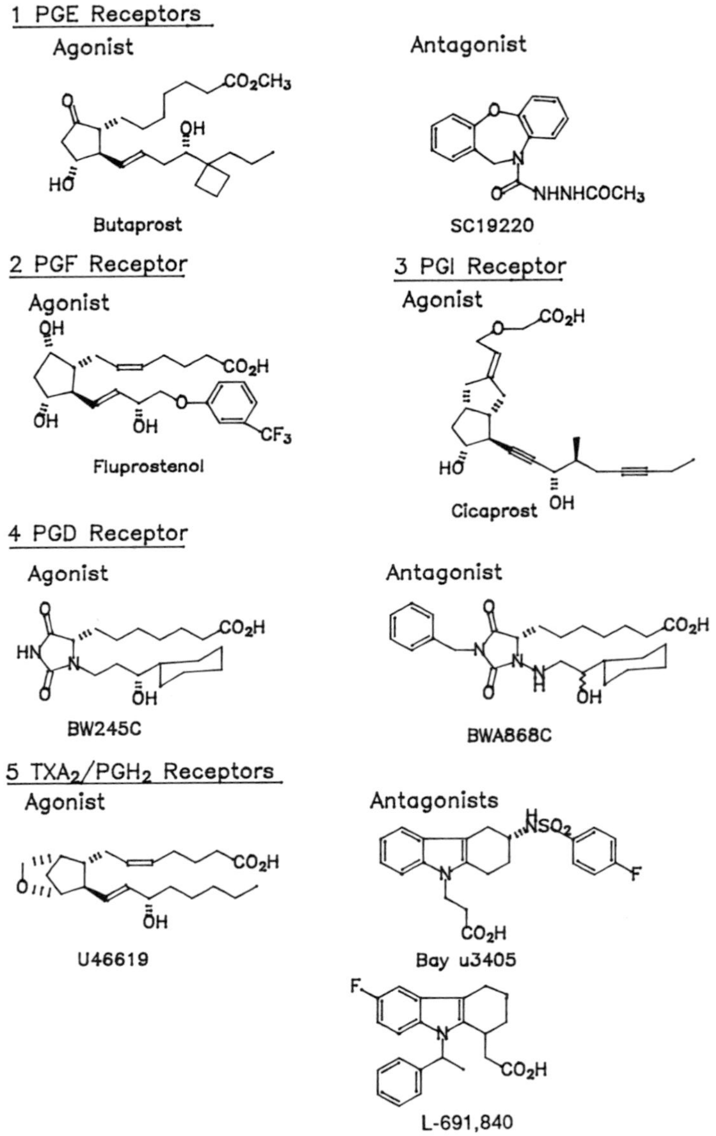

1 PGE Receptors
Agonist

Butaprost

Antagonist

SC19220

2 PGF Receptor
Agonist

Fluprostenol

3 PGI Receptor
Agonist

Cicaprost

4 PGD Receptor
Agonist

BW245C

Antagonist

BWA868C

5 TXA$_2$/PGH$_2$ Receptors
Agonist

U46619

Antagonists

Bay u3405

L-691,840

Fig.1.   Selective Agonists and Antagonists
of Prostanoid Receptors.

CURRENT CLASSIFICATION OF PROSTANOID RECEPTORS

PGE Receptors

It was initially suggested using the functional classification system that PGE receptors comprised of a subtype of the contractile/stimulant receptor X_3 and a subtype of the relaxant/inhibitory receptor ψ_1. Butaprost (Fig 1) was identified as a highly selective agonist of the latter subtype with no activity at X_3 or any of the other prostanoid receptors (7).

Additional PGE selective receptor agonists have been identified and evaluated on a range of tissues on which PGE_2 is the predominant agonist (Table 1). It can be seen that these agonists have different patterns of activity, strengthening the earlier suggestion from the butaprost study that subdivisions of the PGE receptor exist (7,8). It has been proposed that three PGE subtypes exist. The third of these PGE-3 is responsible for contractile/stimulant actions on some tissues and relaxant/inhibitory on others. If this subtype can be confirmed with a selective antagonist it seems unlikely that the classification based upon functional activity can continue to be used.

Table 1. Subtypes of the PGE Receptor

Receptor (Sub) Type	Tissues	Selective Agonist	Selective Antagonist
PGE-1	Guinea Pig Ileum (L)*, Dog Fundus	Sulprostone	SC 19220
PGE-2	Cat Trachea, Guinea Pig Ileum (C)+	Butaprost AY 23636	None
PGE-3	Chick Ileum Rat Gastric Mucosa (Inhibition of acid secretion)	AY 23636 Sulprostone	None

* (L) - longitudinal, + (C) - circular smooth muscle.

Butaprost is the only agonist which acts at one PGE subtype, AY 23636 and rioprostil act at PGE-2 and PGE-3

whereas sulprostone acts on the PGE-1 and PGE-3 subtypes. It
was suggested that another PGE analogue, misoprostil had a
similar profile to sulprostone on the PGE receptor, however,
its activity on cat trachea, a tissue with only the PGE-2
receptor subtype present, suggests that misoprostil is a
general PGE receptor agonist (9,10). Unlike natural PGE_2,
however, misoprostil has little or no activity on other
prostanoid receptor types.

All of these studies involved PGE agonists and as such are
only preliminary confirmation of the original classification.
Fortunately a weak but selective PGE antagonist SC19220 (Fig
1) was identified some years ago and has provided additional
support for the agonist studies. The PGE-1 actions of
sulprostone are antagonised by SC19220 whereas the actions of
butaprost and AY23626 are unaffected as is the activity of
sulprostone on PGE-3 receptors (Gardiner, unpublished, 8).
AH6809 was also identified as a PGE antagonist but has since
been shown to act as an antagonist of both TXA_2/PGH_2 and PGD_2
receptors and as an inhibitor of phosphodiesterase,
questionning its value as a tool for classification studies
(11).

PGF Receptors

In support of the preliminary classification that a PGF
receptor type exists a number of $PGF_{2\alpha}$ analogues (e.g.,
fluprostenol see Fig 1) which were originally chosen for their
luteolytic activity have proved to be highly potent and very
selective agonists at the $PGF_{2\alpha}$ receptor (3).

Despite early interest in an antagonist for $PGF_{2\alpha}$ only one
such antagonist $PGF_{2\alpha}$ dimethylamine/amide has been reported
although its selectivity and potency are largely unknown (12).

PGI Receptors

The low metabolic and chemical stability of PGI_2 led to a
large amount of effort being devoted to the production of
stable PGI_2 derivatives. Probably the most widely studied of
these are iloprost, cicaprost (Fig 1) and 6 α carba PGI_2.
Evaluation of these analogues on a range of tissues/platelets
has demonstrated that only cicaprost has good selectivity for
the PGI_2 receptor (13). Although the other analogues are
potent agonists at the PGI_2 receptor they are also potent
agonists of a PGE receptor subtype. Based upon studies with
iloprost and other PGI_2 analogues, it was suggested that
subtypes of the PGI_2 receptor exist (4). These analogues were
anti-aggregatory but antagonised PGI_2 on the vasculature. It
seems more likely, however, that the unexpected antagonist

activity on the vasculature is due to the additional activity of these analogues on PGE contractile receptors. Such activity will functionally antagonise PGI_2-induced relaxations.

At present no PGI_2 antagonist exists to confirm or refute the agonist studies.

PGD Receptors

Although preliminary studies suggested that distinct PGD_2 receptors exist little support can be found for this using selective agonists. As yet only one selective PGD_2 agonist BW 245C has been reported but recent studies suggest that this hydantoin PGD_2 analogue (Fig 1) is also active at PGE and TXA_2/PGH_2 receptors (14). It seems surprising that as yet no tissue has been identified in which PGD_2 or BW 245C are the most potent agonists.

Although a number of PGD_2 antagonists with low selectivity have been reported NO164, AH6809 etc. confirmation of the existence of this receptor type came only recently with the discovery of the potent and selective PGD_2 antagonist BW A868C (14). BW A868C has been shown to antagonise what are thought to be the PGD receptor mediated effects of PGD_2 and BW 245C but it has no activity on all of the other prostanoid receptor types. It is interesting that on the platelet BW A868C antagonises the anti-aggregatory activity of BW 245C without revealing a pro aggregatory TXA_2/PGH_2 receptor mediated effect as occurs with PGD_2. In contrast, however, BW 245C is known to contract some vascular tissues via a TXA_2/PGH_2 receptor and to antagonise U46619 actions on such tissues. Such conflicting data for BW 245C in two systems known to contain TXA_2/PGH_2 receptors may strengthen suggestions (see later) that subtypes of the TXA_2/PGH_2 receptor exist.

TXA_2/PGH_2 receptors

Following the preliminary classification of TXA_2/PGH_2 receptors with U46619, a large number of additional agonists have been evaluated to determine whether subtypes of this receptor exist. EP171 (Fig 1) is both more potent and more selective than U46619 for TXA_2/PGH_2 receptors however its slow onset and long duration of action make it impractical for routine studies (15). All of the selective TXA_2/PGH_2 agonists confirm the preliminary receptor classification but do not suggest that subtypes of this TXA_2/PGH_2 receptor exist.

A large number of TXA_2/PGH_2 antagonists have been identified e.g. SQ30741, EP092, AH23848, GR32191, ICI192666,

S-145 and BAY u3405 (Fig 1). Most are highly selective for this receptor but their different profiles of activity in a number of tissues/platelets have led to controversial suggestions that subtypes of TXA_2/PGH_2 receptors exist (4).

In our studies we suspected that such subtypes might exist when we demonstrated that two selective antagonists, EP092 and AH23848, had significantly lower potencies against U46619 on some tissues (human bronchial muscle, ferret trachea) than on others (human platelets, guinea-pig lung strip, human lung strip) (16). Our suspicion seems to have been strengthened by a recent report using another TXA_2/PGH_2 antagonist, GR32191 (17). This compound has a significantly lower antagonist potency on rat lung and rabbit aorta against U46619 than on most of the other test tissues. One possibility for these findings is the existence of a TXA_2/PGH_2 receptor subtype at which GR 32191 is less active.

We have probed this area further using another compound L691840 which was reported to selectively antagonise TXA_2/PGH_2 receptors on platelets but not smooth muscle (18). This compound proved to be an antagonist of U46619 on human platelets but had a much lower potency on the rat aorta and guinea-pig trachea. It had good activity on human bronchial muscle and ferret trachea (Table 2).

Taken together, our studies suggest that at least two TXA_2/PGH_2 receptor subtypes exist. It is possible however to antagonise all subtypes of the TXA_2/PGH_2 receptors using the novel highly potent and selective antagonist BAY u3405 (19).

Table 2. Evidence for the subclassification of the TXA_2/PGH_2 receptor

TXA_2/PGH_2 antagonist	pA_2/pK_B			
	Guinea pig trachea	Rat Aorta	Human Washed Platelets	Human Bronchial Muscle
EP092	8.7	8.1	8.0	6.8
AH23848	8.5	7.9	8.3	6.9
L 691840	6.0	6.0	8.6	7.7
BAY u3405	8.9	9.2	8.6	8.5

SUMMARY

Although still at a preliminary stage the original working hypothesis that five distinct prostanoid receptor types exist (3) has been strengthened by studies testing a number of selective agonists and/or antagonists.

Such compounds can be systematically used to probe the involvement/presence of prostanoid receptor types in tissues/disease processes to identify the desired profile of new drugs (Table 3). Although this classification will probably be modified in the light of new pharmacological tools, it seems apparent that the use of such an approach is likely to lead to new therapeutic products in the prostanoid field.

Table 3. Classification of Prostanoid Receptors

PG Receptor	Tissue with Homogenous Population	Selective Agonist	Selective Antagonist	Nomenclature (3)
PGE	Guinea pig Ileum (L), Dog Fundus	Sulprostone	SC19220	EP_1
PGE	Cat trachea, Guinea pig Ileum (C)	Butaprost	–	EP_2
PGE	Chick Ileum	Sulprostone	–	EP_3
PGF	Dog/Cat Iris	Fluprostenol		FP
PGI	–	Cicaprost	–	IP
PGD	–	BW 245C	BW A868C	DP
TXA_2/ PGH_2	Guinea pig Lung, Rat Aorta	U46619	BAY u3405	TP_{1-3}

REFERENCES

1. Gardiner, P.J., Collier, H.O.J. (1980) Prostaglandins, 19; 819-841.
2. Black, J., Gerskowitch, V.P., Leff, P. (1982) In: Ganellin, C.R., Parsons, M.E. eds, Pharmacology of histamine receptors, London, Wright P.S.G., 1.
3. Coleman, R.A., Humphrey, P.P.A., Kennedy, I. (1985) In: Kelsner, S. ed, Trends in Autonomic Pharmacology, Vol.3, Taylor and Francis, London and Philadelphia, 35-49.
4. Halushka, P.V., Mais, D.E., Mayeux, P.R. et al. Ann.Rev.Pharm.Tox., (1989) 10; 213-239.
5. Whittle, B.J.R., Moncada, S., Vane, J.R. (1978) Prostaglandins, 16; 373-388.
6. Miller, O.V., Gorman, R.R. (1979) J.Pharmacol. Expt.Ther., 210; 134-140.
7. Gardiner, P.J. (1986) Br.J.Pharmac, 87; 45-56.
8. Coleman, R.A., Kennedy, I., Sheldrick, R.L.G. (1987) Br.J.Pharmacol., 91; 323P.
9. Eglen, R.M., Whiting, R.L. (1988) Br.J.Pharmacol., 94; 591-601.
10. Coleman, R.A., Humphrey, J.M., Sheldrick, R.L.G. et al. (1988) Br.J.Pharmacol., 95; 724P.
11. Kiery, R.J., Lumley, P. (1988) Br.J.Pharmacol., 94; 745-754.
12. Stringer, R.B., Fitzpatrick, T.M., Corey, E.J. et al. (1982) J.Pharmacol.Expt.Ther., 220; 521-525.
13. Armstrong, R.A., Lawrence, R.A., Jones, R.L. et al. (1989) Br.J.Pharmacol., 97; 657-668.
14. Giles, H., Leff, P., Bolofo, M.L. et al. (1989) Br.J.Pharmacol., 96; 291-300.
15. Jones, R.L., Wilson, N.H., Lawrence, R.A. (1989) Br.J.Pharmacol., 96; 875-887.
16. McKenniff, M., Rodger, I.W., Norman, P. et al. (1988) Eur.J.Pharmacol., 153; 149-159.
17. Lumley, P., White, B.P., Humphrey, P.P.A. (1989) Br.J.Pharmacol., 97; 783-794.
18. Guindon, Y., Yoakim, C., Gillard, J.W. (1987) European Patent Application, EP234708A.
19. Seuter, F., Perzborn, Fiedler, U.H., et al. (1989) Abstracts XIIth Int.Congress Int.Soc.Thrombosis and Haemastasis, Page 112: 355.

Advances in Prostaglandin, Thromboxane, and Leukotriene Research, Vol. 20, edited by B. Samuelsson et al. Raven Press, Ltd., New York © 1990.

PEPTIDE LEUKOTRIENE RECEPTORS AND ANTAGONISTS

R. D. Krell, D. Aharony, C. K. Buckner and E. J. Kusner

Department of Pharmacology
Pulmonary Section
ICI Pharmaceuticals Group
Division of ICI Americas Inc.
Wilmington, DE 19897

The structural elucidation of the peptide leukotrienes (LT) (16, 17) was the most significant event in the science of slow-reacting substance of anaphylaxis since its discovery (5). The appreciation that slow-reacting substance of anaphylaxis was a family of products derived from arachidonic acid metabolism, i.e., LTC_4, LTD_4 and LTE_4, permitted the synthesis of pure materials by medicinal chemists for biologists to evaluate. Soon after their chemical synthesis it was confirmed that these materials were capable of producing the series of biological effects, i.e., bronchoconstriction, pulmonary edema and mucus secretion, common to allergic asthma. These findings led to the hypothesis that peptide leukotrienes may be the long sought mediators of this disease (19). In pursuit of this hypothesis, the pharmaceutical industry launched a major effort to modulate the activity of this family of products by either inhibiting the biosynthetic pathway or by antagonizing LT receptors at the end organ. The success of the receptor antagonist effort will be the focus of this communication.

Heterogeneity of Peptide Leukotriene Receptors

The first biologic studies carried out with synthetic leukotrienes were designed to determine if they exerted their potent biologic activities by interacting with specific membrane receptors. Two pieces of evidence suggested that receptor activation was the mechanism of action for the leukotrienes. 1) Biological responses to the LT demonstrated a strong chiral preference for the naturally occurring 5(S) 6(R) configuration of LTD_4 (3, 23). 2) The biological effects, in most systems, were competitively antagonized by FPL 55712, the first peptide LT antagonist discovered by Augstein et al. (2). Later, ligand binding studies would directly demonstrated the existence of membrane receptors for both LTD_4 and LTE_4 (15, 18). The unequivocal demonstration of a receptor for LTC_4 by ligand binding techniques has yet to be described, although functional studies have demonstrated an LTC_4 receptor in guinea pig trachea (20). The major concern with previous $^3H-LTC_4$ binding studies is the ability of this ligand to bind to the ubiquitous glutathione transferase (22).

Some of the first quanitative pharmacological studies carried out with FPL 55712, suggested the potential for LT receptor heterogeneity. Fleisch et al. (6) postulated, based on differences in the apparent affinity constant for FPL 55712 in antagonizing the contractile activity of LTD_4, that LT receptors in guinea pig ileum were not identical to guinea pig tracheal and lung parenchymal strip receptors which appeared similar. These findings were later confirmed with another, newer, LT antagonist from the same chemical series as FPL 55712, i.e., LY 171,883 (7). Schild analysis of the antagonism of LTD_4-induced tracheal contractions in guinea pig tracheal strips by FPL 55712 consistently failed to demonstrate that the compound was a competitive antagonist. This observation led Krell et al. (12) to provide circumstantial evidence that LTD_4 receptors in this tissue were of two subtypes: FPL 55712 demonstrate a half log unit lower affinity for one type than the other. LTE_4 appears to preferentially interact with the subtype with higher affinity for FPL 55712. Recently, Aharony et al. (1) have suggested that in guinea pig lung parenchymal membranes $^3H-LTE_4$ may bind to a subset of LTD_4 receptors. This proposal is, however, not supported by the studies of (15) which suggested that both LTD_4 and LTE_4 interacted with identical sites, which were of equal density.

FPL 55712, in addition to antagonizing LTD_4 and LTE_4, also antagonized LTC_4-induced contractions in most tissues. In guinea pig trachea, antagonism of LTC_4-induced contractions by FPL 55712 were not independent of the concentration of the antagonist, as should be the case for a competitive antagonist. This enigma was finally solved when it was determined that guinea pig tracheal and parenchymal smooth muscle were able to metabolize LTC_4, first to LTD_4 by the action of γ-glutamyltranspeptidase and subsequently to the less potent (10 fold) LTE_4 by an aminopeptidase (20). When the ability of FPL 55712 to block the contractile activity was evaluated in the presence of L-serine borate, an inhibitor of γ-glutamyltranspeptidase, FPL 55712 no longer provided antagonism of the contractile effects of LTC_4. On the basis of these findings it was postulated that LTC_4 interacted with a receptor that was distinct from the two, high and low affinity for FPL 55712, in guinea pig trachea with which LTD_4/E_4 interact. These functional pharmacologic findings have been confirmed (9, 10) and extended to lung parenchyma by ligand binding assays (11). In summary, guinea pig tracheal smooth muscle appears to contain three peptide leukotriene receptors viz, two with which LTD_4/E_4 interact, and a third with which LTC_4 interacts.

The major questions arising from these studies was -- what are the pharmacologic characteristics of peptide LT receptors in human airway smooth muscle? Obviously, if human airway receptors differ substantially from those in guinea pig trachea, the primary preclinical pharmacologic test system, then antagonists discovered with this preparation may lack activity in human tissue. To answer this question an extensive series of experiments were carried out using human intralobar airway smooth muscle (4). Both FPL 55712 and LY 171,883, peptide LT antagonists from the hydroxyacetophenone series, demonstrated identical affinities versus LTC_4 and LTD_4, in the presence or absence of metabolic inhibitors. The apparent dissociation constant (K_B) for FPL 55712 was approximately one-half log unit lower in human as compared to guinea pig airway smooth muscle. Similar results were obtained with the more potent and selective peptide LT antagonist ICI 198,615 (13, 21). These results were confirmed and extended to LTE_4 using ICI 204,219, an analog of ICI 198,615 (Table 1, Figure 1).

TABLE 1. Apparent dissociation constants (K_B) for ICI 204,219 (3×10^{-8}M) against peptide leukotrienes in human intralobar airway smooth muscle

Agonist	$-$Log Molar K_B Values for ICI 204,219	n^a	$-$Log Molar EC_{50} for LT's
LTC_4	8.56 ± 0.26^b	9	8.54 ± 0.33
LTD_4	8.57 ± 0.16	8	8.62 ± 0.17
LTE_4	8.53 ± 0.23	7	8.25 ± 0.11

[a] Number of tissues from different patients.
[b] Values are means $\pm$ SEM.

This antagonist demonstrates a $-$log K_B value of 8.5 versus LTC_4, LTD_4 and LTE_4. This value is approximately 10-fold lower than that determined against LTD_4 and LTE_4 in guinea pig tissue. These results indicate that the three peptide leukotrienes interact with the same receptor in human airway smooth muscle which is similar, but not identical to, guinea pig tracheal LTD_4/LTE_4 receptors. It is also noteworthy that LTC_4, D_4 and E_4 are equipotent in human tissue (Table 1).

Current Status of Leukotriene Antagonists

Figure 1 depicts several distinct chemical classes of peptide leukotriene antagonists presently available that have been, or are believed to be, in clinical trials. FPL 55712 and LY 171,883 and are hydroxyacetophenones ONO-RS-1048 is a derivative of hydroxyacetophenone, SKF 104,353 and SKF S-106,203 are analogs of the peptide leukotrienes, L-660,711, RG 12,525, SR 2640 and WY 48,252 are napthylene derivatives, ICI 198,615 is an indazole and ICI 204,219 an inverted indole. Potency ranges for these compounds from pK_B values of 7 (FPL 55712, LY 171,883) to a high of 10 (ICI 198,615) on guinea pig airway smooth muscle. SR 2640, RG 12,525, SKF 104,353, SKF S-106,203, L-660,711, and ICI 204,219 are all currently in, or about to enter, clinical trials. WY 48,252, LY 171,883 and FPL 55712 have been withdrawn from trials with no, or equivocal, results. With this large number of chemically diverse, potent and selective antagonists, it appears highly likely that the hypothesis that peptide leukotrienes are involved in the etiology of asthma will be strongly tested within the next few years. It should be borne in mind that asthma is a complex disease with a multitude of potential mediators. It may indeed be too much to expect any single therapeutic class of agents to be "the magic bullet". Rather, the use of combinations of drugs, and not necessarily combinations from the same therapeutic classes, may provide the best clinical results.

Proposal for the Provisional Classification of LT Receptors

The heterogeneity of leukotriene receptors has been appreciated for many years. It is highly probable that we have little more than a superficial understanding of how diverse a family they really represent. Within the next few years more detailed functional and biochemical experiments with the new antagonists depicted in Figure 1 along with the powerful techniques of molecular biology will undoubtly offer a fuller appreciation as to the actual size and diversity of this family of proteins. These caveats not withstanding it was considered worthwhile, at least to attempt, to classify these receptors according to what is presently known in an effort to provide a working framework for the future.

Based on these considerations the receptor classification system illustrated in Table 2 is being put forth for consideration.

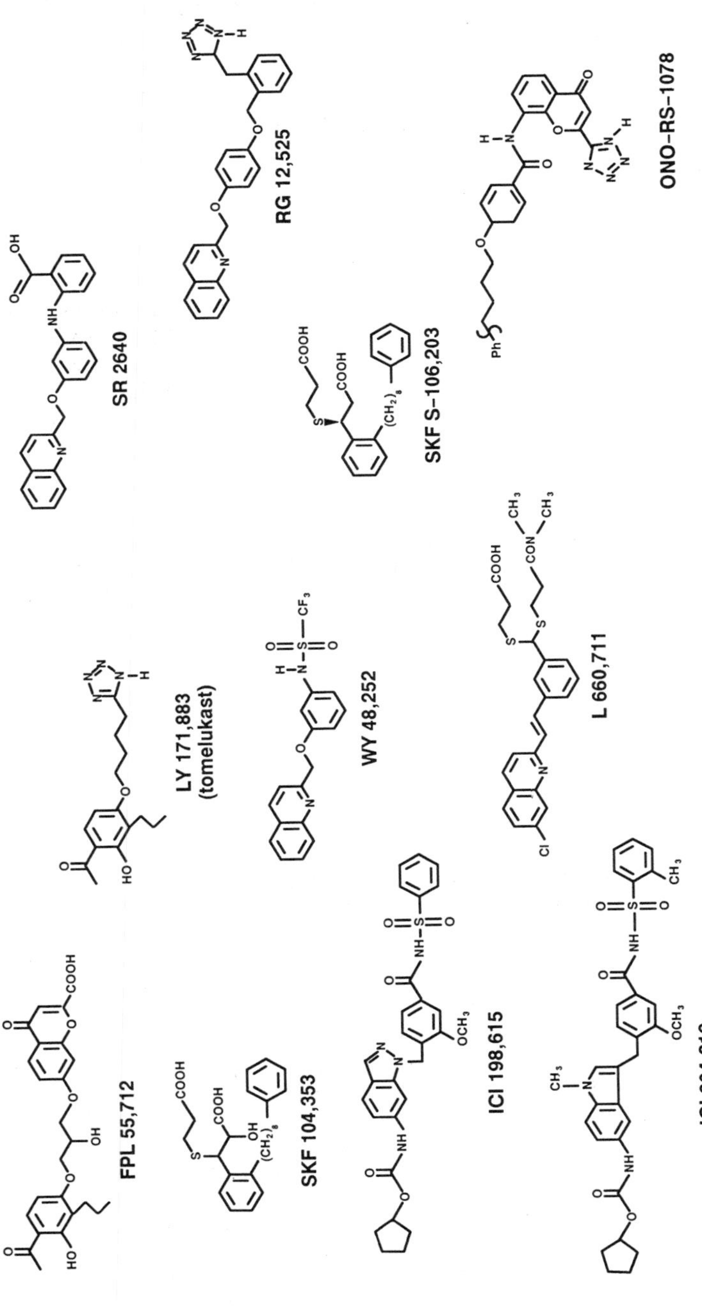

FIG. 1. Structures of Peptide Leukotriene Antagonists in Clinical Trials

TABLE 2. <u>Proposed provisional classification of leukotriene receptors</u>

Receptor	Tissue	Agonist(s)	Antagonists
a) Peptide LT's			
pLT_1	GP Trachea	LTC_4	None
pLT_{2a}	GP Trachea	LTD_4/E_4	High affinity for FPL 55712 (Also, LY 171,883, SKF 104,353, L 660,711, ICI 198,615, ICI 204,219)
pLT_{2b}	GP Trachea	LTD_4/E_4	low affinity for FPL 55712
pLT_{2c}	Human Bronchial Smooth Muscle	$LTC_4/D_4/E_4$	FPL 55712, SKF 104,353, ICI 204,219, ICI 198,615
pLT_{2d}	GP Ileum	LTD_4/E_4	FPL 55712, LY171,883
b) Nonpeptide LT (LTB_4)			
LTB_{4Ia}	PMN	LTB_4 (high affinity)	
LTB_{4Ib}	PMN	LTB_4 (low affinity)	

The abbreviation pLT has been adopted for the peptide
leukotriene receptors. A two receptor system, with multiple
subtypes of one of the two is proposed. The pLT_1 receptor
exists in guinea pig tracheal smooth muscle, interacts with
LTC_4 and is not antagonized by any of the presently
available antagonists. The second leukotriene receptor,
pLT_2, appears to exist in a variety of subtypes (Table 2).
The agonists appear to be either LTD_4 or LTE_4, with one
exception <u>viz</u>, pLT_{2c}, where LTC_4 interacts as well, and all
are antagonized by at least some of the currently available
antagonists. The antagonists do not demonstrate similar
affinity for these classes, thus there designation as
subclasses of the pLT_2 receptor. Antagonists uniformly
demonstrate highest affinity in guinea pig ileum, followed
by guinea pig airway smooth muscle and then human airway
smooth muscle. It is recognized that several tissues which
are responsive to the peptide LT have been omitted, perhaps

most notably guinea pig lung parenchyma. In this instance, the complexity of the cell types giving rise to the contractile response makes appropriately quantitative pharmacologic analysis difficult and thus, classification precarious indeed. For others which have been omitted (viz, pulmonary artery/vein, mydocardium, segments of gastrointestinal smooth muscle, uterus, etc.) not enough information is presently available, particularly concerning the ability of the newer, more potent antagonists to inhibit responses to peptide LT's, to consider classification at this time. This proposed classification is based solely on functional studies. However, in many instances ligand binding studies do lend support to the proposed classification.

In addition to the spasmogenic peptide leukotrienes, the nonpeptide leukotriene, LTB_4, is another product of the lipoxygenase pathway of arachidonic acid metabolism. LTB_4 is a potent chemotatic, chemokinetic autacoid which as well can induce degranulation of polymorphonuclear leukocytes (PMN). Lin et al. (14) demonstrated the existance of high and low affinity receptors for LTB_4 on PMN's. The high affinity sites appear to mediate chemokinesis, chemotaxis and increased adherence while the low affinity sites mediate enzyme release and oxidative bursts (8). Potent, seemingly selective antagonists for LTB_4 are currently being disclosed; however, detail reports of their biochemical pharmacology have not yet been made available. On this basis, it is proposed (Table 2) that the high and low affinity LTB_4 receptors be termed LTB_4 I_a and LTB_4 I_b, respectively.

This proposed classification for LT's is undoubtly over simplified; however, it is hoped that it can be a useful framework for those studying the biochemistry and pharmacology of leukotrienes and their antagonists in the future.

Acknowledgements. The authors extend their sincere appreciation to Ms. Sharon Roberts for her assistance in the compilation of this manuscript. We also express our appreciation to Dr. Sven-Erik Dahlén for helpful discussions regarding the classification of leukotriene receptors.

REFERENCES

1. Aharony, D., Catanese, C. A. and Falcone, R. C. (1989): J. Pharmacol. Exp. Ther. 248:581-588.
2. Augstein, J., Farmer, J. B., Lee, T. B., Sheard, P. and Tattersall, M. L. (1973): Nature (Lond). 245:215-.
3. Baker, S. R., Boot, J. R., Jamieson, W. B., Osborne, D. J. and Sweatman, W. J. F. (1981): Biochem. Biophy. Res. Comm. 103:1258-1264.

4. Buckner, C. K., Krell, R. D., Laravuso, R. B., Coursin, D. B., Bernstein, P. R. and Will, J. A. (1986): J. Pharmacol. Exp. Ther. 237:558-562.

5. Feldberg W. and Kellaway, C. H. (1938): J. Physiol. (Lond.). 94:187-226.

6. Fleisch, J. H., Rinkema, L. E. and Baker, S. R. (1982): Life Sciences. 31-577-581.

7. Fleisch, J. H., Rinkema, L. E., Haisch, K. D., Swanson-Bean, D., Goodson, T., Ho, P. K. P. and Marshall W. S. (1985): J. Pharmacol. Exp. Ther. 233:148-157.

8. Goldman, D. W., Gifford, L. A., Marotti, T., Koo, C. H. and Goetzel, E. J. (1987): Fed. Proc. 46:200-203.

9. Hand, J. M. and Schwalm, S. F. (1987): Prostaglandins. 33:709-716.

10. Hand, J. M. Schwalm, S. F., Englebach, I. M., Auen, M. A., Musser, J. H. and Kreft A. F. (1989): Prostaglandins. 37:181-191.

11. Hogaboom, G. K., Mong, S., Wu, H-L. and Crooke, S. T. (1983): Biochem. Biophy. Res. Comm. 116:1136-1143.

12. Krell, R. D., Tsai, B. S., Berdoulay, A., Barone, M. and Giles, R.E. (1983): Prostaglandins. 25:171-178.

13. Krell, R. D., Giles, R. E., Yee, Y. K. and Snyder, D. W. (1987): J. Pharmacol. Exp. Ther. 243:557-564.

14. Lin, A. H., Ruppel, P. L. and Gorman, R. R. (1984): Prostaglandins. 29:837-849.

15. Mong, S., Scott, M. O., Lewis, M. A., Wu, H-L., Hogaboom, G. K., Clark, M. A. and Crooke, S. T. (1985): Europ. J. Pharmacol. 109:183-192.

16. Morris, H. A., Taylor, G. W., Piper, P. J. and Tippins, J. R. (1980): Nature. 285:104.

17. Murphy, R. C., Hammarström, S. and Samuelsson, B. (1979): Proc. Natl. Acad. Sci. 76:4275-4279.

18. Pong, S-S. and DeHaven, R. N. (1983): Proc. Natl. Acad. Sci. 80:7415-7419.

19. Samuelsson, B. (1983): Science (Wash, D.C.). 220:568-575.

20. Snyder, D. W. and Krell, R. D. (1984): J. Pharmacol. Exp. Ther. 231:616-622.

21. Snyder, D. W., Giles, R. E., Keith, R. A., Yee, Y. K. and Krell, R. D. (1987): J. Pharmacol. Exp. Ther. 243:548-556.

22. Sun, F. F., Chau, L. Y. and Austen, K. F. (1987): Fed. Proc. 46:204-207.

23. Tsai, B-S., Bernstein, P. R., Macia, R. A., Conaty, J. and Krell, R. D. (1982): Prostaglandins. 23:489-506.

*Advances in Prostaglandin, Thromboxane,
and Leukotriene Research,* Vol. 20,
edited by B. Samuelsson et al.
Raven Press, Ltd., New York © 1990.

SIGNAL TRANSDUCTION PROCESSES
FOR THE LTD₄ RECEPTOR

Stanley T. Crooke[1], Henry Sarau[2], David Saussy[3],
James Winkler[2] and James Foley[2]

[1]ISIS Pharmaceuticals, 2280 Faraday Avenue, Carlsbad, CA 92008
[2]Smith Kline & French Laboratories, King of Prussia, PA 19406
[3]Eli Lilly & Company, Indianapolis, IN 46285

BACKGROUND

Although many studies suggested the existence and heterogeneity of leukotriene receptors, it was not until direct radioligand binding studies were performed that they were conclusively demonstrated. Initially, these studies employed the radiolabeled agonists, LTB_4, LTC_4 and LTD_4. More recently, an LTD_4 radiolabeled antagonist (ICI 198615) has been synthesized and is available commercially.

The receptors and signal transduction processes about which most is known are the LTD_4 receptors. Studies in our laboratory and by Pong and Dehaven demonstrated LTD_4 binding sites in guinea pig lung (22,33,34,43). We subsequently characterized the LTD_4 receptors in other tissues and species, demonstrated that binding sites observed were indeed receptors, studied the effects of cations and guanine nucleotides on the receptors and solubilized and partially characterized the LTD_4 receptors (30,35,36,38,39). We also reported evidence suggesting that there may be tissue specific isotypes of LTD_4 receptors (23).

The critical step in delineating the LTD_4 signal transduction process was the identification of LTD_4 receptors in smooth muscle cells and the demonstration that some cell lines displaying LTD_4 receptors contracted in response to LTD_4 (6). This has allowed the study of the receptors and signal transduction processes in clonally derived cells. Employing cells of various types, we have dissected the signal transduction processes employed by the LTD_4 receptors and characterized the genetic and epigenetic processes that regulate the receptors and signalling (7,9,10,11,12,15,32,37,40,41,46,47,59).

A key observation that helped focus attention on several of the later steps in the LTD_4 signal transduction process was that approximately 4 minutes after the LTD_4 receptors are stimulated, arachidonic release is increased (9). This phenomenon is receptor driven, dependent on RNA and protein synthesis and liberates various metabolites of arachidonic acid that have profound physiological consequences. Thus, the controversy about the effects of LTD_4 that are dependent or independent of cyclooxygenase products (7,10) was resolved at least at the cellular level.

Although LTC_4 binding sites have been identified in a variety of cells and tissues (24,29,44,53), their physiological role is far less clear. In fact, studies in our laboratory suggested that most of the specific LTC_4 binding sites identified are not receptors (38) and studies in Austen's laboratory demonstrated that the majority of LTC_4 binding sites identified are guatathione-S-transferase (53,54). Nevertheless, there may be specific LTC_4 receptors and their characteristics are obscured by the specific binding of LTC_4 to guatathione-S-transferase (49,50).

Similarly, a number of studies have suggested that LTE_4 receptors may exist (17,55). In contrast to LTC_4 binding sites, however, we have found no evidence for the existence of specific LTE_4 binding sites in any cell line or tissue studies, and we have shown that LTE_4 is a partial agonist at the LTD_4 receptor (48,59).

LTB_4 receptors and their signal transduction mechanisms have also been studied extensively. These receptors are clearly different than LTD_4 receptors. In human blood polymorphonuclear leukocytes (PMNs), there are two classes of LTB_4 receptors based on differences in affinity for ^3H-LTB_4 (18,20). Occupancy of the low affinity state receptor class has been associated with release of lysosomal enzymes and superoxide generation, while occupation of high affinity state receptors appears to induce chemotaxis (21,27). The signal transduction processes of LTB_4 receptors have been studied and shown to be similar but far from identical to those employed by LTD_4 receptors (27,47). Comparisons of the LTB_4 and LTD_4 receptors, signal transduction processes, genetic and epigenetic regulation have been greatly facilitated by the identification of a clonally derived cell line that displays both types of receptors and transduction systems (47).

Inasmuch as the leukotrienes are not stored and a number of cell lines that display LTD_4 and LTB_4 receptors also express the enzymes required for leukotriene biosynthesis, we consider the key enzyme in the pathway, 5-lipoxygenase, a part of the signal transduction process. Recently, significant advances in understanding 5-lipoxygenase and its regulation have been reported (2,16,25,28,31,45,62). The recent cloning of the gene for 5-lipoxygenase and other proteins involved in signal transduction will greatly facilitate future studies. The involvement of 5-LO in LTD_4 signal transduction has been recently reviewed (13) and will not be discussed here.

CURRENT STATUS

The Receptors

Table I compares the properties of LTB_4 and LTD_4 receptors and signalling processes in U-937 cells (14,47). The receptors in guinea pig lung are comparable to those in human fetal and adult lung and a variety of tissues and cell lines including RBL-1 cells and U-937 cells (14). LTD_4 receptors are glycoproteins that are located in the plasma membranes of all cells and tissues displaying the receptors. The receptors can be solubilized as a complex containing guanine nucleotide binding proteins and possibly phospholipase C using various detergents (39).

**Comparison of Properties of Basal and
DMSO Differentiated U937 Cells**

	Basal		DMSO	
	LTB_4	LTD_4	LTB_4	LTD_4
Membrane Receptors				
K_d	N.D.	$.42 \pm .12$	$.15 \pm .06$	$.35 \pm .12$
B_{max}	N.D.	170 ± 56	300 ± 86	480 ± 76
Divalent Cations Stimulation	Stimulation			
Na^+	N.D.	Inhibition	Inhibition	
Guanine Nucleotides	Transition of Affinity State			
-SH Alkylating Reagents	Inhibition			
Calcium Mobilization				
EC_{50}	N.D.	3.0 ± 0.6	2.4 ± 0.4	3.3 ± 0.6
Maximum Mobilization	16 ± 11	342 ± 36	334 ± 45	1554 ± 136
% of Ca^{++} from Intracellular Release	N.D.	40-50%	25-35%	20-25%
% Inhibited by Pertussis Toxin	N.D.	40-60%	95-100%	40-60%

N.D. = Not Determined (insufficient signal for quantitative results)

Table 1

Signal Transduction

Figure 1 shows the most recent iteration of our model explaining LTD_4 receptors and signal transduction processes. LTD_4 interacts with highly selective and specific LTD_4 receptors located in the plasma membrane. When activated by LTD_4, the LTD_4 receptors can interact with at least two G-proteins. The extent to which LTD_4 receptors use G-proteins that are insensitive to pertussis toxin varies as a function of the cell type and perhaps as a function of differentiation (8,48). Via interactions with the G-proteins, the LTD_4 receptors mobilize Ca^{++} by at least three mechanisms (Figure 2). These include a G-protein modulated phosphoinositide-specific phospholipase C (PI-PLC), a receptor operated calcium channel (ROC), and an as yet unidentified process. Resulting from the interactions described above, several second messengers are elaborated. There is a rapid, transient increase in intracellular calcium derived from both internal stores and extracellular calcium (47). Inositol phosphate metabolism is enhanced resulting in rapid increases in the intracellular signalling inositol phosphates.

Subsequent to the liberation of DAG, inositol phosphates and Ca^{++}, protein kinase C (PKC) is activated and appears to play two pivotal roles. First, it is clearly involved in propagating the signal as it activates various intracellular proteins including topoisomerase I (32). Second, PKC activation is involved in both heterologous desensitization of LTD_4 receptors (56,57) and in modulating the normal activity of LTD_4 signal transduction.

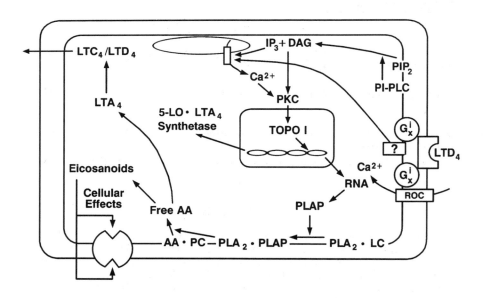

Fig. 1 Model of LTD_4 Signal Transduction

Activation of topoisomerase I is essential for LTD_4 receptor-initiated induction of transcription of at least one gene involved in the second phase of the signalling process. Activation of topoisomerase I is blocked by selective receptor antagonists and a PKC inhibitor, staurosporine (32). If topoisomerase I is inhibited by selective inhibitors such as camptothecin, the second phase in the signal transduction process is inhibited (32). This second phase of the signalling process is initiated with the increased transcription of a gene for a protein that activates a PC-specific PLA_4, phospholipase activating protein (PLAP) (11,12). PLAP increases PLA_2 activity either through direct interactions with the enzyme, the substrate or an inhibitor of the enzyme. PLA_2 activation increases the release of arachidonic acid that is metabolized via the cyclooxygenase and lipoxygenase pathways in a variety of ways, depending on the phenotype of the cell and other factors. If the predominant metabolites are contractile, e.g. thromboxane A_2, the cells display increased contractile activity. If the predominant metabolites are relaxant, e.g. prostacyclin, the cells may relax (6,9,10).

Figure 2 presents the LTD_4 signal transduction clock. Within the first 5-20 seconds after interaction of LTD_4 with its receptors, key intracellular mediators are released or formed (phosphoinositides, DAG, Ca^{++}). Within 20-30 seconds, PKC is translocated and activated, and after approximately 60 seconds, topoisomerase I is activated. By 120 seconds, transcription of the gene for PLAP is enhanced and after approximately 400 seconds, arachidonic acid release is enhanced and active metabolites are formed. Thus, the process is rapid, coordinated, complex and driven by the interaction of the agonist with the receptor. Figure 2 also shows sites at which various compounds may inhibit steps in the process. SK&F 104353, a selective LTD_4 receptor antagonist, inhibits interactions with the receptor. Pertussis toxin inhibits some components of the initial signalling event. Staurosporine inhibits PKC, preventing both signal propagation and heterologous desensitization. Camptothecin inhibits topoisomerase I, inhibiting PLAP production. Inhibitors of RNA synthesis (actinomycin D) and protein synthesis (cyclohexamide) inhibit production of PLAP. Steroids may inhibit PLA_2 and aspirin and nonsteroidal anti-inflammatory agents inhibit cyclooxygenase mediated metabolism of arachidonic acid.

Calcium Mobilization

As much as 80% of the increased intracellular Ca^{++} induced by LTD_4 is derived from extracellular sources (15,48). Pertussis toxin inhibits the influx of extracellular Ca^{++} with only little effect on LTD_4-induced release of intracellular Ca^{++}. Thus, in Figure 2, we suggest that a pertussis toxin-sensitive, G-protein-coupled, receptor-operated Ca^{++} channel (ROC) is involved in the Ca^{++} influx. This channel may also be stimulated by inositol tetrakisphosphate.

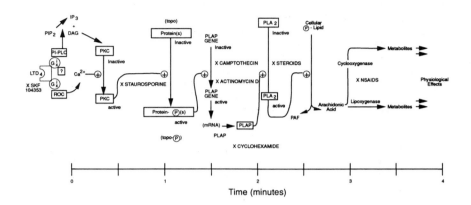

FIG. 2. A cellular clock for the LTD₄ receptor signal transduction process.

+ = positive effect; x = inhibitor of process.

Phosphoinositide Metabolism

LTD$_4$ receptors are coupled to a PI-PLC via at least two G-proteins, one sensitive to pertussis toxin (Figure 2). Although we have not yet identified the PI-PLC that is associated with LTD$_4$ receptors, we have identified and characterized a signalling PI-PLC coupled to vasopressin V$_1$ receptors (1). This enzyme or a member of its family may be associated with the LTD$_4$ receptors. This PI-PLC, PI-PLC I, is located in and associated with the cell membrane (3). PI-PLC I is phosphorylated in vivo and in vitro by PKC, and upon phosphorylation, appears to be translocated from the cell membrane to the cytosol (3). The sequence of the cDNA for this PI-PLC is now known (4) and it differs from other PI-PLCs that have been cloned (4,5,51,52). Its most interesting feature is the presence at the amino and carboxy termini of two regions that are homologous to thioredoxin. We have proposed that the enzymatic mechanism involved in phosphoinositide metabolism may be a phospho-transferase reaction such as that employed by thioredoxin in which an inositol phosphothiol intermediate may be formed.

The Role of Topoisomerase I

The "elbow" in the signal transduction process is the enhanced transcription of PLAP. To achieve enhanced transcription, topoisomerase I is activated. Activation is induced by LTD$_4$ interactions with the LTD$_4$ receptor, resulting in activation of protein kinase C. LTD$_4$ receptor antagonists and a protein kinase C inhibitor, staurosporine, inhibit topoisomerase I activation, PLAP production and release of arachidonic acid (32).

Moreover, the concept that activation of membrane-localized receptors may induce gene transcription as a part of their signalling process appears to be a more general principle. Angiotensin II receptor activation (26) and vasopressin V_1 (42) receptor activation have recently been shown to induce c-fos gene transcription. Additionally, tumor necrosis factor has been shown to induce PLAP via interactions with its cell surface located receptors (12). However, the coupling of LTD_4 receptor-activation to enhanced transcription of the PLAP gene is extraordinarily rapid. The demonstration of several steps, e.g., PKC and topoisomerase I activation before enhanced transcription and several post transcriptional steps that flow in the order predicted by the model, enhances our confidence that indeed such rapid induction of transcription is feasible.

Mechanisms of Regulation of the LTD₄ Transduction Pathway

We have recently reviewed progress in understanding the regulation of LTD_4 signal transduction (13). We have shown that when U937 cells are differentiated with dimethyl sulfoxide (DMSO), the numbers of LTD_4 and LTB_4 receptors increases and there is suggestive evidence that other components in the signal transduction process, including G-proteins and PLC, are altered as well. Table I compares the receptors and calcium mobilization in basal and differentiated U937 cells. The increased coupling efficiency of LTD_4 receptors in differentiated U937 cells suggests coordinate genetic regulation of receptors and components of the signalling system.

The receptors and signal transduction processes are also subject to complex epigenetic regulation (13,59). Highly specific tachyphylaxis of Ca^{++} mobilization in response to LTD_4 occurs. Within 30 seconds after an LTD_4 induced Ca^{++} transient, cells are refractory to an additional LTD_4 dose. Recovery is observed within a few minutes when the agonist is removed and the cells rechallenged with LTD_4. Tachyphylaxis appears to occur with regard to both extracellular and intracellular Ca^{++}. We are currently exploring the possibility that tachyphylaxis results from depletion of receptor-coupled intracellular Ca^{++} pools, depletion of "extracellular" Ca^{++} pools or refractoriness of Ca^{++} channels.

LTD_4 receptors are also subject to homologous desensitization. Prior exposure of RBL-1 cells to LTD_4 resulted in a concentration and time dependent reduction in calcium mobilization. The maximum decrease was 40%. The EC_{50} for desensitization was 1-3 nM LTD_4 and the time required to observe 50% of the decrease was 7.5 minutes (58). Thus, this process is obviously different from the Ca^{++} tachyphylaxis previously discussed. Inasmuch as the density of the LTD_4 receptors decreased by 23% while Ca^{++} mobilization decreased by 40%, factors other than loss of receptors may also be involved. Decreased responsiveness to LTD_4 upon repeated exposure has also been reported from experiments employing strips of guinea pig ilium (17).

We have extended our studies on homologous desensitization to include the U937 cell line. This cell line is particularly important as it displays both LTD_4 and LTB_4 receptors and both are under genetic as well as epigenetic regulation. In this cell line, we have demonstrated that the two clearly distinct receptors with similar signalling processes are independently regulated (59,61). Moreover, using a partial agonist, LTE_4 and the changes in responsiveness after desensitization, we have shown that a substantial receptor reserve exists for LTD_4 in both the basal and differentiated U937 cells (59).

Although the level of receptor reserve was approximately equal in basal and differentiated cells, the homologous desensitization induced by LTD_4 was greater in the basal cells, providing additional data suggesting that differentiation of U937 cells alters components of the signal transduction system in addition to the receptors (29).

LTD_4 receptors and signalling processes are also affected by heterologous desensitization (8,56). Thus, LTD_4 receptor stimulation results in activation of PKC which is involved in propagating signal transduction and in regulating the process (57). Phorbol esters induce heterologous desensitization of LTD_4 receptors and this is prevented by pretreatment with the PKC inhibitor staurosporine (57). Additionally, PMA-induced desensitization of LTD_4 signal transduction can be reversed with staurosporine (60).

LTD_4 Receptors are Coupled to Increases in PIP_3 Levels and to IP_4 Production

Studies designed to determine the identity of the question mark in Figure 1 have resulted in the demonstration that LTD_4 induces production of IP_4 which cannot be accounted for by metabolism of IP_3. The production of IP_4 is receptor mediated, partially inhibited by pertussis toxin and blocked by antagonists of the LTD_4 receptor. Our tentative conclusion is that LTD_4 receptors are coupled through a pertussis toxin sensitive and pertussis toxin insensitive G-proteins to a PIP_3-PLC and produce IP_4 directly via this mechanism.

Additionally, LTD_4 induces a rapid relatively transient increase in PIP_3 levels in the membrane. This increase is entirely blocked by pretreatment with pertussis toxin. The increase in PIP_3 content is receptor mediated and blocked by LTD_4 antagonists. It occurs in the presence or absence of extracellular calcium. Thus, we believe that simultaneously with increasing production of IP_4, PIP_3 levels are increased in a receptor mediated fashion. The precise mechanisms accounting for the increase in PIP_3 are not delienated. Nor is the role of the increase in PIP_3 levels in signal transduction. For example, we have not rigorously excluded the possibility that the increase in IP_4 might result from the increase in substrate (PIP_3) for a PLC. These and other questions are the subject of current investigations.

Conclusions

LTD_4 receptors and the signal transduction pathway have been partially dissected. The signalling system is complex and the LTD_4 receptors can employ several signalling devices. The information gained from studying the LTD_4 signal transduction process may provide insights into signal transduction in general.

REFERENCES

1. Aiyar, N., Bennett, F., Nambi, P., Valinski, W., Angioli, M., Stassen, F.L. and Crooke, S.T. Biochem. J. 261:63-70, 1989.
2. Balcarek, J.M., Theisen, T., Varrichio, A. and Crooke, S.T. J. Biol. Chem. 263:13937-13941, 1988.
3. Bennett, C.F. and Crooke, S.T. J. Biol. Chem. 262:13789-13797, 1987.
4. Bennett, C.F., Balcarek, J., Varrichio, A. and Crooke, S.T. Nature 334:268-270, 1988.
5. Bloomquist, B.T., Shortridge, R.D., Schneuwly, S., Perdew, M., Montell, C., Steller, H., Rubin, G., and Pak, W.L. Cell 54:723-733, 1988.
6. Clark, M.A., Cook, M., Mong, S. and Crooke, S.T. Eur. J. Pharmacol. 116:207-220, 1985.
7. Clark, M., Bomalaski, J.S., Conway, T., Wartell, J. and Crooke, S.T. Prostaglandins 32:703-708, 1986.
8. Clark, M., Conway, T.M., Bennett, C.F., Crooke, S.T. and Stadel, J.M. Proc. Natl. Acad. Sci. 83:7320-7324, 1986.
9. Clark, M.A., Littlejohn, D., Conway, T.M., Mong, S., Steiner, S. and Crooke, S.T. J. Biol. Chem. 261:10713-10718, 1986.
10. Clark, M.A., Littlejohn, D., Mong, S. and Crooke, S.T. Prostaglandins 31:157-166,1986.
11. Clark, M., Conway, T., Shorr, R. and Crooke, S.T. J. Biol. Chem. 262:4402-4406, 1987.
12. Clark, M.A., Chen, M-J., Crooke, S.T. and Bomalaski, J.S. Biochem. J. 250:125-132, 1988.
13. Crooke, S.T., Mattern, M., Sarau, H.M., Winkler, J.D., Saussy, D.L., Balcarek, J., Wong, A. and Bennett, C.F. Trends in Pharm. Sciences 10:103-107, 1988.
14. Crooke, S.T., Mong, S., Clark, M., Sarau, H., Wong, A., Vegesna, R., Winkler, J.D., Balcarek, J. and Bennett, C.F. In Cellular and Molecular Aspects of Inflammation. (S.T. Crooke and G. Poste, Eds.) 1988; pp. 321-333. Plenum Press, New York.
15. Crooke, S.T., Mong, S., Sarau, H.M., Winkler, J.D. and Vegesna, V.K. Ann. N.Y. Acad. Sci. 524:153-161, 1988.
16. Dixon, R.A.F., Jones, R.E., Diehl, R.D., Bennett, C.D., Kargman, S., and Rouzer, C.A. Proc. Natl. Acad. Sci. USA 85:416-420, 1988.
17. Fleisch, J.H., Rinkema, L.E. and Marshall, W.S. Biochem. Pharmacol. 33:3919-3922, 1984.
18. Goldman, D.W. and Goetzl, E.J. J. Exp. Med. 159:1027-1041, 1984.
19. Goldman, D.W., Gifford, L.A., Young, R.N. and Goetzl, E.J. Fed Proc. 44:781, 1985.
20. Goldman, D.W., Olson, D.M., Gifford, L.A. and Goetzl, E.J. Fed. Proc. 44:736, Abs. a1898, 1985.
21. Goldman, D.W., Gifford, L.A., Marotti, T., Koo, C.H., and Goetzl, E.J. Fed. Proc. 46:200-203, 1987.
22. Hogaboom, G.K., Mong, S., Wu, H-L. and Crooke, S.T. Biochem. Biophys. Res. Commun. 116:1136-1143, 1983.
23. Hogaboom, G.K., Mong, S., Stadel, J.M. and Crooke, S.T. J. Pharmacol. Exp. Ther. 233:686-693, 1985.

24. Hogaboom, G.K., Mong, S., Stadel, J.M. and Crooke, S.T. Mol. Pharmacol. 27:236-245, 1985.
25. Hogaboom, G.K., Cook, M., Newton, J., Varrichio, A., Shorr, R., Sarau, H. and Crooke, S.T. Mol. Pharmacol. 30:510-519, 1986.
26. Kawahara, Y., Sunako, M., Tsuda, T., Fukuzaki, H., Fukumoto, Y., and Takai, Y. Biochem. Biophys. Res. Commun. 150:52-59, 1988.
27. Koo, C.H., Baud, L., Sherman, J.W., Harvey, J.P., Goldman, D.W. and Goetzl, E.J. In Cellular and Molecular Aspects of Inflammation (G. Poste and S.T. Crooke, Eds.) 1988; pp. 305-316. Plenum Press, New York.
28. Kretsigner, RH., and Creutz, C.E. Nature 320:573-574, 1986.
29. Lewis, M.A., Mong, S., Vessella, R.L., Hogaboom, G.K., Wu, H-L. and Crooke, S.T. Prostaglandins 27:961-974, 1984.
30. Lewis, M.A., Mong, S., Vessella, R.L. and Crooke, S.T. Biochem. Pharmacol. 34:4311-4317, 1985.
31. Matsumoto, T., Fund, C.D., Radmark, O., Hoog, J-O., Jornvall, H. and Samuelsson, B. Proc. Natl. Acad. Sci. USA 85:26-30, 1988.
32. Mattern, M.R., Mong, S., Mong, S-M, O'Leary Bartus, J., Sarau, H.M., Clark, M.A., Foley, J.J. and Crooke, S.T. Biochem. J., 1989. In press.
33. Mong, S., Wu. H.-L., Clark, M.A., Stadel, J.M., Gleason, J.G. and Crooke, S.T. Prostaglandins 28:805-824, 1984.
34. Mong, S., Wu, J-L., Hogaboom, G.K., Clark, M.A. and Crooke, S.T. Eur. J. Pharmacol. 192:1-11, 1984.
35. Mong, S., Wu, H-L., Hogaboom, G.K., Clark, M.A., Stadel, J.M. and Crooke, S.T. Eur. J. Pharmacol. 106:241-253, 1985.
36. Mong, S., Wu, H-L., Scott, M.O., Lewis, M.A., Weichman, B.M., Kinzig, C.M., Gleason, J.G. and Crooke, S.T. J. Pharmacol. Exp. Ther. 234:316-325, 1985.
37. Mong, S., Hoffman, K., Wu, H-L. and Crooke, S.T. Mol. Pharmacol. 31:35-41, 1986.
38. Mong, S., Hogaboom, G.K., Clark, M.A. and Crooke, S.T. In Receptors in Drug Research (R. O'Brien, Ed.) Marcel Dekker, Inc., New York, 1986; 205-230.
39. Mong, S., Wu, H-L., Stadel, J.M. and Crooke, S.T. Mol. Pharmacol. 29:235-243, 1986.
40. Mong, S., Miller, J., Wu, H-L. and Crooke, S.T. J. Pharmacol. Exp. Ther. 244:508-515, 1987.
41. Mong, S., Wu, H-L, Wong, A., Sarau, H.M. and Crooke, S.T. J. Pharmacol. Exp. Ther. 247:803-813, 1988.
42. Nambi, P., Watt, M., Whitman, M., Aiyar, N., Moore, J.P., Evan, G.I. and Crooke, S.T. FEBS Lett. 245:61-61, 1989.
43. Pong, S-S. and DeHaven, R.N. Proc. Natl. Acad. Sci, USA 80:7415-7419, 1983.
44. Pong, S-S., DeHaven, R.N., Kuehl, F.A. and Egan, R.W. J. Biol. Chem. 258:9616-9619, 1983.
45. Rouzer, C. and Kargman, S. J. Biol. Chem. 263:10980-10988, 1988.
46. Sarau, H., Mong, S., Foley, J., Wu, H-L. and Crooke, S.T. J. Biol. Chem. 262:4034-4041, 1987.
47. Sarau, H.M., Foley, J.J., Wu, H-L., Crooke, S.T. and Mong, S. Submitted.

48. Saussy, D.L., Sarau, H.M., Foley, J.J., Mong, S. and Crooke, S.T. J. Biol. Chem., 1989. In press.
49. Snyder, D.W. and Krell, R.D. J. Pharmacol. Exp. Ther. 231:616-622, 1984.
50. Snyder, D.W. and Bernstein, P.R. Eur. J. Pharmacol. 138:397-405, 1987.
51. Stahl, M.L., Ferenz, C.R., Kelleher, K.L., Kriz, R.W., and Knopf, J.L. Nature 332:269-272, 1988.
52. Suh, P-G., Ryu, S.H., Moon, K.H., Suh, H.W., and Rhee, S.G. Cell 54:161-169, 1988.
53. Sun, F.F., Chau, L-Y., Spur, B., Corey, E.J., Lewis, R.A. and Austen, K.F. J. Biol. Chem. 261:8540-8546, 1986.
54. Sun, F.F., Chau, L.Y., and Austen, K.F. Fed. Proc. 46:204-207, 1987.
55. Takayanagi, I., Ohashi, M., and Sato, T. J. Pharmacobio-Dyn. 9:829-835, 1986.
56. Vegesna, R.V.K., Mong, S. and Crooke, S.T. Eur. J. Pharmacol. 147:387-396, 1988.
57. Vegesna, R.V., Wu, H-L., Mong, S. and Crooke, S.T. Mol. Pharmacol. 33:537-542, 1988.
58. Winkler, J.D., Mong, S. and Crooke, S.T. J. Pharmacol. Exp. Ther. 244:449-455, 1988.
59. Winkler, J.D., Sarau, H.M., Foley, J.J. and Crooke, S.T. J. Pharmacol. Exp. Ther. 247:54-62, 1988.
60. Winkler, J.D., Sarau, H.M., Foley, J.J., and Crooke, S.T. Biochem. Biophys. Res. Commun. 157:521-529, 1988.
61. Winkler, J.D., Sarau, H.M., Foley, J.J., Mong, S. and Crooke, S.T. J. Pharm. Exp. Ther. 246:204-210, 1988.
62. Wong, A., Hwang, S.M., Cook, M., Hogaboom, C.K. and Crooke, S.T. Biochem. 27:6763-6769, 1988.

Advances in Prostaglandin, Thromboxane,
and Leukotriene Research, Vol. 20,
edited by B. Samuelsson et al.
Raven Press, Ltd., New York © 1990.

EICOSANOID RECEPTORS OF THE GASTROINTESTINAL TRACT

K.-Fr. Sewing and M. Beinborn

Abteilung Allgemeine Pharmakologie
Medizinische Hochschule Hannover
Konstanty-Gutschow-Str. 8
D-3000 Hannover 61, FRG.

Eicosanoids have been described to have several physiological and pharmacological functions in different areas of the gastrointestinal tract: regulation of mucosal blood flow, inhibition of gastric acid secretion, maintenance of gastric mucosal integrity, stimulation of intestinal fluid and electrolyte secretion and although I believe that the word should be banned, gastric mucosal "cytoprotection". The data suggest some of them are receptor-mediated. It is surprising to realize that although many eicosanoids are around and have been thoroughly investigated, research on gastrointestinal eicosanoid receptors has started only recently. Our work began in 1985 when we realized that a report in the literature on the existence of prostacyclin receptors in the gastric mucosa was based upon some pitfalls (2,12). So we developed a radioligand binding assay using ^{3}H-labelled prostaglandin E_2 with a high specific activity as radioligand (3). With this radioligand binding assay we addressed the following questions:

1. Does the gastric mucosa contain binding sites for one or more naturally occurring eicosanoids?
2. Which cell types do eicosanoid binding sites - if detectable - belong to?
3. Do gastric mucosal eicosanoid binding sites serve any function?
4. Do gastric mucosal eicosanoid binding sites change their characteristics under pathological conditions?
5. Are prostanoid binding sites of the gastric mucosa different from those in other tissues?

In a first attempt to spot and to characterize specific binding of prostaglandins, we prepared subcellular particles from mucosal cells of various segments of the porcine gastrointestinal tract and performed radioligand binding assays using ^{3}H-prostaglandin E_2 as radioligand. The results were analyzed by Scatchard plots and can be summarized as follows:
1. Each part of the gastrointestinal mucosa contains

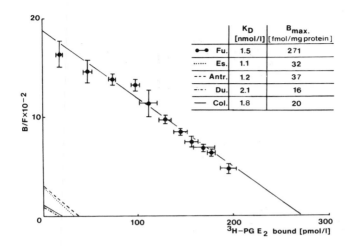

FIG. 1. Scatchard plots of ^{3}H-prostaglandin E_2 binding to plasma membranes of different parts of the porcine gastrointestinal mucosa.

specific prostaglandin E_2 binding sites (Fig 1).
2. The number of binding sites per unit protein is highest in the fundic mucosa (Fig. 1).
3. The affinity of prostaglandin E_2 to the binding sites in the different parts of the gastrointestinal mucosa is more or less identical (Fig 1).
4. There is no indication that in any of the different areas of the gastrointestinal mucosa there is more than one binding site although one has to admit that due to the small number of binding sites in some areas the results do not allow a clearcut decision.
5. From the subcellular distribution of relevant marker enzymes and binding sites it has to be concluded that the binding sites are associated with the plasma membranes (data not shown).

Based upon the finding that the fundic mucosa contains the highest number of prostaglandin E_2 binding sites we focussed our interest on the next question which of the fundic cells contain prostaglandin E_2 binding sites. The fundic glands contain at least four different cell types: parietal cells, chief cells, mucous cells and endocrine cells. Therefore, when using as starting material the homogenate of the total gatric mucosa allocation of biochemical findings to specific cell types is impossible. Therefore, we had to isolate and to enrich different cell types of the fundic mucosa (11).

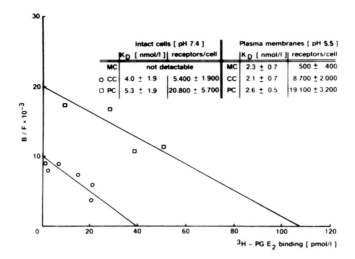

FIG. 2. Scatchard plots of ^{3}H-prostaglandin E_2 binding
to intact parietal and chief cells and their plasma
membranes of the porcine fundic mucosa.

Cell isolation was achieved by incubation of the fundic mucosa with collagenase and pronase which resulted
in an inhomogeneous cell suspension. This cell suspension was subjected to counterflow elutriation by using
the Beckman elutriation system. This procedure allows
separate enrichment of parietal cells, chief cells and
mucous cells which were identified by specific cyto-
logical staining. These different cell populations can
be used to carry out radioligand binding studies with
enriched cell populations or with plasma membranes
prepared from them. These studies can be summarized as
follows:

1. Each of the three cell types, parietal cells, chief
cells and mucous cells contain specific prostaglandin
E_2 binding sites (Fig 2).
2. The rank order of binding site density was parietal
cells > chief cells > mucous cells (Fig 2).
3. The affinity of prostaglandin E_2 to the binding sites of the different cell types is more or less identical (Fig 4).
4. Again there is no indication that in any of the
different cell types there is more than one binding
site.
5. From the rank order of potency of various eicosanoids to displace ^{3}H-prostaglandin E_2 from its binding

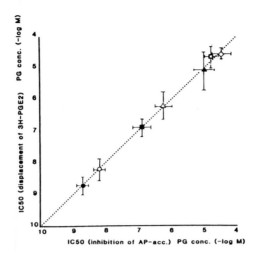

FIG. 3. Correlation between the ^{14}C-aminopyrine accumulation and displacement of ^{3}H-prostaglandin E₂ (●), 16-16-dimethylprostaglandin E₂ (○), prostaglandin F₂α (▲), iloprost (■) prostaglandin D₂ (□), BW 245c (▲), and U 46619 (◇) $y = 0.99 x + 0.08$, $r = 0.948$ (8).

site we have to conclude that the parietal cells contain only a binding site for prostaglandin E₂. In logical consequence the next series of experiments served the question whether or not the binding sites characterized have receptor function. It is well known that in particular natural and synthetic E-type prostaglandins are inhibitors of parietal cell acid secretion. Therefore, we compared several natural and synthetic prostaglandin analogues for their potency to displace ^{3}H-prostaglandin E₂ from its binding site and to inhibit parietal cell acid production. The method for measuring acid production (6) requires brief explanation. A fixed number of isolated and enriched parietal cells are exposed under standardized conditions to the weak base ^{14}C-aminopyrine which due to its physicochemical properties upon stimulation of acid secretion accumulates in parietal cell tubulovesicles in a concentration-dependent manner. Separation of these cells from the suspension medium - still containing ^{14}C-aminopyrine - is achieved by quick centrifugation of an iloquot of the cell suspension through a cushion of silicon oil into 3 N KOH which is then counted in a liquid scintillation counter (10,11). For our purpose the cells were stimulated by 1 µmol/l histamine which

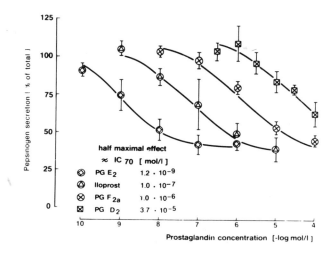

FIG. 4. Inhibition of histamine-stimulated pepsinogen secretion from porcine isolated and enriched chief cells by prostaglandin E_2, iloprost, prostaglandin $F_{2\alpha}$, and prostaglandin D_2.

is approximately the half maximal concentration. All natural and synthetic eicosanoids tested caused a concentration-dependent displacement of ^{3}H-prostaglandin E_2 and a concentration-dependent inhibition of parietal cell acid production. Plotting the individual K_d-values vs the IC_{50}-values to inhibit acid production a straight line is obtained with a slope not significantly different from unity (Fig 3)(8). From these experiments we feel justified to conclude: 1. The parietal cell prostaglandin E_2 binding site has a true receptor function which can be described as inhibition of stimulated acid secretion.
2. The molar range at which binding and inhibition of acid secretion take place favours the hypothesis that for endogenous prostaglandin E_2 of which we know that it can be released from gastric mucosal cells (5) modulation of stimulated gastric acid secretion is a physiological function. Our information on prostaglandins on chief cell function is much less complete. Prostaglandin E_2 - in contrast to the stable choline ester carbachol - has no stimulatory effect on pepsinogen secretion from isolated and enriched chief cells as measured by the modified Anson method. However histamine-stimulated pepsinogen secretion was inhibited in a concentration-dependent manner (Fig. 4).

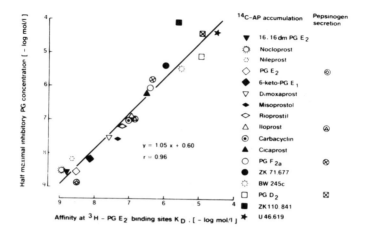

FIG. 5. Correlation between affinity to ^{3}H-prostaglandin E_2 binding sites and antisecretory potency of different prostanoids in porcine fundic mucosa.

The limited number of eicosanoids studied in a comparative manner for chief cell binding and inhibition of histamine-stimulated pepsinogen secretion allows the cautious conclusion that - although smaller in number - chief cells have prostaglandin E_2-receptors (Fig 5) and that their physiological function is to modulate pepsinogen secretion.

Whether the same holds true for mucous cells is currently under investigation.

There are numerous investigations dealing with the role of endogenous eicosanoids for the integrity of the gastrointestinal mucosa all based upon Robert's (9) original observation that minute quantities (doses lower than those which are necessary to inhibit acid secretion) of prostaglandins protect the mucosa from damage caused by noxious agents. Later it was found that immunization of rabbits against prostaglandin E_2 produced gastric lesions (8). In a systematic study in which five rabbits were immunized to produce antibodies against prostaglandin E_2 and five rabbits were sham-immunized, four of the five immunized and only one of the sham-immunized animals developed gastric ulceration. In these animals we studied the prostaglandin E_2-receptor characteristics and found an up-

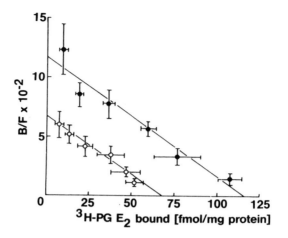

FIG. 6. Binding characteristics of ^{3}H-prostaglandin E_2 in gastric mucosal plasma membranes from immunized (●) and sham immunized (○) rabbits (1).

regulation of these receptors (Fig 6) (1). In the whole context this makes sense in such a way that scavange of endogenous prostaglandin E_2 by antibodies produces prostaglandin E_2 depletion which in turn enhances the power of the remaining prostaglandin E_2 to inhibit acid secretion and thereby to potentially lower the agressiveness of the gastric juice. The properties of prostaglandin E_2 to have a function in mucosal integrity and to inhibit gastric acid secretion have launched numerous research activities to develop synthetic prostaglandin E_2 or other prostaglandin analogues as antiulcer agents. For various reasons they all more or less failed. One of the reasons for failure are so far inevitable side effects predictable from the spectrum of prostaglandin effects. One of the major problems is the fact that the musculature of the uterus, in particular that of the pregnant uterus, very sensitively responds to prostaglandins by contraction. This of course, limits the use of porstaglandins structurally closely related to prostaglandin E_2 as antiulcer agents. Therefore, we were interested in the question whether prostaglandin E_2 receptors in the female reproductive system would differ in their characteristics from those in the gastric mucosa or in other words whether among the numerous prostaglandin derivatives serving as candidates as antiulcer agents there would be one which has a higher affinity to the gastric mucosa than to the female reproductive system. We compared a number of eicosanoids which we had access to in radioligand binding assays in two systems, the gastric fundic mucosa and the uterus muscle. What we found was very disappointing: none of the compounds tested proved to have a higher affinity to the fundic mucosa than to the uterus muscle (4) suggesting that - at least after parenteral administration - all of the analogues tested might have a similar spectrum of side effects.

In summary the picture to be drawn looks as follows: the fundic mucosa has specific binding sites for prostaglandin E_2 which act as receptors on parietal cells for inhibition of stimulated acid and on chief cells possibly for inhibition of stimulated pepsinogen secretion. Gastric mucosal prostaglandin E_2 receptors are up-regulated during prostaglandin E_2 scavange by antibodies. These prostaglandin receptors are indistinguishable from those in the uterus muscle with regard to receptor affinity of different synthetic prostaglandin analogues.

REFERENCES

1. Beinborn, M., Hell, M., Seidler, U. and Sewing, K.-Fr. (1989): Prostaglandins (in press).
2. Beinborn, M., Kromer, W., Staar, U. and Sewing, K.-Fr. (1985): Res. Commun. Chem. Pathol. Pharmacol. 49:337-351.
3. Beinborn, M., Netz, S., Staar, U. and Sewing, K. -Fr. (1988): European J. Pharmacol. 147:217-226.
4. Beinborn, M., Nüstedt, V. and Sewing, K.-Fr. (1988): Scand. J. Gastroenterol. 24 (Suppl. 164):21-25.
5. Hell, M., Bauer, A.C., Schmidt, F.W. and Sewing, K-Fr. (1988). Z. Gastroenterologie 26 (Suppl. 1):31-36.
6. Berglindh, T., Helander, H.F. and Öbrink, K.J. (1976): Acta physiol. Scand. 97:401-414.
7. Olson, G.A., Leffler, C.W. and Fletcher, A.M. (1985): Prostaglandins 19:475-480.
8. Seidler, U., Beinborn, M. and Sewing, K.-Fr. (1989): Gastroenterology 96:314-320.
9. Robert, A., Nezamis, Y.E., Lancaster, C. et al. (1979): Gastroenterology 77:433-443.
10. Sewing, K.-Fr., Beil, W. and Beinborn, M. (1989): Gastroenterology 96:1625.
11. Sewing, K.-Fr., Harms, P., Schulz, G. and Hannemann, H. (1983): Gut 24:557-560.
12. Tepperman, B.L., Soper, B.D., and Emery, S.K. (1984): Prostaglandins 18:477-484.

Advances in Prostaglandin, Thromboxane,
and Leukotriene Research, Vol. 20,
edited by B. Samuelsson et al.
Raven Press, Ltd., New York © 1990.

LEUKOTRIENES IN THE CARDIOVASCULAR SYSTEM

P. J. Piper, A. P. Sampson, H. bin Yaacob and J. M. McLeod

Department of Pharmacology, Hunterian Institute, Royal College
of Surgeons of England, Lincoln's Inn Fields, London WC2A 3PN

INTRODUCTION

Cysteinyl-containing leukotrienes (LTs) have potent actions on various types of smooth muscle and are able to alter the calibre of blood vessels. Usually, LTs C_4 or D_4 increase vascular resistance (see (16,13). For instance, in man, intracoronary injection of LTD_4 produced increased coronary vascular resistance and reduction in mean arterial blood pressure (12). However, in human or porcine skin, LTs C_4 or D_4 cause vasodilatation (2). LTB_4 has little smooth muscle activity but synergises with vasodilator prostaglandins to produce exudation of plasma (23), a property also shared by LTC_4. It is therefore possible that LTs may cause oedema of the vessel wall which would contribute to narrowing of the lumen. Both LTC_4 and LTD_4 caused reduction in coronary flow in guinea·pig working hearts *in vitro* whereas LTB_4 has no apparent action on cardiac function (9). The LTs also cause reduction in ventricular developed tension which appears to be secondary to the impairment of coronary flow. LTs C_4 and D_4 have differing profiles of action in the heart. Leukotriene C_4 is more potent than LTD_4 in reducing coronary flow and cardiac developed tension. Further, the reduction in cardiac developed tension induced by LTC_4 is of slower onset and longer duration than that due to LTD_4.

GENERATION OF LEUKOTRIENES

1. Vascular tissue

Leukotrienes may be generated from vascular tissue by immunological or non-immunological stimuli (see (15)). LTB_4, LTC_4 and its metabolites LTD_4 and LTE_4 are formed from human coronary and pulmonary arteries by challenge with human anti-IgE or calcium ionophore A23187; higher concentrations of LTs are consistently released by A23187 than by immunological challenge. LTs can also be released from a number of porcine blood vessels; the output of LTs varies between blood vessels, with the highest concentration being formed by cerebral arteries (17).

2. Peripheral venous blood

Leukotrienes may also be generated in human whole blood in a dose-related fashion by incubation with A23187 (10-40 µM). We have recently demonstrated the release of LTs C_4, D_4 and E_4 from human peripheral venous blood challenged with A23187 (25µM) (21) and shown that significantly higher concentrations of LTs are released in asthmatic blood. Heparinised samples of peripheral venous blood from normals or asthmatics were incubated with A23187 (25µM) for up to 120 min at 37°C. After centrifugation, $[^3H]$-LTs were added as internal standards and endogenous LTs were extracted with ethanol, partially purified with C_{18} Sep-Pak cartridges and subjected to reverse-phase HPLC. LTs B_4, C_4, D_4 and E_4 were quantitated by means of specific radioimmunoassays.

There was a rapid rise in LTB_4 levels and significantly more LTB_4 was formed in asthmatic blood at all time points, reaching a plateau at 30-60 min. Peak levels at 30 min were 436±73 (asthmatic) and 246±26 (normal) ng ml^{-1}. LTB_4 was metabolised by w- and β-oxidation to 20-carboxy and 20-hydroxy derivatives but, after 120 min, metabolism to those derivatives was less than 20%.

The peak output of LTC_4 in asthmatic blood (106±24.8 ng ml^{-1}) occurred at 10 min and the concentration was significantly higher than in normal blood (39.7±12.7 ng ml^{-1}). Levels of LTC_4 declined from 10-120 min when they were less than 6 ng ml^{-1}. Significantly higher concentrations of LTD_4 (39.8±10 ng ml^{-1}) were generated in asthmatic blood than in normal blood (15.2±1.0 ng ml^{-1}) and again reached a plateau at 20-30 min and declined over 120 min. The concentration of LTE_4 in both normal and asthmatic blood increased rapidly over 120 min; after 30 min, levels were 103±14.0 ng ml^{-1} (asthmatic) and 59.4±9.9 ng ml^{-1} (normal).

^3H-LTC_4 was converted to LTE_4 by both normal and asthmatic blood and there was no difference in metabolism. There was no significant difference in differential cell counts between normal and asthmatic blood.

LEUKOTRIENES IN CARDIAC ANAPHYLAXIS

To investigate the possible role of LTs in the heart in shock conditions, their generation in, and contribution to, cardiac anaphylaxis (10) in guinea pig hearts *in vitro* was studied (see (25)).

Hearts from guinea pigs which had previously been sensitized to ovalbumin were perfused with Tyrode solution via retrograde cannulation of the aorta, by a modification of the Llangendorf technique, to allow measurement of coronary perfusion pressure and ventricular developed tension. Coronary vascular resistance was calculated from the formula:

$$\frac{\text{Peak perfusion pressure}}{\text{Peak coronary flow}} - \frac{\text{Basal perfusion pressure}}{\text{Basal coronary flow}} = \frac{\text{Coronary}}{\text{vascular}} \text{ resistance}$$

When ovalbumin 100 µg was injected into the coronary circulation, there was a rapid, biphasic increase in perfusion pressure accompanied by a fall in cardiac developed tension. The effluent was collected at 1 min intervals for 10 min, subjected to reverse-phase HPLC and the levels of LT B_4, C_4, D_4 and E_4 and of thromboxane (Tx) B_2 were measured by radioimmunoassay (25). TxB_2 was the first eicosanoid to appear in the cardiac effluent and reached a peak in the first minute. When generation of TxA_2 was inhibited by indomethacin (2.8 µM), infused into the hearts 15 min before and during cardiac anaphylaxis, the release of LTs was significantly potentiated and its duration extended beyond 10 min. This was accompanied by a higher-than-normal incidence of post-challenge atrial fibrillation and by exacerbation of cardiac anaphylaxis (Fig.1). Treatment of either normal or indomethacin-treated hearts with the 5-lipoxygenase inhibitor, CGS 8515, inhibited the release of LTC_4 but not that of TxB_2 and lessened the effects of cardiac anaphylaxis (25).

Bolus injection of LTC_4 (30 pmol) into normal hearts caused an increase in coronary perfusion pressure, lasting about 4 min. On the other hand, the increase in coronary perfusion pressure following ovalbumin challenge of sensitized hearts remained elevated for longer than 10 min in hearts, which is longer than the duration of release of LTs following antigen (Fig.1). This suggests

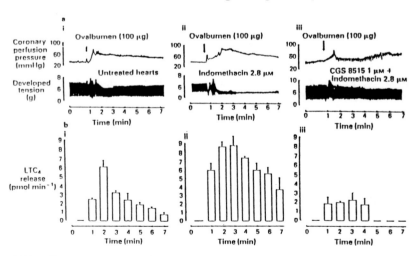

FIG.1. Effects of ovalbumen challenge (100 µg) on coronary perfusion pressure and cardiac developed tension (a) Representative tracings from four separate experiments in untreated hearts (i), indomethacin-treated hearts (ii) and hearts treated with CGS 8515 in the presence of indomethacin (iii). (b) Mean data for the experiments shown in a(i), a(ii) and a(iii). *Reproduced from* Yaacob, H.B. & Piper, P.J. (1988) *Br.J.Pharmacol.*, 95, 1322-1328.

that the protracted increase in coronary perfusion pressure may be mediated by other vasoactive mediators in addition to LTs.

Platelet-activating factor (PAF) is another mediator of cardiac anaphylaxis (11) and has been shown to stimulate release of LTs in isolated hearts from rat or guinea pig (18) (19). LTC_4 then accounts for part of the PAF-induced changes in cardiac function. Treatment of hearts with a 5-lipoxygenase inhibitor, CGS 8515, protects against the increase in perfusion pressure but not the reduction in cardiac developed tension caused by PAF (24).

In sensitized hearts treated with the PAF antagonist WEB 2086 (14,24), there was partial inhibition of the anaphylactic increase in coronary perfusion pressure (Fig.2) but WEB 2086 had less inhibitory effect than the 5-lipoxygenase inhibitor, CGS 8515. WEB 2086 caused 36% reduction in antigen-induced total release of LTs but had no effect on the generation of TXB_2. These results demonstrate that PAF released during cardiac anaphylaxis does not stimulate the release of all the LTs generated during immunological challenge but may contribute, in part, to their release.

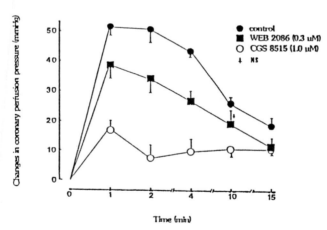

FIG.2. Increase of coronary perfusion pressure in cardiac anaphylaxis in guinea pig isolated hearts is inhibited by CGS 8515 but only attenuated by WEB 2086. *Reproduced from* Piper, P.J. (1989) *Drug Res.& Drug Development in the 21st C.*,pp.162-171.

LEUKOTRIENE ANTAGONISTS

The coronary constriction induced by LTs in guinea pig heart *in vitro* is antagonised by the LT receptor antagonist, FPL 55712 (1). In this study, we have investigated the effects of three LTD_4 receptor antagonists which have been shown to have a high specificity against LTD_4 in airways (7,6,8). The coronary flow and cardiac developed tension were measured in guinea pig hearts as described above.

The LTD$_4$ antagonists Mk-571 5-18.5µM (7), SK&F 104,353 0.01-0.1µM (6) or ICI 198,615 0.003-0.3µM (22) were added to the perfusing Krebs' solution 20 min before and during intracoronary injections of LTC$_4$, LTD$_4$ or the TxA$_2$ mimetic, U-44069. The three receptor antagonists had differing effects against the cardiac actions of LTC$_4$ or LTD$_4$, as shown in Table 1.

Table 1   <u>Comparative actions of LTD$_4$ antagonists</u>
            <u>in guinea pig trachea and heart *in vitro*</u>

	Trachea	Heart
MK-571	antagonises LTD$_4$ and LTC$_4$ in nM range	In µM range antagonises LTD$_4$, LTC$_4$ and U44069
SK+F 104,353	antagonises LTD$_4$ in nM range. Not active against LTC$_4$	active in nM range against LTD$_4$ and LTC$_4$. No effect against U44069
ICI 198,615	antagonises LTD$_4$ in nM range. Little action against LTC$_4$	antagonises LTD$_4$ in nM range. Little action against LTC$_4$

DISCUSSION and CONCLUSIONS

Leukotrienes may be generated from vascular tissue or whole peripheral venous blood, as described above. Leukotrienes may be formed by various leukocytes; for example, see (20), (5). On the other hand, platelets do not form LTs but can convert LTA$_4$ formed by other cells to LTs (4). Challenge of blood from asthmatics consistently resulted in generation of significantly higher levels of LTB$_4$ and cysteinyl LTs C$_4$, D$_4$ and E$_4$. Since the degradation of LTs was the same in normal and asthmatic blood, blood from asthmatics must have an enhanced capacity for generation of LTC$_4$. In our study, there was no difference in differential cell counts between normal and asthmatic blood but granulocytes from asthmatics have been shown to release higher concentrations of LTs than granulocytes from normals (3). There may therefore be an inherent cellular difference in leucocytes or platelets from asthmatics, which results in generation of elevated output of LTs on challenge. Such a variation might occur in LTA$_4$ synthase in leucocytes or in the ability of platelets to convert LTA$_4$ formed by other cells (4) and requires further investigation.

Leukotrienes are generated in guinea-pig isolated hearts during immunological challenge and are potent vasoconstrictors in the coronary circulation of a number of species, including man. This suggests that they may contribute to the fall in cardiac output and resulting hypotension which occurs in various shock conditions. Inhibition of release of LTs in cardiac anaphylaxis and part of its actions in the coronary circulation are due to generation of LTC_4. However, studies with the PAF antagonist, WEB 2086, showed that, although PAF might trigger part of the anaphylactic release of LTC_4, it could not account for the total amount generated. The actions of exogenous LTs in guinea pig isolated hearts were antagonised by the LTD_4 receptor antagonists MK-571, SK&F 104,353 and ICI 198,615. Mk-571 was less active in the heart than had been reported in guinea-pig trachea (7) and, at the doses used, was not specific for LTD_4. SK&F 104,353 antagonised both LTD_4 and LTC_4 in the heart at the same dose range as that reported in guinea pig trachea where it blocked LTD_4 but had little action against LTC_4 (6). ICI 198,615 (8) was active at the same doses against LTD_4 in both heart and trachea and had little action against LTC_4 in either system. These studies suggest that, if LTs have a pathophysiological role in the heart in shock conditions, SK&F 104,353 may be of therapeutic value because it is active against LTC_4 as well as LTD_4, the former being more potent than the latter in the heart.

REFERENCES

1. Augstein, J., Farmer, J.B., Lee, T.B., Sheard, P. and Tattersall, M.L. (1973): *Nat. New Biol.*, 245: 215-217.

2. Camp, R.D.R., Coutts, A.A., Greaves, M.W., Kay, A.B. and Walport, M.J. (1983): *Br. J. Pharmacol.*, 80: 497-502.

3. Damon, M., Chavis, C., Daures, J-P., Crastes de Paulet, A., Michel, F.B. and Godard, Ph. (1989): *Eur. Respir. J.*, 2: 202-209.

4. Edenuis, C., Heidvall, K. and Lindgren, J.A. (1988): *Eur. J. Biochem.*, 178: 81-86.

5. Fels, A.O., Pawlowski, N.A., Cramer, E.B., King, T.K., Cohn, Z.A. and Scott, W.A. (1982): *Proc. Natl. Acad. Sci. USA*, 79: 7866-7870.

6. Hay, D.W.P., Muccitelli, R.M., Tucker, S.S., Vickery-Clark, L.M. and Torphy, T.J. (1987): *J. Pharmacol. Exp. Ther.*, 243: 474-481.

7. Jones, T.R., Guindon, Y., Young, R., Champion, E., Charette, D., Ethier, D., Hamel, R., Ford-Hutchinson, A.W. and Fortin, R. (1988): *Can. J. Physiol. Pharmacol.*, 64: 1532-1542.

8. Krell, R.D., Giles, R.E., Yee, Y.K. and Snyder, D.W. (1987): *J. Pharmacol. Exp. Ther.*, 243: 557-564.

9. Letts, L.G. and Piper, P.J. (1982): *Br. J. Pharmacol.*, 76: 169-176.

10. Levi, R., Allan, G. and Zavecz, J.H. (1976): *Life Sci.*, 18: 1255-1264.

11. Levi, R., Burke, J.A., Guo, Z-G., Hattori, Y., Hoppen, C.M., McManus, L.M., Hanahan, D.J. and Pinckard, R.N. (1984): *Circ. Res.*, 54: 117-124.

12. Marone, G., Giordano, A., Cirillo, R., Triggiani, M. and Vigorito, C. (1988): *Ann. NY Acad. Sci.*, 524: 321-333.

13. Piper, P.J. (1983): *Brit. Med. Bull.*, 39: 255-259.

14. Piper, P.J. (1989), *Drug Research and Drug Development in the 21st Century*, edited by H.P. Wolff, A. Fleckenstein and E.O. Philipp. p. 162-171. Springer-Verlag, Berlin, Heidelberg.

15. Piper, P.J., Antoniw, J.W. and Stanton, A.W.B. (1988): *Ann. NY Acad. Sci.*, 524: 133-141.

16. Piper, P.J. and Samhoun, M.N. (1987): *Brit. Med. Bull.*, 43(2): 297-311.

17. Piper, P.J. and Stanton, A.W.B. (1985): *Adv. Prostaglandin, Thromboxane, Leukotriene Res.*, 15: 333-337.

18. Piper, P.J. and Stewart, A.G. (1986): *Br. J. Pharmacol.*, 88: 595-605.

19. Piper, P.J. and Stewart, A.G. (1987): *Br. J. Pharmacol.*, 90: 771-783.

20. Rankin, J.A., Hitchcock, M., Merrill, W., Bach, M.K., Brashler, J.R. and Askenase, P.W. (1982): *Nature*, 297: 329-331.

21. Sampson, A.P., Evans, J.M., Piper, P.J. and Costello, J.F. (1989): *Br. J. Pharmacol.*, 96: 77P.

22. Snyder, D.W., Giles, R.E., Keith, R.A., Yee, Y.K. and Krell, R.D. (1987): *J. Pharmacol. Exp. Ther.*, 243: 548-564.

23. Wedmore, C.F. and Williams, T.J. (1981): *Nature*, 289: 646-650.

24. Yaacob, H.B. and Piper, P.J. (1988): *Br. J. Pharmacol.*, 95: 521P.

25. Yaacob, H.B. and Piper, P.J. (1988): *Br. J. Pharmacol.*, 95: 1322-1328.

Advances in Prostaglandin, Thromboxane,
and Leukotriene Research, Vol. 20,
edited by B. Samuelsson et al.
Raven Press, Ltd., New York © 1990.

MICROVASCULAR ACTIONS OF EICOSANOIDS IN THE HAMSTER CHEEK POUCH

P. Hedqvist, J. Raud and S.-E. Dahlén

Department of Physiology, and Institute of Environmental Medicine,
Karolinska Institutet, S-10401 Stockholm, Sweden

INTRODUCTION

Ample experimental evidence indicates that eicosanoids can profoundly affect important microvascular functions, notably those related to the inflammatory process. For example, it has long been thought that the antiphlogistic effect of non-steroidal anti-inflammatory drugs (NSAID:s) is a consequence of inhibited formation of prostaglandins, and the more recently discovered leukotrienes provoke microvascular changes that imply a role as inflammatory mediators.

The aim of this chapter is to summarize our recent work on microvascular actions and interactions of some eicosanoids with potential to mediate or modulate significant events in acute inflammation. The results are based on intravital microscopy of the terminal vascular bed of the hamster cheek pouch, which has been adopted for in vivo quantitation of mediator release and dynamic microvascular changes during immunologically induced acute mast cell-dependent inflammation.

MEDIATORS OF ANTIGEN-INDUCED INFLAMMATION

The sequence of microvascular events in early inflammation is with few exceptions characterized by the following partly overlapping reactions; (i) changes in arteriolar diameters (constriction followed by dilatation), (ii) increased venular permeability promoting macromolecular leakage and formation of tissue edema, and (iii) diapedesis and migration of leukocytes into the area of injury. In our model for antigen-provoked inflammation in the hamster cheek pouch (immunization i.p. with 10 μg ovalbumin in 10 mg $Al(OH)_3$, followed by 1 μg ovalbumin in $Al(OH)_3$ four weeks later, and topical challenge of the pouch performed after additional 7-10 days) the process has been documented to be truly mast cell-dependent and presumably triggered via mast cell-bound IgE (19). Analysis of this antigen-induced inflammation revealed that histamine liberated from the mast cells accounted for part of the "immediate" plasma leakage occurring from postcapillary venules. On the other hand, histamine could not be held responsible for any of the following reactions; accumulation and diapedesis of leukocytes, the leukocyte-dependent "delayed" leakage of plasma from postcapillary and larger venules, or the changes in arteriolar caliber.

Two potential chemotactic mediators in allergic inflammation are LTB_4 and platelet activating factor (PAF). Both agents have been shown to be potent inducers of plasma leakage and leukocyte diapedesis in the hamster cheek pouch, with PAF also causing vasoconstriction (5, 1, 2). However, PAF seems to have little or no bearing to the antigen-induced inflammation. Thus, the potent PAF antagonist WEB 2086 (3) failed to reduce antigen-induced vasoconstriction, plasma leakage or leukocyte accumulation, whereas it annulled corresponding reactions of similar magnitude elicited by PAF (19). On the other hand, the lipoxygenase inhibitors L-651392 (10) and BW755C (14) seem to offer some protection against antigen-induced inflammation in the cheek pouch, especially when given together (19).

A reportedly more potent, and possibly also more selective, inhibitor of leukotriene biosynthesis is MK886, also known as L-663,536 (9). It blocks the translocation of cytosolic 5-lipoxygenase to the cell membrane rather than being a direct 5-lipoxygenase inhibitor (22). We have recently tested MK886 for protective effect on mast cell-dependent allergic inflammation in the hamster cheek pouch. Immunized animals were pretreated with indomethacin (6 mg/kg i.v.) in order to uncouple prostaglandin "feedback" inhibition of mediator release, and chlorpheniramine (3 µM topically to the pouch) to block the target action of liberated histamine. Using this protocol, a 5-minute topical challenge with antigen was found to cause extensive leakage of plasma which was almost abolished in animals treated with MK886 (3 mg/kg i.v. and 3 µM topically to the pouch) (Fig. 1). The number of emigrated leukocytes was also substantially reduced (Fig. 1), and the initial vasoconstriction could no longer be demonstrated. Microvascular responses to exogenous leukotrienes were not inhibited by MK886. In additional experiments we used ICI-198,615, a high affinity receptor antagonist for cysteinyl-containing leukotrienes (15). Using the same protocol as above, ICI-198,615 (1 µM topically) inhibited antigen-induced vasoconstriction completely and plasma leakage substantially, without significantly affecting evoked emigration of leukocytes.

Taken together, these observations indicate that endogenous leukotrienes are major mediators of allergic mast cell-dependent inflammation in the hamster cheek pouch. In particular, cysteinyl-containing leukotrienes can be held responsible for the early vasoconstriction, and LTB_4 for at least part of leukocyte emigration. With regard to the antigen-induced extravasation of plasma, it is apparent that leukotrienes as a group account for virtually all leakage that is not due to liberated histamine. At present, the relative importance of LTB_4 versus LTC_4-D_4-E_4 can not be established but the data with ICI-198,615 suggest that cysteinyl-leukotrienes may be of importance also for the the delayed phase of plasma exudation after challenge with antigen. Finally, neither leukotrienes nor histamine seem to have any bearing to antigen-induced vasodilation. Rather, the diminished vasodilation after indomethacin treatment suggests involvement by vasodilating prostaglandins (20).

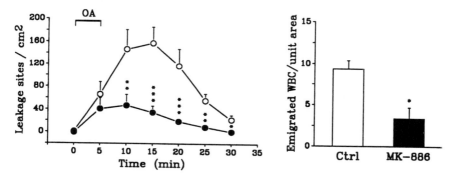

FIG. 1. *Challenge of the hamster cheek pouch with specific antigen (ovalbumin, 10 µg/ml, topically for 5 min) provokes plasma leakage and leukocyte (WBC) emigration (open symbols and column) which are substantially reduced after inhibition of leukotriene biosynthesis with MK886 (3 mg/kg i.v. and 3 µM topically to the pouch)(filled symbols and column. Mean values ± SD, n=5-6. *, P<0.05; **, P<0.01; ***, P<0.001.*

MODULATION OF ANTIGEN-INDUCED INFLAMMATION BY VASODILATING PROSTANOIDS

The vasodilating prostaglandins E_2 and I_2 (PGE_2, PGI_2) are generally considered to be inflammatory agents, notwithstanding they per se provoke little or no edema or pain. A straightforward explanation is that they sensitize pain receptors (7, 8) and enhance the response to edema-producing agents as a consequence of arteriolar dilation and increased blood flow (24). However, there are many reports which indicate that vasodilating prostaglandins also inhibit evoked release of inflammatory mediators, at least in vitro (17, 18, 11). Likewise, NSAID:s sometimes enhance inflammatory reactions, in spite of being potent inhibitors of prostaglandin cyclooxygenase (14, 12). These seemingly discordant reports could indicate that vasodilating prostaglandins operate on more than one level, and with opposite effects, in the inflammatory process. This possibility has recently been explored in detail (19, 20, 21).

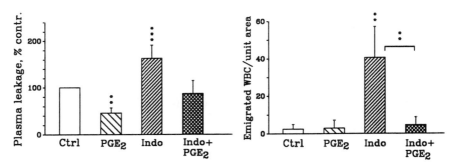

FIG. 2. *Total (0-40 min) leakage of plasma (left panel) and number of emigrated leukocytes (right panel) 40 min after topical challenge with specific antigen (ovalbumin, 10 g/ml for 5 min) either alone (Ctrl) or in the presence of PGE_2 (30 nM topically) or indomethacin (5 mg/kg i.v. and 6 M topically, or indomethacin + PGE_2 in the hamster cheek pouch. Mean values ± SD, n=5-7. *,P<0.05; **,P<0.01 vs. antigen alone.*

Thus, PGE_2 and PGI_2 consistently and markedly enhanced the extravasation of plasma evoked by histamine, LTC_4, and LTB_4, as well as the LTB_4-induced accumulation of leukocytes. Virtually the same potentiation was obtained with two other vasodilators, forskolin and nitroprusside, in concentrations that matched the vasodilative effect of PGE_2 and PGI_2. Per se, none of the four compounds (PGE_2, PGI_2, forskolin, nitroprusside) caused plasma leakage or cell accumulation, indicating that their principal action was to make the terminal vascular bed more responsive to inflammatory mediators.

A different pattern emerged when actively sensitized hamsters were used to characterize the influence of vasodilating prostaglandins and the NSAID prototype, indomethacin, on the sequence of microvascular reactions that ensue challenge with antigen (Fig. 2). In this case, PGE_2 and PGI_2 inhibited the evoked leakage of plasma and the accumulation of leukocytes. Forskolin also acted inhibitory, whereas nitroprusside enhanced the responses. The observed inhibition with PGE_2, PGI_2, and forskolin indicated an action on a plane distinct from the target level for inflammatory mediators, and most likely on the process of mediator release from the mast cells. This interpretation gained confirmation by the finding that PGE_2 substantially inhibited in vivo release of histamine evoked by antigen or compound 48/80 in the cheek pouch (Fig. 3). Furthermore, indomethacin caused substantial enhancement of antigen-provoked release of histamine as well as a marked potentiation of the inflammatory response (Fig. 2, 3). Prostaglandin E_2 reversed the indomethacin-induced potentiation both as regards mediator release and the ensuing inflammatory reactions (Fig. 2, 3). The results summarized here indicate that vasodilating prostaglandins can modulate the inflammatory process at two distinct levels and with opposite effects, namely by inhibition of mediator release and enhancement of mediator action. Furthermore, the differential effect of PGE_2, PGI_2 and forskolin versus that of nitroprosside on mediator release, and on cyclic nucleotide formation, indicates that inhibition of mediator release is distinct from the process of vasodilation. Presumably, the inhibition of mediator release is due to increased tissue levels of cAMP. Finally, indomethacin enhancement of antigen-induced inflammation, and its complete reversal by exogenous PGE_2, advocates a modulatory function on mediator release also by endogenously formed prostanoids.

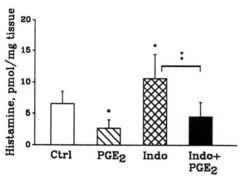

FIG. 3. In vivo histamine release to buffer surrounding hamster cheek pouch after topical antigen challenge (ovalbumin, 10 g/ml for 5 min) either alone (Ctrl) or in the presence of PGE_2 (30 nM topically) or indomethacin (5 mg/kg i.v. and 6 M topically) or indomethacin + PGE_2. Mean values ± SD, n=5-7. *, P<0.05; **, P<0.01.

LIPOXIN A_4 AS AN INHIBITOR OF LEUKOCYTE-DEPENDENT INFLAMMATION

Lipoxin A_4 (LXA_4) is one major representative of a new class of arachidonic acid derivatives whose biosynthesis involves interaction between different lipoxygenases which are abundant in mammalian tissues (23). Lipoxin A_4 has been found to display a number of biological actions suggesting that it may be a modulator of events such as intracellular signal transduction, immunological surveillance, and inflammation (4). In the hamster cheek pouch, LXA_4 elicits vasodilatation and increased blood flow without causing any changes in vascular permeability or leukocyte-endothelium interactions (6).

However, recent observations in the cheek pouch indicate that LXA_4 may be a potent inhibitor of the target actions of the inflammatory mediator leukotriene B_4 (LTB_4)(13). Thus, LXA_4 was found to block LTB_4-induced extravasation of plasma (Fig. 4) and diapedesis of leukocytes. It is unlikely that the inhibition occurred at the level of the LTB_4-receptor, in part because of dissimilar structures, but also because another receptor-mediated effect of LTB_4, contraction of the guinea pig lung strip, is unaffected by LXA_4. On the other hand, LXA_4 did not affect the leukocyte-independent postcapillary leakage of plasma evoked by histamine (Fig. 4). Because the plasma leakage elicited by LTB_4 occurs secondary to accumulation and diapedesis of leukocytes, and since the two effects were inhibited in parallel, it is likely that LXA_4 specifically interferes with mechanisms for leukocyte-dependent alteration of microvascular permeability. In line with this view is a recent report that LXA_4 may inhibit neutrophil chemotaxis stimulated by LTB_4 or fMLP in vitro (16).

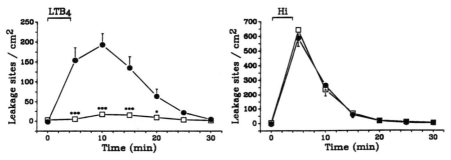

FIG. 4. (Left panel) Leukocyte-dependent "indirect" extravasation of plasma provoked by LTB_4 (300 nM)(filled circles) is inhibited by LXA_4 (3 μM)(open squares). (Right panel) Leukocyte-independent "direct" leakage of plasma induced by histamine (10 μM)(filled circles) is not inhibited by LXA_4 (3 μM)(open squares). Mean values ± SEM, n=4-7. *, P<0.05; **, P<0.01; ***, P<0.001.

CONCLUSIONS

It is obvious that the eicosanoids display a number of biological actions with direct implication to the microvascular bed, and the process of inflammation. With regard to the leukotrienes, it is well established that they may be released from both blood borne and tissue residing cells, and that they in minute concentrations provoke local tissue edema and accumulation of phagocytizing cells and thus mimic cardinal signs of inflammation. The recent findings that selective inhibitors of leukotriene formation or action attenuate or even annul important events in immunologically induced inflammation provide direct evidence for the leukotrienes being significant endogenous inflammatory mediators.

It is generally accepted that also vasodilating prostaglandins contribute to the dynamics of inflammation. Unlike the leukotrienes they seem to function primarily as modulators, with capacity to both enhance and inhibit different events in that process. Judged from cheek pouch model of mast cell-dependent inflammation, the inhibition predominates. However, factors such as the sites of prostaglandin production, including the type preferentially formed, and the degree of local blood flow will influence the final result and may in other instances change the balance in favour of enhancement of inflammation.

Finally, LXA_4 is representative of a third class of eicosanoids with potential to influence inflammation. The microvascular actions of LXA_4 (vasodilatation, inhibition of leukocyte migration, and restriction of leukocyte-dependent extravasation of plasma) imply that LXA_4 may be a modulator of inflammation that is different from that exerted by vasodilating prostaglandins. If present, it could represent a mechanism for down-regulation of inflammation.

ACKNOWLEDGEMENTS

Supported by grants from the Swedish Medical Research Council (14X-4342, 14X-09071), the Wallenberg Foundation, the National Environment Protection Board (5324069-3), the Institute of Environmental Medicine, the Lars Hierta Foundation, the Magn. Bergvall Foundation, and Karolinska Institutet.

REFERENCES

1. Björk, J., Hedqvist, P. and Arfors, K.-E. (1982): *Inflammation*, 6:189-200.

2. Björk, J. and Smedegård, G. (1983): *Eur. J. Pharmacol.*, 96:87-94.

3. Casals-Stenzel, J. (1987): *Immunopharmacology*, 13:117-124.

4. Dahlén, S.-E. (1989): *Adv. Prostaglandin Thromboxane Leukotriene Res.*, 19:122-127.

5. Dahlén, S.-E., Björk, J., Hedqvist, P., Arfors, K.-E., Hammarström, S., Lindgren, J.-Å. and Samuelsson, B. (1981): *Proc. Natl. Acad. Sci. USA*, 78:3887-3891.

6. Dahlén, S.-E., Raud, J., Serhan, C.N., Björk, J. and Samuelsson, B. (1987): *Acta Physiol. Scand.*, 130:643-648.

7. Ferreira, S.H. (1972). *Nature New. Biol.*, 240:200-203.

8. Ferreira, S.H., Nakamura, M. and Abreu-Castro, M.S. (1978): *Prostaglandins*, 16:31-37.

9. Ford-Hutchinson, A.W. (1990): *Adv. Prostaglandin Thromboxane Leukotriene Res.*, Vol. 20.

10. Guindon, Y., Girard, Y., Maycock, A., Ford-Hutchinson, A.W., Atkinson, J.G., Bélanger, P.C., Dallob, A., DeSousa, D., Dougherty, H., Egan, R., Goldenburg, M.M., Ham, E., Fortin, R., Hamel, P., Hamel, R., Lau, C.K., Leblanc, Y., McFarlane, C.S., Piechuta, H., Thérien, M., Yoakim, C. and Rokach, J. (1987): *Adv. Prostaglandin Thromboxane Leukotriene Res.*, **17**:554-557.

11. Ham, E.A., Soderman, D.D., Zanetti, M.E., Dougherty, H.W., McCauley, E. and Kuehl Jr, F.A. (1983): *Proc. Natl. Acad. Sci. USA*, **80**:4349-4353.

12. Hedqvist, P., Dahlén, S.-E. and Palmertz, U. (1984): *Prostaglandins*, **28**:605-608.

13. Hedqvist, P., Raud, J., Palmertz, U., Haeggstöm, J., Nicolaou, K.C. and Dahlén, S.-E. (1989): *Acta Physiol. Scand.*, **237**:571-572.

14. Higgs, G.A., Eakins, K.E., Mugridge, K.G., Moncada, S. and Vane, J.R. (1980): *Eur. J. Pharmacol.*, **66**:81-86.

15. Krell, R.D., Aharony, D., Buckner, C.K. and Kusner, E.J. (1990): *Adv. Prostaglandin Thromboxane Leukotriene Res.*, Vol. 20.

16. Lee, T.H., Horton, C.E., Kyan-Aung, U., Haskard, D., Crea, A.E.G. and Spur, B.W. (1989): *Clin. Sci.*, **77**:195-203.

17. Lichtenstein, L.M. and Bourne, H.R. (1971): In: *Biochemistry of Acute Allergic Reactions*, edited by K.F. Austen and E.L. Becker. pp. 161-174, Blackwell Scientific Publications, Oxford.

18. Loeffler, L.J., Lovenberg, W. and Sjoerdsma, A. (1971): *Biochem. Pharmacol.*, **20**:2287-2297.

19. Raud, J. (1989): *Acta Physiol. Scand.*, **135**(Suppl 578):1-58.

20. Raud, J., Dahlén, S.-E., Sydbom, A., Lindbom, L. and Hedqvist, P. (1988): *Proc. Natl. Acad. Sci. U.S.A.*, **85**:2315-2319.

21. Raud, J., Sydbom, A., Dahlén, S.-E. and Hedqvist, P. (1989): *Agents Actions*, **28**:108-114.

22. Rouzer, C.A. and Kargman, S. (1989): In: *Leukotrienes and Prostanoids in Health and Disease*, edited by U.Zor, Z.Naor and A.Danon. New Trends in Lipid Mediators Research, vol.3, pp. 25-29, Karger, Basel.

23. Serhan, C.N. and Samuelsson, B. (1988): *Adv. Exp. Med. Biol.*, **229**:1-14.

24. Williams, T.J. (1983):. *Br. Med. Bull.*, **39**:239-242.

Advances in Prostaglandin, Thromboxane, and Leukotriene Research, Vol. 20,
edited by B. Samuelsson et al.
Raven Press, Ltd., New York © 1990.

MODIFICATION OF THE LIPOXYGENASE PATHWAY
OF ARACHIDONIC ACID METABOLISM

Anthony W. Ford-Hutchinson

Merck Frosst Centre for Therapeutic Research,
Department of Pharmacology, P.O. Box 1005,
Pointe Claire-Dorval, Québec, H9R 4P8, Canada

INTRODUCTION

Leukotrienes are products of the metabolism of arachidonic acid through the 5-lipoxygenase enzyme pathway (8, 22). The peptidolipid leukotrienes, leukotrienes C_4, D_4 and E_4, have been considered as potential meditors of human bronchial asthma and other allergic diseases because of the potent effects of these compounds on smooth muscle contraction, vascular permeability changes, mucous production and their potential involvement in bronchial hyperreactivity (3, 11, 17, 23, 25). Leukotriene B_4 has been considered as a potential mediator of inflammatory diseases such as inflammatory bowel disease and psoriasis, because of its role as a chemotactic agent for polymorphonuclear leukocytes (8, 9). The regulation of either the action or production of leukotrienes can be achieved in man through the use of either specific, potent, selective leukotriene D_4 receptor antagonists or effective leukotriene biosynthesis inhibitors. Examples of such drugs currently in clinical trials in man are the leukotriene D_4 receptor antagonist, MK-571 (12), and the leukotriene biosynthesis inhibitor, MK-886 (10), the structures of which are shown below.

MK-571

MK-571

Pharmacological Studies

MK-571 (also known as L-660,711; (3-(((3-(2-(7-chloro-2-quinolinyl)ethenyl)phenyl)((3-dimethyl amino-3-oxo-propyl)thio) methyl)thio)propanoic acid) is a member of a new class of potent leukotriene D_4 receptor antagonists (12). The activity of this compound can be demonstrated in vitro through the selective and competitive inhibition of the binding of [^{3}H]-leukotriene D_4 binding to both guinea-pig (IC_{50} value 0.9 nM) and human (IC_{50} value 8.5 nM) lung homogenates and through the failure to inhibit the binding of [^{3}H]-leukotriene C_4 to the same homogenates (IC_{50} values > 20 μM) (12). The receptor binding activity can also be demonstrated functionally in tissue bath experiments through competitive antagonism of contractions of the guinea pig trachea and ileum induced by leukotriene D_4 (pA_2 values respectively of 9.4 and 10.5) and leukotriene E_4 (pA_2 values of 9.1 and 10.4 respectively). MK-571 is also a competitive inhibitor of contractions of human trachea induced by leukotriene D_4 (pA_2 value 8.5). Evidence that leukotriene D_4 is a major mediator of IgE-induced contractions on human tracheal strips was obtained through inhibition of this, presumably mast cell mediated event, by MK-571 with an approximate IC_{50} of 2 μM (complete inhibition at 20 μM). Leukotriene D_4 receptor antagonism was also observed in vivo in the anesthetized guinea pig where MK-571 (either administered by the i.v. or i.d. route) inhibited bronchoconstriction induced by the intravenous administrations of leukotrienes C_4 and D_4 (12). The selectivity of MK-571 for the leukotriene D_4 receptor was shown by the failure to block contractions of the guinea-pig trachea induced by histamine, acetylcholine, 5-hydroxytryptamine, prostaglandin $F_{2\alpha}$, U-44069 and prostaglandin D_2 and the failure to inhibit bronchoconstriction in vivo in the guinea pig induced by either arachidonic acid, U-44069, histamine, acetylcholine or 5-hydroxytryptamine.

Before testing a compound such as MK-571 in man, it was important to show significant in vivo acitivity in a number of animal models following administration by a variety of routes (i.v., p.o. or aerosol). Studies in man were expected to involve antagonism of leukotriene D_4-induced bronchoconstriction to test intrinsic potency, followed by inhibition of antigen-induced bronchoconstriction (both early and late phase) and thus animal models representative of both types of studies were used. With regard to inhibition of leukotriene D_4-induced bronchoconstriction in anesthetized guinea pigs, MK-571 (10 μg/kg i.v.) inhibited the bronchoconstriction induced by either bolus i.v. injections or continuous infusions of leukotrienes D_4 and C_4 (12, Masson et al., submitted for publication). In addition, at a dose of 3 μg/kg i.v. the drug shifted the dose response curve to i.v. leukotriene D_4 38-fold. In a model more close to man, in the conscious squirrel monkey, oral pretreatment with MK-571 produced dose-related inhibition of bronchoconstriction induced by an aerosol of leukotriene D_4, with complete inhibition seen at a dose of 1 mg/kg p.o. (12). MK-571 was also effective in a number of models of antigen-induced bronchoconstriction. In a rodent model using an inbred line of rats with nonspecific bronchial hyperreactivity, MK-571 inhibited the immediate bronchoconstrictor response when combined with an anti-serotonin agent, methysergide, with an ED_{50} of 0.1 mg/kg (4 hours pretreatment p.o.). The compound was also effective in a primate model in which squirrel monkeys were challenged with aerosols of ascaris antigen (MK-571 given at 0.5 mg/kg p.o. 2 hours pretreatment) (12). The late response to antigen has been studied in ascaris-sensitive sheep and in this model a continuous infusion of MK-571 (25 μg/kg/min), starting 1 hour prior to antigen challenge, resulted in a significant attenuation of the immediate bronchoconstriction and a complete inhibition of the late response (1). In addition to its effects on antigen-induced bronchoconstriction, MK-571 has also been shown to be effective against antigen-induced changes in vascular permeability. This has been demonstrated in a guinea pig model of allergic conjunctivitis where the vascular permeability changes to challenge with either leukotriene D_4 or antigen were monitored through the accumulation of intravenously administered (^{99m}technicium)-labelled albumin (6). Following either a single or two antigen challenges, MK-571 produced similar inhibition to that observed with a combination of H_1 and H_2 antagonists. Combinations of MK-571 together with H_1 and H_2 antagonists resulted in almost complete suppresion of the response (6).

Clinical Studies

Clinical trials with less potent leukotriene D_4 receptor antagonists such as L-649,923, L-648,051 and LY-171883 showed that these compounds were only able to partially antagonize bronchoconstriction induced by either leukotriene D_4 or allergen in man (3-5, 16). Thus, it was not possible to determine the true role of leukotriene D_4 in allergen-induced bronchoconstriction using these agents and these studies indicated the need for more functionally efficacious compounds that would induce at least a 50-fold shift in the dose response curve to bronchoconstriction induced by leukotriene D_4 in either normal volunteers or mildly asthmatic subjects. The preclinical data outlined above suggested that MK-571 might be able to meet this need. Safety assessment, which has included two weeks intravenous and fourteen week oral toxicological studies in dogs and rats with high doses of MK-571, has revealed no toxicological abnormalities. Thus MK-571 was

administered intravenously to normal men in single doses
ranging from 15 to 1500 mg (24). No significant side effects
were observed and no laboratory abnormalities were found
indicating that MK-571 was well tolerated at doses likely to be
effective in the treatment of asthma. Preliminary
pharmacokinetic data estimated peak plasma concentrations of
the [+] and [-] enantiomers in excess of 300 μg/ml at the
1500 mg dose with a half life of approximately 3 hours. MK-571
was then tested in 6 healthy male volunteers against
leukotriene D_4-induced bronchoconstriction at intravenous
doses producing approximately 110, 6 and 1 μg/ml plasma
concentrations [13]. During placebo treatment, LTD_4 caused
bronchoconstriction in all subjects whereas during the three
active drug treatments, all MK-571 administrations completely
inhibited LTD_4-induced bronchoconstriction. Similar studies
were carried out in six asthmatic men [14]. These studies
demonstrated, first, that when compared to placebo, intravenous
MK-571 (277 mg) increased baseline airway caliber as measured
by sGaw. Secondly, in a three period, placebo controlled study
the ability of two doses of MK-571 to inhibit LTD_4-induced
bronchoconstriction was studied. Both 28 and 277 mg of MK-571
inhibited the leukotriene D_4-induced bronchoconstriction
significantly. Thus it was concluded that intravenous MK-571
was well tolerated in asthmatics, that MK-571 was a potent
antagonist of leukotriene D_4-induced bronchoconstriction in
asthmatics and the results also suggested that leukotriene D_4
may contribute to basal airway tone in asthmatics [14]. Having
established that MK-571 is a potent leukotriene D_4 antagonist
in either normal or asthmatic subjects, current studies are
aimed at assessing the effects of this compound on
provocation-induced bronchoconstriction as well as its effects
in ongoing asthma.

MK-886

MK-886

Pharmacological Studies

MK-886 (also known as L-663,536; (3-[-(4-chlorobenzyl)-3-t-butyl-thio-5-isopropylindol-2-yl]-2,2-dimethyl propanoic acid) is a potent inhibitor of leukotriene biosynthesis in a variety of intact leukocyte preparations, including human polymorphonuclear leukocytes, where it shows an IC_{50} of 2.5 nM (10). The compound also inhibits leukotriene biosynthesis in human whole blood with a higher IC_{50} (1.1 μM) reflecting the protein binding of this compound. At this concentration no effect was seen on cyclooxygenase or 12-lipoxygenase, an effect also observed in washed human platelets. The compound had no effect on either rat or porcine 5-lipoxygenase indicating that MK-886 is not a direct 5-lipoxygenase inhibitor (10). As has been demonstrated for MK-571, when administered in vivo, MK-886 was a potent inhibitor of antigen-induced dyspnea in inbred rats pretreated with methysergide (ED_{50} 0.036 mg/kg p.o.) and also inhibited the ascaris-induced immediate bronchoconstriction in squirrel monkeys at a dose of 1 mg/kg p.o. (10). The compound was an effective inhibitor of leukotriene biosynthesis in vivo in a variety of models including a rat pleurisy model (ED_{50} 0.2 mg/kg p.o.), an inflamed rat paw model (ED_{50} 0.8 mg/kg), a model in the guinea pig ear where leukotriene synthesis was induced by topical challenge with ionophore A23187 (ED_{50} 0.6 μg topically and 2.5 mg/kg p.o.) and a model analogous to the antigen-induced bronchoconstriction in inbred hyperreactive rats where leukotriene excretion was monitored in rat bile following intratracheal installation of antigen (10). These results indicate that MK-886 is a potent inhibitor of leukotriene biosynthesis both in vitro and in vivo, that it shows similar inhibition of immediate bronchoconstriction to the leukotriene D_4 receptor antagonist MK-571 and that the compound is suitable for studying the role of leukotrienes in a variety of pathological situations.

Mechanism of Action Studies on MK-571

As indicated above, MK-886 is a potent inhibitor of leukotriene synthesis in intact cells but shows no activity in either broken cell preparations or purified 5-lipoxygenase preparations (10). As MK-886 has no effect on the immobilization of arachidonic acid, a number of studies have been initiated to examine the effects of the compound on the activation of 5-lipoxygenase. A number of suggestions have been made in the literature that 5-lipoxygenase, an enzyme normally thought to be present in the cytosol, might undergo an activation step. Such evidence include the facts that the activity of 5-lipoxygenase is highly dependent on calcium and that it is stimulated by both ATP and phosphatidlcholine micelles. In addition, the human enzyme has been shown to be stimulated by a number of undefined protein fractions and a membrane preparation (20, 21). These early results have suggested that there may be a regulatory process for the activation of 5-lipoxygenase which is consistent with the fact that leukotriene synthesis only occurs in cells following exposure to stimuli which result in a considerable elevation in intracellular calcium, a very different situation to that observed with the cyclooxygenase enzyme. The fact that membranes might be involved in this activation process has been suggested from a number of observations. These include the fact that the substrate, arachidonic acid, is derived from membrane phospholipids through the actions of specific phospholipase A_2, the fact that the enzyme is stimulated by either membrane or phosphatidalcholine vesicles and that the cloning studies with human 5-lipoxygenase have shown sequence homologies with the interfacial binding domains of lipases suggestive of membrane interactions. Other calcium dependent enzymes, such as protein kinase C and phospholipase C, are thought to undergo a translocation to the membrane following cellular activation (7,15). Evidence has been obtained that 5-lipoxygenase may undergo a similar activation step, in that following activation of human polymorphonuclear leukocytes with ionophore A23187, 5-lipoxygenase enzyme activity and 5-lipoxygenase protein disappears from the cytosol and inactivated 5-lipoxygenase protein appears in the 100,000 xg membrane preparations (18). These results can be interpreted to indicate that enzyme inactivation involves translocation to the membrane where the enzyme becomes activated, synthesizes leukotrienes and undergoes inactivation. Evidence in support of this was the fact that varying the ionophore concentration resulted in varying amounts of leukotriene synthesis which could be correlated with the varying amounts of enzyme translocation. In addition the cytosolic 5-lipoxygenase pool retains its biological activity indicating that this enzyme pool has not been used for leukotriene synthesis. Also, termination of leukotriene synthesis during ongoing cell activation by addition of excess chelating agent (EDTA) resulted in the termination of enzyme translocation (18).

As 5-lipoxygenase translocation was thought to be an important facet of leukotriene biosynthesis in intact polymorphonuclear leukocytes it was an obvious step to study the effects of MK-886 on this process. In fact MK-886 caused a dose-dependent inhibition of the translocation of 5-lipoxygenase to the membrane, an effect which could be correlated with the inhibition of leukotriene biosynthesis (19, Rouzer et al., submitted for publication). Further evidence in support of this was the fact that a range of structural analogues of MK-886 showed an excellent correlation between their potency as inhibitors of 5-lipoxygenase translocation and their ability to inhibit leukotriene biosynthesis in intact polymorphonuclear leukocytes. It could be argued that translocation has nothing to do with cell activation but simply reflects the removal and deposition of inactive enzyme after leukotriene biosynthesis. An important piece of evidence against this was that addition of MK-886, after activation of the cells with ionophore A23187, and thus after enzyme translocation had occurred, resulted in the release back into the cytosol of inactive enzyme which presumably had previously undergone translocation. Therefore, these experiments with MK-886 provide important support for the theory that 5-lipoxygenase translocation is an obligatory step for cellular leukotriene biosynthesis. Further studies are aimed at defining the nature of this translocation event, where 5-lipoxygenase translocates to and exactly how MK-886 interferes with this process.

CONCLUSIONS

Leukotrienes have been postulated to be important mediators of a number of human diseases, in particular bronchial asthma. However, it has been impossible until recently to test these theories in man as no drugs were available which either produced effective antagonism of leukotriene D_4 or were shown to be biochemically effective as leukotriene biosynthesis inhibitors in the human lung. This situation is now changed and the use of compounds such as MK-571 and MK-886 will provide definitive evidence for a role for leukotriene D_4 in diseases such as human bronchial asthma.

REFERENCES

1. Abraham, W.M. and Stevenson, J.S. 1988. FASEB J. 2:A1057.

2. Arm, J.P., Spur, B.W. and Lee, T.H. 1988. J. Allergy Clin. Immunol. 82:654-660.

3. Barnes, N., Evans, J., Zakrzewski, J., Piper, P. and Costello J. 1988. Prog. Clin. Biol. Res. 263:393-403.

4. Barnes, N., Piper, P.J. and Costello, J. 1987. J. Allergy Clin. Immunol. 79:816-821.

5. Britton, J.R., Hanley, S.P. and Tattersfield, A.E. 1987. J. Allergy Clin. Immunol. 79:811-816.

6. Chan, C., Dagenais, F., Firby, P., Foster, A. and Ford-Hutchinson, A.W. 1989. Can. J. Physiol. Pharmacol., In press.

7. Creutz, C.E., Dowling, L.G., Kyger, E.M. and Franson, R.C.
    1985. J. Biol. Chem. 260:7171-7173.

8. Ford-Hutchinson, A.W. 1985. Fed. Proc. 44:25-29.

9. Ford-Hutchinson, A.W., Bray, M.A., Doig, M.V., Shipley,
    M.E. and Smith, M.J.H. 1980. Nature 286:264-265.

10. Gillard, J., Ford-Hutchinson, A.W., Chan, C., Charleson,
    S., Denis, D., Foster, A., Fortin, R., Leger, S.,
    McFarlane, C.S., Morton, H., Piechuta, H., Riendeau, D.,
    Rouzer, C.A., Rokach, J., Young, R., MacIntyre, D.E.,
    Peterson, L., Bach, T., Eiermann, G., Hopple, S., Humes,
    J., Hupe, L., Luell, S., Metzger, J., Meurer, R., Miller,
    D.K., Opas, E. and Pacholok, S. 1989. Can. J. Physiol.
    Pharmacol. 67:456-464.

11. Jones, T.R., Davis, C. and Daniel, E.E. 1982 Can. J.
    Physiol. Pharmacol. 60:638-643.

12. Jones, T.R., Zamboni, R., Belley, M. Champion, E.,
    Charette, L., Ford-Hutchinson, A.W., Frenette, R.,
    Gauthier, J.-Y., Leger, S., Masson, P., McFarlane, C.S.,
    Piechuta, H., Rokach, J., Williams, H., Young, R.N.,
    DeHaven, R.N. and Pong, S.S. 1989. Can. J. Physiol.
    Pharmacol. 67:17-28.

13. Kips, J.C., Joos, G., Margolskee, D., Delepeleire, I.,
    Rogers, J.D., Pauwels, R. and Van Der Staeten, M. 1989a.
    Am. Rev. Resp. Dis. In press.

14. Kips, J.C., Joos, G., Margolskee, D., Delepeleire, I.,
    Pauwels, R. and Van Der Straeten, M. 1989b. In:
    Proceedings of the 8th Congress of the European Pediatric
    Respiratory Society, Freiburg, West Germany, Sept. 10-14,
    1989.

15. Melloni, E., Pontremoli, S., Michetti, M., Sacco, O.,
    Sparatore, B., Salamino, F. and Horecker, B.L. 1985. Proc.
    Natl. Acad. Sci. U.S.A. 82:64356439.

16. Phillips, G.D., Rafferty, P. Robinson, C. and Holgate,S.T.
    1988. J. Pharmacol. Exp. Ther. 246:732-738.

17. Piper, P.J. 1984. Physiol. Rev. 64:744-761.

18. Rouzer, C.A. and Kargman, S. 1988. J. Biol. Chem.
    263:10980-10988.

19. Rouzer, C.A. and Kargman, S. 1989. In: "New Trends in
    Lipid Mediators Reserch", edited by Zor, U., Noar, Z. and
    Danon, A., Karger, Basel, vol. 3, In press.

20. Rouzer, C.A. and Samuelsson, B. 1985. Proc. Natl. Acad. Sci. U.S.A. 82:6040-6044.

21. Rouzer, C.A., Shimizu, T. and Samuelsson, B. 1985. Proc. Natl. Acad. Sci. U.S.A. 82:7505-7509.

22. Samuelsson, B. 1983. Science 220:568-575.

23. Smith, L.J., Greenberger, P.A., Patterson, R., Krell, R.D. and Bernstein, P.R. 1985. Am. Rev. Respir. Dis. 131:368-372.

24. Van Hecken, A., DeSchepper, P.J., Margolskee, D.J., Hsieh, J.Y.K., Robinette, R.S., Buntinx, A. and Rogers, J.D. 1989. Eur. J. Clin. Pharmacol., In press.

25. Weiss, J.W., Drazen, J.M., McFadden, E.R., Weller, P., Corey, E.J., Lewis, R.A. and Austen, K.F. 1983. JAMA 249:2814-2817.

Advances in Prostaglandin, Thromboxane, and Leukotriene Research, Vol. 20, edited by B. Samuelsson et al. Raven Press, Ltd., New York © 1990.

INTERACTIONS OF EICOSANOIDS AND CYTOKINES IN IMMUNE REGULATION

Robert A. Lewis

Syntex Research, Syntex Corporation
Palo Alto, CA 94304

INTRODUCTION

With regard to immune responsiveness as it may be regulated by eicosanoids, relatively few generalizations can be made for the human. Although lymphocytes, like all other somatic cells, have the genomic sequences for dioxygenases and other enzymes of the cyclooxygenase and various lipoxygenase pathways (1). the functional gene products are normally not expressed (27). On the other hand, at least some T lymphocytes do have apparent receptors for certain eicosanoids (13,26) through which the transduced signals can be immunoregulatory. In contrast, mono-cytes and macrophages have the capacities to generate functional gene products from both cyclooxygenase and 5-lipoxygenase path-ways; in the case of macrophages, the specific eicosanoid products depend upon the specific microenvironment -- e.g. pulmonary alveolar versus peritoneal -- in which the cell resides (4).

In order to appreciate the biological impact of eicosanoids in their rather modestly explored relevance to immunology, it is first critical to review some of the presently understood general rules governing maturation, activation, and regulation of mononuclear leukocytes.

AN IMMUNOLOGIC OVERVIEW

Specific humoral immune responses are dependent upon the secretion from B lymphocytes of antigen-specific immunoglobulin molecules, including IgG (four subclasses), IgA (two sub-classes), IgM, and IgE. The antigen specificity (more properly in the case of each antibody molecule, specificity for a very small set of molecular domains of the antigen, termed an "epitope") resides in geometrically interfacing "hypervariable regions" at one end of the Ig molecule. With the exception of humoral immune responses to certain "helper-independent antigens," which elicit IgM responses, production of antibody requires additional peptide signals from "helper" T lymphocytes (Th cells). These signals are generically included among molecules termed "cytokines"; when they originate from lymphocytes, they are more specifically termed "lymphokines," and a number that have been sequenced in the past decade are designated as "interleukins" (IL). Both Th cells and B cells must mature in order that the full spectrum of Ig synthesis occur, and both must clonally proliferate so that the Ig response be at a biologically meaningful level. Specific cellular immune responses are the province of the cytotoxic subset of T lymphocytes (Tc), as well as of IgG receptor (IgG-FcR)-bearing leukocytes armed with specific antibodies for antibody-dependent cellular cytotoxicity (ADCC).

The maturation of all lymphocytes begins in the bone marrow with their differentiation from the ultimate (and, for the human, as yet uncharacterized) stem cells, via mononuclear precursors. T cell pregenitors that are morphologically lymphoid move to the thymus and take up residence before they have acquired either CD_4 or CD_8 surface markers -- and are termed "double negative" or CD_4 $^-CD_8$ $^-$ cells. Early in thymic T cell differentiation, those double negative T lymphocytes (immunochemically identifiable as T cells because they bear the surface CD_3 marker) which also have begun to bear low levels of the heterodimeric interleukin 2 receptor (IL-2R) can be activated by IL-1 (probably of thymic epithelial origin) to express more IL-2R, independent of their expression of IL-2 (9). The subsequent differentiation of so-called suppressor CD_4 $^+CD_8$ $^-$ helper-inducer Th cells and of CD_4 $^-CD_8$ $^+$ (Ts) and cytotoxic (Tc) lymphocytes is regulated by as-yet uncharacterized thymic signals as a two-stage event, in which double negative cells first become double positive (CD_4 $^+CD_8$ $^+$) and then lose one or the other marker.

Full thymic maturation of T cells includes the genomic rearrangement of each of the two chains of the heterodimeric antigen-specific "T cell receptor" (TCR), a member of the immunoglobulin gene superfamily, prior to its expression on the cell surface. This occurs independent of antigen and prepares the wide variety of T cell clones that will recognize all foreign antigens. The genomic rearrangements that select variable (v) diversity (d), and joining (j) regions of the αβ TCR chains to spatially proximitate the constant region (as well as rearrangements of the less common γδ TCR) are like rearrangements of the genomic sequences for immunoglobulin gene regions in B cells.

The exodus of differentiated T cells of each class from the thymus is an active, rather than a passive, event. "Negative selection" destroys self-reactive $CD_4{}^+CD_8{}^+$ T cell clones (and thus generally prevents autoimmunity) and "positive selection" is believed to specifically mandate the exit of non self-reactive clones from the thymus; both are apparently antigen-driven and mediated by presentation of denatured antigen in association with major histocompatibility complex (MHC) proteins of antigen-presenting cells (APC), such as the thymic epithelial cells. Both negative and positive selection events are suggested to have a subspecificity, in that antigen can be presented to $CD_4{}^-CD_8{}^+$ T cells only when it is bound to MHC Class I molecules (alleles of HLA-A, -B and -C in the human) and to $CD_4{}^+CD_8{}^-$ T cells when it is bound to MCH Class II molecules (alleles of DP, DQ, and DR in the human). Later, presentation of a given antigen in the extra-thymic periphery (e.g. lymph nodes and Peyer's patches) will be similarly restricted to the context of host MHC Class I and Class II alleles for the $CD_8{}^+$ and $CD_4{}^+$ T cells, respectively, so as to allow clonal expansion of the antigen-specific T cells and attendant production of lymphokines. These latter events require the transduction of a signal from the multimeric T cell class surface molecule CD_3, which is tightly associated with the TCR. Thus, binding of TCR to processed antigen and MHC Class I or II, as cooperatively regulated by the binding of CD_8 to Class I or CD_4 to Class II, induces a geometric alteration in CD_3, such that the intracellular biochemical cascade is initiated.

Despite the complexity of these events, even they are alone insufficient to allow a normal response of T cell differentiation and proliferation to antigen. There is an additional requirement of the activated T cell for IL-1, produced from the APC in response to antigen processing and/or presentation. Beyond these early events, the activation of a given clone of T cells provides a complex set of lymphokine signals which have stepwise, synergistic, or opposing effects on the complete functional maturation of themselves (autocrine) and the recruitment of other T cells (paracrine). That this should be necessary makes teleologic sense, in that those clones which are less efficiently activated (due, for instance, to weaker avidity of antigen-binding) can be recruited and expanded in a paracrine fashion. Similarly, the activation and subsequent differentiation of B cells to undergo Ig class switching (e.g. from IgM to an IgG subclass) and Ig secretion is also conditioned by T cell lymphokines. These are produced not only in response to T cell-macrophage interactions, but also by T cell-B cell interactions, wherein the B cell acts as the APC, as well as the responder to subsequent T cell peptide signals. These cytokine-mediated signalling events will be discussed below, in the context of additional signals provided by eicosanoids. Whereas both $CD_4{}^+$ Th cells and $CD_8{}^+$ Tc lymphocytes are clearly activated by antigen-mediated binding to a (now) "classical"

TCR in the context of MHC on an APC or target cell (in the latter case, e.g., host cell presenting Class I and viral antigen), the parallel events for CD_8 $^+$ suppressor (Ts) cells, especially with regard to the TCR, are presumed to occur based upon far fewer proven examples.

The maturation of B cells, prior to their interactions with Th cells is conditioned by a series of unidentified signals in the bone marrow. Maturation of pro-B cells to pre-B cells to B cells is evidenced by the appearance of intracellular (cytoplasmic) μ heavy chain and later by non-secreted cell surface IgM, followed by both surface IgM and IgD. It is only after cell activation that the Ig class switch occurs, with further differentiation of the B cells to "plasma cells" and Ig secretion of the same isotype as the surface-bound molecules. In the process, enhanced mutation of the genomic v region hypervariable sequences allows further selection for production of antibodies with high antigen affinity. Still less is known about the regulation of the stepwise maturation of monocytes, and the subsequent differentiation to macrophages (see below).

This overview will not deal with the biology of the less phenotypically-defined mononuclear cells such as natural killer (NK) cells and natural cytotoxic (non T-) lymphocytes (NC), except to note the respective enhancing and inhibitory effects of LTB_4 and PGE_2 on their functions (31).

CYTOKINES AND EICOSANOIDS IN IMMUNOLOGY

In consideration of the maturation of the monocytic/ macrophage subset of APCs, it is well established that human peripheral blood monocytes can be activated by the calcium ionophore A23187 and by the more physiologic stimuli of the FMLP tripeptide in the presence of cytochalasin B or aggregated Ig to produce nanogram quantities of both 5-lipoxygenase products, LTB_4 and $LTC_4/10^6$ cells (11,41,42), as well as to generate the cyclooxygenase products PGE_2 and TxA_2. The conversion of the monocyte to a macrophage clearly requires more than adherence to a substratum, since the latter does not preserve the capacity of the cell to generate 5-lipoxygenase products (3), whereas the human tissue macrophage in both pulmonary alveolar and peritoneal compartments is competent for leukotriene generation, when appropriately activated. Furthermore, additional (undefined) signals in one or both of these compartments result in a clearly enhanced (relative to blood monocytes) generation of only LTB_4 in the alveolar cells but of both LTB_4 and LTC_4 in the peritoneal cells (10,18,19,23). Human pulmonary alveolar macrophages, when activated for 24 hours with as little as 10 U/ml IFN-γ, will express additional IgG-Fc_1 receptors and greatly enhance the transduction of an aggregated IgG signal to produce more LTB_4 (28). Of less certain relevance to the human, is the demonstration that primitive myelomonocytic cells in the chicken can be matured (in the presence of an inserted temperature-sensitive transforming virus) to express the capacity to synthesize leukotrienes before they express certain cellular markers associated with monocyte maturation (14). Human monocytes and macrophages respond to particulate stimuli (e.g. zymosan) and bacterial lipopoly-saccharide (LPS) with production of several monokines, including IL-1α (at least some of which may remain membrane-associated) and IL-1β (which is clearly secreted), tumor necrosis factor-alpha (TNF-α), and several unsequenced or partially sequenced acidic monokines (7,20,38). In nanomolar concentrations, LTB$_4$ enhances monocyte IL-1 generation as stimulated by either LPS or zymosan (32). Also IFN-γ, produced by activated Th cells, not only induces increased expression of IgG-FcR$_1$, but also of MHC II on monocytes/ macrophages (4,40), while producing suppression of IL-1 biosynthesis (33). These effects relate to leukotriene biosynthesis, since, as will be discussed, production of IFN-γ by the Th cell is up-regulated by LTB$_4$ (33,34) and, if analogy holds with murine cells, by LTC$_4$ (15). Thus, leukotrienes can influence both up-regulation and down-regulation of IL-1 biosynthesis.

LTB$_4$, at picomolar concentrations, induces both the pro-liferation of Ts cells and their suppressive effects on the proliferation of Th cells (2,30), and thus inhibits Ig synthesis in cultures of mixed peripheral blood mononuclear cells (2). LTC$_4$, at nanomolar concentrations, also suppresses Ig synthesis, but possibly by direct action on the B cells.[1] Activation of the Th cell in the extra-thymic (peripheral) lymphoid tissues requires (at least) two signals: that transduced from CD$_3$ in response to the activation of the associated antigen-specific TCR (in the "context" of MHC II and with the cooperative interaction of CD$_4$ with MHC II) and APC-derived IL-1β (and possibly APC-associated IL-1α). As previously noted, IL-1β enhances the expression of IL-2 receptor (IL-2R) and, in concert with the CD$_3$ signal, increases the generation of IL-2. IL-2 has a major positive feedback effect in inducing more of its own receptor (6,16). When IL-2 occupies a number of IL-2R, the Th produces IFN-γ, and this enhancement is augmented by LTB$_4$ and perhaps by LTC$_4$, as noted above. That the former occurs is quite likely, in view of the demon-stration that certain CD$_4$[+] T cells have LTB$_4$ receptors (26). That this type of process may also activate CD$_8$[+] Tc or Ts cells (substituting MHC I for MHC II) is also likely, in that some of these cells also have IL-2R and LTB$_4$ receptors (26). However, it is not clear as to whether they produce their own IL-2 or receive this signal only from Th cells. As to the sources of leukotrienes which affect this cooperativity, they are almost surely derived from cells other than lymphocytes, as previously noted. PGE$_2$, likewise provided by non-lymphoid cells, inhibits the IL-1-dependent portion of lymphocyte activation, including the generation of IL-2 (5,29). Biological suppressive effects of PGE_2, as mediated by Ts cells, include inhibition of cell-mediated cytotoxicity, and of Ig biosynthesis (17,43).

The sources of IL-1, as well as of antigen presentation to Th cells by "APC" are not limited to monocyte/macrophages. In the extrathymic periphery, these functions can be occasionally carried out by other cell types, among which are prominently included B cells. The B cell, which is not yet secreting antibody, is matured sequentially by the "helper" interleukins, which sequentially include IL-2, IL-4, IL-5, and IL-6; each of these derive from Th cells. Whereas in the murine system, there appears to be a clear separation of those Th cells producing IL-2 and IFN-γ ("Th 1 cells") and those generating IL-4, IL-5, and IL-6 ("Th 2 cells") (22), the cellular Th sources and their regulation is probably more complicated in the human (24,25). Based upon studies of human CD_4^+ Th clones, it appears that the major difference among human Th cells is in their responsiveness to IL-4 as an additional signal to proliferation along with that of IL-2 (25). Furthermore, those Th cells that proliferate to only IL-2 and not IL-4 have their proliferation blocked by TNF-α, whereas those that proliferate to both signals are unaffected by TNF-α (25). Thus the monocyte/macrophage can modulate the proliferation of some Th cells via both augmentatory (IL-1) and inhibitory (TNF-α) signals, but can only up-regulate other Th cells.

When Th cells produce IL-2, IL-4, IL-5, and IL-6 in response to activation by processed antigen, these lymphokines sequentially advance the differentiated state of the B cells all the way to active Ig secretion. However, during the antigen-driven immunologic event, the B cell is also affected by a direct activation. Indeed, the binding of antigen to B cell surface Ig (once expressed) allows the internalization of antigen and its subsequent cell surface presentation in association with MHC II to Th cells. Thus functioning as an APC, the B cell primes the Th cell to produce IL-4, IL-5, and IL-6 and thus collaborates in its own maturation. Furthermore, in the presence and binding of antigen and these interleukins, the B cell facilitates its isotype switching and somatic hypermutation to produce higher affinity antibody. It should be additionally noted that some positive feedback of IL-6 in synergism with IL-1 on T cell proliferation has been suggested, although the biological significance of this IL-6 effect may vary with conditions of T cell activation (21).

In B cells and T cells, most, if not all, of the proliferative signals are transduced with critical intermediate steps of both serine-threonine protein phosphorylation (as by protein kinase C) and tyrosine protein phosphorylation. This is particularly exemplified for the actions of IL-2 (8,12).

CONCLUDING COMMENTS

That the effects of PGE_2, LTB_4, and LTC_4 cannot be be said to be strictly proinflammatory or antiinflammatory for any single eicosanoid mediator is neither remarkable nor contradictory. The set of immunological regulatory events described above involve sequential segments of a biochemical cascade in each responding cell and, often, sequential interactions between cells. Thus, mediation of both positive and negative regulation of the same biological or biochemical event as separate effects of a single eicosanoid do not nullify each other, but can rather provide stepwise activation and deactivation of the event. Under conditions of homeostasis, the provision of regulatory eicosanoids to responding lymphocytes and/or monocytes presumably derives from a quite limited number of cell types in their microenvironments. However, during inflammatory processes, granulocytes may infiltrate tissue spaces; when pathobiologic activation of these cells occurs, additional eicosanoids can be produced. These events are also expected to be continuously varied by ongoing cytokine-dependent regulation of each cell source. It has been shown, for example, that certain acidic monokines, as well as T cell-derived IL-3 and GM-CSF can up-regulate the capacities of eosinophils to produce LTC_4 ((7,35,37). Additionally, IL-1 has been suggested to stimulate production of LTB_4 by by neutrophils (39), and IFN-γ concentrations of less than 1 U/ml can effect a doubling of LTC_4 generation by antigen-challenged mixed leukocytes of allergic patients (36).

Although the data being developed presently on eicosanoid-cytokine interplay in immunology are clearly instructive about mechanisms at the cellular level, the recognition that all inflammatory diseases are continuously evolving should caution those who wish to draw conclusions which impact therapeutic decisions until some appropriate clinical studies are accomplished.

REFERENCES

1. Ambrus, J. L., Jr., Jurgensen, C. H., Witzel, N. L., Lewis, R. A., Butler, J. L., and Fauci, A. S. (1988): J. Immunol., 140:2382-2388.
2. Atluru, D. and Goodwin, J. S. (1984): J. Clin. Invest., 74:1444-1450.
3. Balter, M. S., Toews, G. B., and Peters-Golden, M. (1989): J. Immunol., 142:602-608.
4. Basham, T. Y. and Merigan, T. C. (1983): J. Immunol. 130:1492-1494.

5. Chouaib, S. and Fradelizi, D. (1982): J. Immunol.,
    129:2463-2468.
6. Cleveland, J. L., Rapp., U. R., and Farrar, W. L. (1987): J.
    Immunol., 138:3495- 3504
7. Dessein, A. J., Lee, T. H., Elsas, P., Ravalese, J. III,
    Silberstein, D., David, J. R., Austen, K. F., and Lewis,
    R. A. (1986): J. Immunol., 137:3290-3294.
8. Evans, S. W. and Farrar, W. L. (1987): J. Cell. Biochem.,
    34:47-59.
9. Falk, W., Männel, D. N., Darjes, H., and Krammer, P. H.
    (1989): J. Immunol., 143:513-517.
10. Fels, A. O., Pawlowski, N. A., Cramer, E. B., King, T. K.
    C., Cohn, Z. A., and Scott, W. A. (1982): Proc. Natl.
    Acad. Sci. USA, 79:7866-7870.
11. Ferreri, N. R., Howland, W. C., and Spiegelberg, H. L.
    (1986): J. Immunol., 136:4188-4193.
12. Ferris, D. K., Willette-Brown, J., Ortaldo, J. R., and
    Farrar, W. L. (1989): J. Immunol., 143:870-876.
13. Fischer, A., LeDeist, F., Durandy, A., and Griscelli, C.
    (1985): J. Immunol., 134:815-819.
14. Habenicht, A. J., Goerig, M., Rothe, D. E., Specht, E.,
    Ziegler, R., Glomset, J. A., and Graf, T. (1989): Proc.
    Natl. Acad. Sci. USA, 86:921-924.
15. Johnson, H. M. and Torres, B. A. (1984): J. Immunol.,
    132:413-416.
16. Kronke, M., Leonard, W. J., Depper, J. M., and Greene, W. C.
    (1983): J. Exp. Med., 161:1593-1598.
17. Kurland, J. I., Kincade, P. W., and Moore, M. A. S. (1977):
    J. Exp. Med., 146:1420-1435.
18. Laviolette, M., Carreau, M., Coulombe, R., Cloutier, D.,
    Dupont, P., Rioux, J., Braquet, P., and Borgeat, P.
    (1988): J. Immunol., 141:2104-2109.
19. Martin, T. R., Altman, L. C., Albert, R. K., and Henderson,
    W. R. (1983): Am. Rev. Respir. Dis., 129:106-111.
20. Matthews, N. (1981): Immunol., 44:135-142.
21. Mizutani, H., May, L. T., Sehgal, P. B., and Kupper, T. S.
    (1989): J. Immunol., 143:896-901.
22. Mosmann, T. R., Cherwinski, H., Bond, M. W., Giedlin, M. A.,
    and Coffman, R. L. (1986): J. Immunol., 136:2348-2357.
23. Ouwendijk, R. J., Zijlstra, F. J., van den Broek, A. M.,
    Brouwer, A., Wilson, J. H., and Vincent, J. E. (1988):
    Prostaglandins 35:437-446.
24. Paliard, X., DeWaal Malefijt, R., Yssel, H., Blanchard, D.,
    Chretien, I., Abrams, J., DeVries, J., and Spits, H.
    (1988): J. Immunol., 141:849-855.
25. Pawelec, G. P., Rehbein, A., Schaudt, K., and Busch, F. W.
    (1989): J. Immunol., 143:902-906.
26. Payan, D. G., Missirian-Bastian, A., and Goetzl, E. J.
    (1984): Proc. Natl. Acad. Sci. USA, 81:3501-3505.
27. Poubelle, P. E., Borgeat, P., and Rola-Pleszczynski, M.
    (1987): J. Immunol., 139:1273-1277.

28. Rankin, J. A., Schrader, C. E., Smith, S. M., and Lewis, R. A. (1989) J. Clin. Invest., 83:1691-1700.
29. Rappaport, R. S. and Dodge, G. R. (1982): J. Exp. Med., 155:943-948.
30. Rola-Pleszczynski, M. (1984): J. Immunol., 135:1357-1360.
31. Rola-Pleszczynski, M., Gagnon, L., Bolduc, D., and LeBreton, G. (1985): J. Immunol., 135:4114-4119.
32. Rola-Pleszczynski, M. and Lemaire, I. (1985): J. Immunol., 135:3958-3961.
33. Rola-Pleszczynski, M., Chavaillaz, P. A., and Lemaire, I. (1986): Prostaglandins Leukotrienes Med., 23:207-210.
34. Rola-Pleszczynski, M., Bouvrette, L., Gingras, D., and Girard, M. (1987): J. Immunol., 139:513-517.
35. Rothenberg, M. E., Owen, W. F., Jr., Silberstein, D. S., Woods, J., Soberman, R. J., Austen, K. F., and Stevens, R. L. (1988): J. Clin. Invest., 81:1986-1992.
36. Saito, H., Hayakawa, T., Mita, H., Yui, Y. S., and Shida, T. (1988): Int. Arch. Allergy Appl. Immunol., 87:286-293.
37. Silberstein, D. S., Owen, W. F., Gasson, J. C., DiPersio, J., Golde, D. W., Bina, J. C., Soberman, R. J., Austen, K. F., and David, J. R. (1986): J. Immunol., 137:3290-3294.
38. Silberstein, D. S., Ali, M. H., Baker, S. L., and David, J. R. (1989): J. Immunol., 143:979-983.
39. Smith, R. J., Epps, D. E., Justen, J. M., Sam, L. M., Wynalda, M. A., Fitzpatrick, F. A., and Yein, F. S. (1987): Biochem. Pharmacol., 36:3851-3858.
40. Steeg, P. S., Moore, R. N., Johnson, H. M., and Oppenheim, J. J. (1982): J. Exp. Med., 156:1780-1793.
41. Williams, J. D., Czop, J. K., and Austen, K. F. (1984): J. Immunol., 132:3032-3040.
42. Williams, J. D., Robin, J. L., Lewis, R. A., Lee, T. H., and Austen, K. F. (1986): J. Immunol., 168:642-648.
43. Wolf, M. and Droege, W. (1982): Cell. Immunol., 72:286-293.

Advances in Prostaglandin, Thromboxane,
and Leukotriene Research, Vol. 20,
edited by B. Samuelsson et al.
Raven Press, Ltd., New York © 1990.

LEUKOTRIENES IN SHOCK SYNDROMES: METABOLISM AND DETECTION IN VIVO

D. Keppler, A. Guhlmann, M. Huber, H.A. Ball,
I. Leier, and G. Jedlitschky

Division of Tumor Biochemistry, Deutsches Krebsforschungszentrum,
D-6900 Heidelberg 1, Federal Republic of Germany

Studies on the metabolism of leukotrienes are a prerequisite for their analysis under *in vivo* conditions. The measurement of systemic or whole body production of LTC_4 has been achieved by analyses in bile (6,7,9-11) into which the major part of the cysteinyl leukotrienes released into the blood circulation are eliminated (1,6,7,9-11,18). In man (15,20) and monkey (6) measurements of endogenous cysteinyl leukotrienes, particularly of LTE_4, in urine provide a reasonable alternative since renal excretion of cysteinyl leukotrienes is more pronounced in primates than in other species (6,22). Species-characteristic index metabolites have been defined for the measurement of systemic cysteinyl leukotriene production in bile or urine (20).

LTC_4 CATABOLISM IN MONKEY AND MAN

Following the intravenous administration of $[^3H]LTC_4$ in the monkey *Macaca fascicularis*, about 40 % of the administered dose were recovered as metabolites in bile and 20 % in urine within 5 hours (6). Similar percentages were reported more recently in the Cynomolgus monkey (26). In monkey blood circulation $[^3H]LTC_4$ (6), as well as $[^3H]LTC_3$ (12), are rapidly converted to $[^3H]LTE$. $[^3H]LTE_4$ is the predominant cysteinyl leukotriene in monkey bile, corresponding to about 11 % of the administered dose after 4 hours (Fig. 1). About 4 % are excreted as LTD_4, in addition, the following ω-oxidation products were identified (Fig. 1 and refs. 2,26): ω-hydroxy-LTE_4, ω-carboxy-LTE_4, ω-carboxy-dinor-LTE_4, and ω-carboxy-tetranor-dihydro-LTE_4. In urine ω-carboxy-tetranor-dihydro-LTE_4 was the predominant LTC_4 metabolite in the monkey (Fig. 1). However, tracer studies in human urine after intravenous $[^3H]LTC_4$ showed that $[^3H]LTE_4$ is the predominant urinary cysteinyl leukotriene in man (22). Therefore, LTE_4 is considered as the most useful index metabolite in human urine.

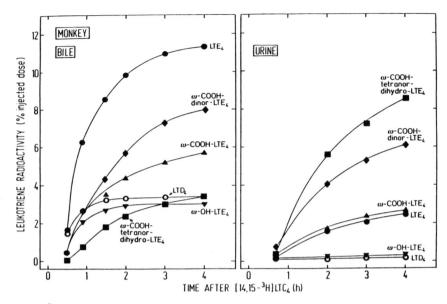

FIG. 1. [³H]Leukotriene metabolites accumulated in bile and urine of the monkey after intravenous [³H]LTC₄. Methods were based on previous studies (2,6) and samples were separated by RP-HPLC as described (4). Biliary and urinary leukotriene metabolites were defined by their retention times and co-elution with synthetic leukotriene standards (obtained from Cascade Biochem, Reading, UK). Mean values from 3 animals.

The capacity of *human liver* for ω-oxidation of cysteinyl leukotrienes was studied in human hepatocyte cultures exposed to [³H]LTE₄ (Fig. 2). [³H]LTE₄ was chosen as the predominant [³H]LTC₄ metabolite reaching and taken up by the liver. The ω-oxidation products derived from LTE₄ included ω-hydroxy-LTE₄, ω-carboxy-LTE₄, ω-carboxy-dinor-LTE₄, and ω-carboxy-tetranor-dihydro-LTE₄ (Fig. 2). It is remarkable that N-acetylation of LTE₄ did not occur in these human hepatocytes. Moreover, LTF₄, which was never detected in bile or urine *in vivo*, was identified under these *in vitro* conditions, suggesting the presence of a sufficient concentration of glutathione.

ENDOGENOUS LTE₄ IN BILE AND URINE OF MONKEY AND MAN

Systemic LTC₄ production was elicited in Cynomolgus monkeys by oral staphylococcal enterotoxin B (6,23) which induces emesis, diarrhoea, and a shocklike reaction in primates (5). *Biliary cysteinyl leukotrienes* were measured after implantation of a subcutaneously looped biliary bypass; tapping of the loop allowed access to bile and prevented interference by

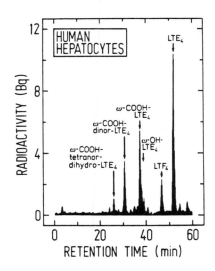

FIG. 2. HPLC separation of [^{3}H]LTE$_4$ metabolites formed by human hepatocytes. Adult human hepatocytes were prepared from surgical liver biopsies (3) and suspended in HAM's F12 medium (3 × 10^9 cells/l). Incubation with [^{3}H]LTE$_4$ (18.5 MBq/l, corresponding to 12.5 nmol/l) was conducted at 37°C with 95 % O$_2$ and 5 % CO$_2$ for 1 hour. After deproteinization leukotriene metabolites were separated by RP-HPLC using a linear gradient of 40 - 80 % aqueous methanol within 35 min followed by 30 min of 80 % aqueous methanol (4). The identification of [^{3}H]leukotriene metabolites was based on co-chromatography with synthetic unlabeled leukotriene standards (Cascade Biochem, Reading, UK) in different HPLC systems.

leukotrienes produced by surgical trauma (7). Endogenous cysteinyl leukotrienes were analyzed by the sequential use of HPLC and a radioimmunoassay that was optimized for LTE$_4$ (6). LTE$_4$ was the major single cysteinyl leukotriene in bile and its concentration rose from 0.2 to 9 nmol/l after a shock-inducing dose of staphylococcal enterotoxin B. In addition, LTD$_4$ at concentrations up to 6 nmol/l, was detected in monkey bile after toxin treatment (6,23).

Analysis of human bile, obtained during enteral retrograde cholangiography in patients with acute pancreatitis, indicated that LTE$_4$ is the predominant endogenous cysteinyl leukotriene (21). The concentration of LTE$_4$ in human bile varies considerably, but in some cases the LTC$_4$ production reflected by the biliary LTE$_4$ may be sufficient to induce known phenomena associated with acute pancreatitis including the shocklike reaction.

In *human urine* LTE$_4$ is the major cysteinyl leukotriene as measured by the combination of HPLC with radioimmunoassay (15,20). The concentration of LTE$_4$ in normal subjects is at 0.3 nmol/l of urine, corresponding to 0.02 μmol/mol of creatinine (Table 1 and ref. 15). Comparable methods for the analysis of urinary LTE$_4$ have been described more recently (25,27). Increased urinary LTE$_4$ has been described in atopic subjects after antigen challenge (27) and in patients with cardiac ischemia (25). In liver cirrhosis and in hepatorenal syndrome, where hepatic uptake, ω-oxidation, and hepatobiliary elimination of cysteinyl leukotrienes may be

TABLE 1

Cysteinyl Leukotrienes in the Urine of Normal Subjects, Patients with Liver Cirrhosis, and Patients with Hepatorenal Syndrome and Liver Cirrhosis

	Normal Subjects (n = 7)	Liver Cirrhosis (n = 8)	Hepatorenal Syndrome and Liver Cirrhosis (n = 5)
		mean (range)	
LTE_4 (nmol/l)	0.3 (0.1 - 0.5)	0.8 (0.1 - 2.6)	7.8 (4.1 - 14)[a]
LTE_4/creatinine (μmol/mol)	0.02 (0.01 - 0.03)	0.11 (0.01 - 0.23)[a]	1.2 (0.6 - 1.9)[a]
LTE_4 production rate (pmol/h)	10 (4 -18)	40 (4 - 131)	350 (33 - 658)[a]

[a]Values differ from those in normal subjects and from those in liver cirrhosis by $p \leq 0.01$ (Wilcoxon-Mann-Whitney test for the one-sided problem).

impaired, we observed a manifold increase in concentration and excretion rate of LTE_4 in urine (15). Based on urinary creatinine, LTE_4 increased from 0.02 in normal subjects to 0.11 and 1.2 μmol/mol in patients with cirrhosis of the liver and with hepatorenal syndrome, respectively (Table 1). It is of interest, that N-acetyl-LTE_4 was below our detection limit in normal urine, but was present at significant concentrations (mean: 1.5 nmol/l) in urine of patients with hepatorenal syndrome (15). The action of increased cysteinyl leukotriene concentrations on the kidneys and their vasculature may contribute to the functional renal failure which can develop in patients with cirrhosis and other severe diseases of the liver.

SYSTEMIC CYSTEINYL LEUKOTRIENE GENERATION AND ITS INHIBITION IN ANAPHYLACTIC SHOCK

A quantitative estimate of systemic cysteinyl leukotriene production by analyses in bile has been achieved in the guinea pig model of ovalbumin-induced anaphylactic shock (9,18). LTC_4 underwent rapid elimination from the circulating blood and was predominantly converted to LTD_4 within the vascular space of the guinea pig (9). To mimic the elimination and metabolism of endogenous LTC_4 generated during anaphylaxis, ^{3}H-labeled LTC_4 was infused intravenously over a period of 15 min, leading to a recovery in bile of 85 % of the infused leukotriene radioactivity within

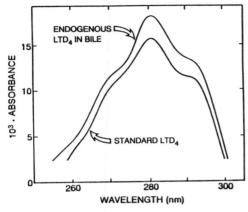

FIG. 3. Absorbance spectra of endogenous LTD_4 from bile during anaphylactic shock and of standard LTD_4 recorded with a photodiode array detector. Bile fractions collected from 5 sensitized guinea pigs 0 - 15 min after ovalbumin challenge were pooled and spiked with $[^3H]LTD_4$ (0.4 KBq, corresponding to 0.25 pmol) to determine the retention time on HPLC (76 min) and the total recovery (48 %) of LTD_4. For comparison, the UV spectrum of 0.1 nmol of synthetic LTD_4 is shown. Spectra were recorded during HPLC using a linear gradient from 0 - 80 % methanol in water with constant 3.3 mmol/l ammomium acetate (pH 4.5) for 60 min followed by 30 min of 80 % aqueous methanol.

2 hours. $[^3H]LTD_4$ was by far the predominant biliary metabolite amounting to 46 % of the infused dose within 30 min. In accordance with previous studies (18) and in line with the tracer studies, LTD_4 also was the major endogenous immunoreactive LTC_4 metabolite in guinea pig bile during anaphylaxis. Antigen challenge was followed within 15 min by a 30-fold increase in the biliary LTD_4 concentration from 2.1 ± 0.6 nmol/l to 63 ± 7 nmol/l (n=10) (9). The endogenous LTD_4 gave a UV spectrum characteristic for cysteinyl leukotrienes and identical with synthetic LTD_4, as recorded during HPLC with a photodiode array detector (Fig. 3). The total amount of LTC_4 produced during guinea pig anaphylaxis within a 30 min-period was calculated to be 0.8 ± 0.2 nmol/kg body weight (n = 10). This estimate is based on the finding that within 30 min 46 % and 18 % of the infused $[^3H]LTC_4$ were recovered in bile as $[^3H]LTD_4$ and $[^3H]LTC_4$, respectively (9). This amount of systemically produced endogenous LTC_4 is sufficient in the guinea pig to evoke signs indicative of systemic anaphylaxis including bronchoconstriction and widespread plasma extravasation (9,13,16). The remarkable sensitivity of the guinea pig to intravenously administered LTC_4 or LTD_4 may be due to the slow intravascular conversion of LTD_4 to LTE_4 (9), to the lack of intrahepatic N-acetylation of LTE_4 (18), and to the slow and limited ω-oxidation of LTE_4 (9) as compared to other species such as the rat (14,19).

The novel inhibitor of leukotriene biosynthesis, MK-886, which acts by interfering with the translocation and activation of arachidonate 5-lipoxygenase (8), was used to suppress leukotriene formation during

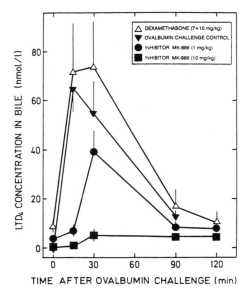

FIG. 4. Time course of LTD_4 levels in bile from ovalbumin-challenged, pyrilamine-pretreated guinea pigs with or without pretreatment with the leukotriene biosynthesis inhibitor MK-886 or dexamethasone (9). The inhibitor was given 15 min prior to challenge at the indicated doses; dexamethasone was administered over a period of 7 days (10 mg/kg daily). Each LTD_4 value was determined by reversed-phase HPLC and subsequent radioimmunoassays and is presented as the mean ± SEM (n = 4-10 animals per group).

anaphylactic shock. At a dose of 10 mg/kg, administered intravenously 15 min before antigen challenge, MK-886 completely inhibited the systemic production of cysteinyl leukotrienes during anaphylaxis (Fig. 4). This inhibition of systemic LTC_4 formation was associated with a complete protection against lethal anaphylactic shock in animals pretreated in addition with the histamine receptor antagonist pyrilamine maleate (1 mg/kg) (P<0.005). Pretreatment with either the inhibitor of leukotriene synthesis or the histamine receptor antagonist reduced the lethality during anaphylactic shock from 100 % to 60 % (P<0.05) and 78 %, respectively (9). Dexamethasone (10 mg/kg daily over 7 days) and pyrilamine pretreatment of guinea pigs reduced the lethality from anaphylactic shock from 100 % to 33 % (P<0.05). However, this glucocorticoid did not suppress the anaphylactic LTC_4 production *in vivo*, neither after a single dose of 10 mg/kg (17) nor after treatment for 7 days (Fig. 4). This remarkable finding may be explained by the differential action of dexamethasone on mast cells, which are the likely source for LTC_4 generation in anaphylaxis, and macrophages. While anti-IgE-induced LTC_4 release by mast cells is not affected by the steroid (24), macrophages do respond to dexamethasone treatment by a reduced release of prostanoids and cysteinyl leukotrienes (9). Our studies in the guinea pig provide direct evidence that cysteinyl leukotrienes play a key role in the lethality from anaphylactic shock and that selective inhibition of *in vivo* leukotriene generation is protective.

ACKNOWLEDGMENTS

We are indebted to Dr. J. Gillard, Dr. A.W. Ford-Hutchinson, and Dr. J. Rokach, Merck Frosst Canada, for providing the leukotriene biosynthesis inhibitor MK-886. Prof. C. Herfarth and Dr. G. Otto, Department of Surgery of Heidelberg University, kindly provided human liver samples obtained during surgery. We thank Ms J. Müller for expert assistance in the leukotriene identifications.

REFERENCES

1. Appelgren, L.-E., and Hammarström, S. (1982): *J. Biol. Chem.* 257: 531-535.

2. Ball, H.A., and Keppler, D. (1987): *Biochem. Biophys. Res. Commun.* 148:664-670.

3. Ballet, F., Bouma, M.E., Wang, S.R., Amit, N., Marais, J., Infante, R. (1984): *Hepatology* 4:849-854.

4. Baumert, T., Huber, M., Mayer, D., and Keppler, D. (1989): *Eur. J. Biochem.* 182:223-229.

5. Bergdoll, M.S. (1979): In: *Foodborne Infections and Intoxications*, edited by H. Riemann and F.L. Bryan; pp.443-494. Academic Press, Orlando, FL.

6. Denzlinger, C., Guhlmann, A., Scheuber, P.H., Wilker, D., Hammer, D.K., and Keppler, D. (1986): *J. Biol. Chem.* 261:15601-15606.

7. Denzlinger, C., Rapp, S., Hagmann, W., and Keppler, D. (1985): *Science* 230:330-332.

8. Gillard, J., Ford-Hutchinson, A.W., Chan, C., Charleson, S., Denis, D., Foster, A., Fortin, R., Leger, S., McFarlane, C.S., Morton, H., Piechuta, H., Riendeau, D., Rouzer, C.A., Rokach, J., Young, R., MacIntyre, D.E., Peterson, L., Bach, T., Eiermann, G., Hopple, S., Humes, J., Hupe, L., Luell, S., Metzger, J., Meurer, R., Miller, D.K., Opas, E., and Pacholok, S. (1989): *Can. J. Physiol. Pharmacol.* 67:456-464.

9. Guhlmann, A., Keppler, A., Kästner, S., Krieter, H., Brückner, U.B., Messmer, K., and Keppler, D. (1989): *J. Exp. Med.* 170:1905-1918.

10. Hagmann, W., Denzlinger, C., and Keppler, D. (1984): *Circ. Shock* 14:223-235.

11. Hagmann, W., Denzlinger, C., and Keppler, D. (1985): *FEBS Lett.* 180:309-313.

12. Hammarström, S., Bernström, K., Örning, L., Dahlén, S.-E., and Hedquist, P. (1981): *Biochem. Biophys. Res. Commun.* 101:1109-1115.

13. Hua, X.-Y., Dahlén, S.-E., Lundberg, J.M., Hammarström, S., and Hedqvist, P. (1985): *Naunyn-Schmiedeberg's Arch. Pharmacol.* 330:136-141.

14. Huber, M., and Keppler, D. (1987): *Eur. J. Biochem.* 167:73-39.

15. Huber, M., Kästner, S., Schölmerich, J., Gerok, W., and Keppler, D. (1989): *Eur. J. Clin. Invest.* 19:53-60.

16. Jones, T.R., Letts, G., Chan, C.-C., and Davies, P. (1989): In: *Leukotrienes and Lipoxygenases: Chemical, Biological and Clinical Aspects*, edited by J. Rokach; pp. 309-403. Elsevier, Amsterdam.

17. Keppler, A., Guhlmann, A., Kästner, S., and Keppler, D. (1989): In: *Leukotrienes and Prostanoids in Health and Disease*, edited by U. Zor, Z. Naor, and A. Danon; pp. 204-209. Karger, Basel.

18. Keppler, A., Örning, L., Bernström, K., and Hammarström, S. (1987): *Proc. Natl. Acad. Sci. USA* 84:5903-5907.

19. Keppler, D., Huber, M., Baumert, T., and Guhlmann, A. (1989): *Advan. Enzyme Regul.* 28:307-319.

20. Keppler, D., Huber, M., Hagmann, W., Ball, H.A., Guhlmann, A., and Kästner, S. (1988): *Ann. NY Acad. Sci.* 524:68-74.

21. Keppler, D., Huber, M., Weckbecker, G., Hagmann, W., Denzlinger, C., and Guhlmann, A. (1987): *Advan. Enzyme Regul.* 26:211-224.

22. Örning, L., Kaijser, L., and Hammarström, S. (1985): *Biochem. Biophys. Res. Commun.* 130:214-220.

23. Scheuber, P.H., Denzlinger, C., Wilker, D., Beck, G., and Keppler, D., and Hammer, D.K. (1987): *Eur. J. Clin. Invest.* 17: 455-459.

24. Schleimer, R.P., Schulman, E.S., MacGlashan, D.W., Jr., Peters, S.P., Hayes, E.C., Adams III, G.K., Lichtenstein,8 L.M., and Adkinson, N.F., Jr.(1983): *J. Clin. Invest.* 71:1830-1835.

25. Tagari, P., Ethier, D., Carry, M., Korley, V., Charleson, S., Girard, Y., and Zamboni, R. (1989): *Clin. Chem.* 35:388-391.

26. Tagari, P., Foster, A., Delorme, D., Girard, Y., and Rokach, J. (1989): *Prostaglandins* 37:629-640.

27. Taylor, G.W., Taylor, I., Black, P., Maltby, N.H., Turner, N., Fuller, R.W., and Dollery, C.T. (1989): *Lancet* I:584-588.

Advances in Prostaglandin, Thromboxane,
and Leukotriene Research, Vol. 20,
edited by B. Samuelsson et al.
Raven Press, Ltd., New York © 1990.

BINDING SITES FOR HISTAMINE AND SULFIDOPEPTIDE LEUKOTRIENES IN NORMAL AND HYPERSENSITIZED HUMAN LUNG FRAGMENTS

Teresa Vigano', Simonetta Nicosia, Maria Rosa Accomazzo, Maria Teresa Crivellari, Daniela Oliva, Alberto Verga*, Maurizio Mezzetti§, and Giancarlo Folco[oo]

Inst. of Pharmacological Sciences, School of Pharmacy, Univ. of Milano, Via Balzaretti 9, 20133 Milano, Italy.
* Bayer Italia, Garbagnate Milanese 20024, Italy.
§ IV Clinic of Surgery, Policlinico di Milano, Via F. Sforza, 20122 Milano
[oo] Inst. of Pharmacology and Pharmacognosy, School of Pharmacy, Univ. of Parma, Via M. D'Azeglio 75, 43100 Parma, Italy.

INTRODUCTION

Airway hyperresponsiveness is generally defined as an increased contractile response of the airway smooth muscle to a variety of stimuli and represents the most common characteristic of bronchial asthma. The mechanisms leading to airway narrowing in the presence of non specific stimuli are, however, unknown, but a role of airway inflammation cannot be excluded (6, 8).

Bronchial hyperreactivity can be modulated directly or indirectly by a variety of mediators that include histamine (H), prostaglandin D_2 (PGD_2) and platelet-activating factor (PAF) (5, 11). Among leukotrienes (LTs), an increased airway responsiveness has been shown in the dog for LTB_4; moreover, the airways of asthmatic patients seem to be more reactive than those of non atopic subjects to LTD_4 (7, 3), although this finding still represents a controversial issue (13).

Atopic subjects are characterised by high circulating levels of IgE and show a marked tendency to develop allergic diseases such as asthma, rhinitis, urticaria etc. (9). Although atopy should not be regarded as a synonym of allergic disease, the atopic subject is genetically susceptible to this type of diseases and show enhanced bronchial reactivity towards specific allergens (specific bronchial

187

hyperreactivity) as well as to non-allergenic substances such as H, methacoline, mist of H_2O etc. (aspecific bronchial hyperreactivity) (2).

The purpose of the present work was to evaluate whether a condition of IgE hypersensitization "in vitro" was associated with changes in binding of sulfidopeptide leukotrienes and H.

METHODS

Macroscopically normal human lung parenchyma from patients undergoing surgery for bronchial carcinoma was minced into fragments of approx. 100 mg each and divided into two aliquots. The tissue was extensively washed with Tyrode's buffer, pH 7.4, and incubated for 3 h at $37^{\circ}C$ in buffer with (passively sensitized, S) or without (control, C) hyperimmune serum, 5 mg/ml. At the end of the incubation both C and S lung fragments were washed again and aliquots (500 mg) frozen for binding and IgE assay. The remaining C and S parenchyma was preincubated for 10' at $37^{\circ}C$ in Tyrode's (1g/10ml, w/v) and subsequently challenged with an anti human IgE antibody kindly provided by Dr. S. Ahlstedt, Pharmacia, Uppsala. 15' later the reaction was stopped and aliquots of the supernatant frozen for enzyme-immunoassay of PGD_2. Binding to LTC_4, LTD_4 and H sites was carried on using crude membrane preparations from C and S parenchymal fragments before immunological challenge. Binding was evaluated at $25^{\circ}C$ for 40' in the presence of 2 nM $^3H\text{-}LTD_4$ (10) and 5 μM ^3H-mepyramine (4) and at $4^{\circ}C$ for 20' in the presence of 50 nM $^3H\text{-}LTC_4$ (12).

Assay of Tissue bound IgE

The tissue was homogenized in Tyrode's buffer (1g/10 ml, w/v) and an aliquot (0.35 ml) centrifuged for 10' at 10.000 g at $4^{\circ}C$; pellets and supernatants were separated and processed separately.

3 different aliquots of 100 ml of each supernatant were incubated for 3 h at room temperature with paper discs covalently saturated with sheep anti-human IgE (Pharmacia IgE PRIST paper discs); after the incubation each sample was washed 3 times with saline solution (2.5 ml) containing 2% Tween 20, freshly prepared, waiting 10' between each wash. 100 ml of rabbit anti-human ^{125}I-IgE (approx 0.05 mCi) were then added to each tube and incubated for 10 h at room temperature. Each sample was then washed again as described, and radioactivity counted using a Packard gamma counter for 2'. Results are expressed as percentage of the mean count of the "Total Activity" added to each tube.

Each pellet obtained from the first centrifugation was resuspended using 300 ml of the rabbit anti human IgE solution, divided in 3 different aliquots and incubated for 3 h at room temperature under vigorous shaking (1200 rpm). Each tube was then washed 3 times with 2.5 ml of the washing buffer mentioned above and centrifuged at 10.000 g for 10' at 4^oC, waiting 10' between each wash.

RESULTS AND DISCUSSION

We have studied the immunological release of PGD_2 and LTC_4-like activity from C and S human lung parenchymal fragments from 23 individuals upon in vitro challenge with an anti-human IgE antibody. The results reported in Fig. 1 indicate that the process of passive sensitization has indeed enriched the lung tissue of IgE: in fact, tissue immunoglobulin levels are approx. 10 folds higher in S than in C fragments. However, no significant increase in mediator releasability takes place.

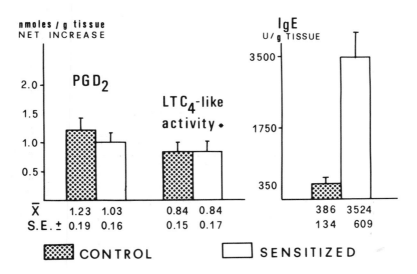

Fig. 1: Release of PGD_2 and of LTC_4-like activity from normal (C) and passively sensitized (S) human lung parenchyma.

This apparent lack of correlation between tissue bound IgE and the release of eicosanoids that takes place after passive sensitization might be explained by the fact that the amount of IgE detectable in C fragments is sufficient to trigger mast cell degranulation followed by massive mediator release. This would not be surprising since all our

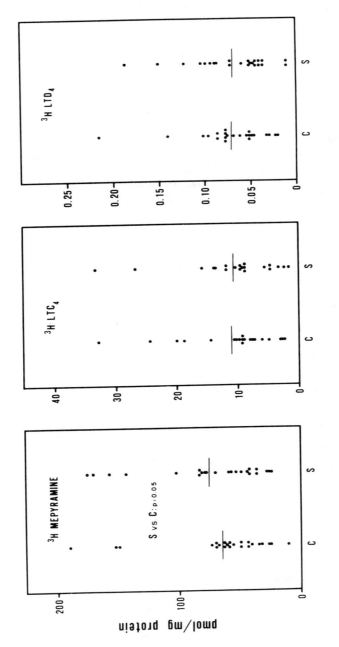

Fig. 2: Binding of ^{3}H-LTC$_4$, ^{3}H-LTD$_4$ and ^{3}H-mepyramine in control (C) and passively sensitized (S) human lung parenchyma. Values are expressed as pmoles/mg protein, $\bar{X} \pm$ S.D., N= 23

patients suffered from bronchial carcinoma, and tumours removed at surgery were characterized by a marked mononuclear cell infiltration suggestive of an active host resistance of immunological nature.

Since a marked difference in lung IgE levels can be demonstrated between C and S fragments, it was of interest to study whether comparable modifications in sulfidopeptide leukotrienes and H receptors might occur. For this purpose we evaluated binding of ^3H-LTC_4, ^3H-LTD_4 and ^3H-mepyramine at a fixed ligand concentration. Such a "single point" binding analysis is able to reveal changes in affinity and/or number of binding sites.

The results reported in Fig. 2 show that the number of pmoles of either LTC_4 or LTD_4 bound/mg protein does not differ in membranes of C vs S fragments. On the other hand, the process of passive sensitization causes a small but statistically significant ($p < 0.02$) increase in ^3H-mepyramine binding. This increase ranges between 3.3 and 156% and tooks place in 18 out of 23 specimens.

Although we cannot discriminate between changes in receptor affinity or density, the length of the incubation would be sufficient even for some receptor neosynthesis.

The different behavior of LTC_4 and LTD_4 binding sites as compared to H sites might lend support to the findings of Adelroth et al. (1) who showed that these sulfidopeptide leukotrienes are unique bronchoconstrictors.

The difference in binding parameters of ^3H-mepyramine might indicate that the process of passive sensitization represents an "in vitro" model for the study of human airway hyperresponsiveness; in this respect it will be important to show if the binding data are matched by an increased contractile effect of H in sensitized human lung parenchyma.

REFERENCES

1. Adelroth, E., Morris, M.M., Hargreave, F.E., and O'Byrne, P.M. (1986): N. Engl. J. Med., 315: 480-484.
2. Allegra, L., and Bianco, S. (1980): Eur. J. Resp. Dis., 61/S106: 41-49.
3. Bisgaard, H., Groth, S., and Madsen, F. (1985): Br. Med. J.,290:1468-1471.
4. Casale, T.B., Rodbard, D., and Kaliner, M. (1985): Biochem. Pharmacol., 34: 3285-3292.
5. Chung, K.F., Aizawa, H., Leikanf, G.D., Ueki, I.F. Evans, T.W. and Nadel, J.A. (1986): J. Pharmacol. Exp.Ther., 236: 580-584

6. Fabbri, L.M., Boschetto, P., Zocca, E., De Marzo, N., Crescioli, S., Maestrelli, P., and Mapp, C.E. (1988): Respiration, 54/S1: 90-94.
7. Griffin, M., Woodrow Weiss, J., Leitch, A.G., McFadden, E.R. Jr., Corey, E.J., Austen, K.F., and Drazen, J.M. (1983): N. Engl. J. Med., 308: 436-439.
8. Hargreave, F.E., Ryan, G., Thomson, N.C., O'Byrne, P.M., Latimer, K., Juniper, E.F., and Dolovic, J.(1981): J. Allergy. Clin. Immunol., 68: 347-352.
9. Ishizaka, K., Ishizaka, T., and Hornbrook, M.M. (1966): J. Immunol., 97: 75-87.
10. Lewis, M.A., Mong, S., Vessella, R.L., and Crooke, S.T. (1985): Biochem, Pharmacol., 34: 4311-4317.
11. Page, C.P., and Robertson, D.N. (1988): In: Ginkgolides Chemistry, Biology, Pharmacology and Clinical Perspectives, edited by P. Braquet vol. 1, pp. 305-312. J.R. Prous Science Publishers, Barcelona.
12. Rovati, G.E., Oliva, D., Sautebin, L., Folco, G.C., Welton, A.F., and Nicosia, S. (1985): Biochem. Pharmacol., 34: 2831-2837.
13. Smith, L.J., Greenberger, P.A., Patterson, R., Krell, R.D., and Bernstein, P.R. (1985): Am. Rev. Respir. Dis., 131: 368-372.

Advances in Prostaglandin, Thromboxane,
and Leukotriene Research, Vol. 20,
edited by B. Samuelsson et al.
Raven Press, Ltd., New York © 1990.

STUDIES OF LEUKOTRIENES AS MEDIATORS IN THE HUMAN LUNG *IN VITRO*

Sven-Erik Dahlén, Thure Björck, Maria Kumlin*,
Elisabeth Granström** and Per Hedqvist

Departments of Physiology, Physiological Chemistry*, Reproductive
Endocrinology** and Institute of Environmental Medicine,
Karolinska Institutet, S-104 01 Stockholm, Sweden

INTRODUCTION

Since the isolation of leukotriene (LT) C_4 from a mouse mastocytoma preparation ten years ago (1), there has been an extraordinary progression in research about leukotrienes and airway function. Specifically, the enigmatic biological principle slow reacting substance of anaphylaxis (SRS-A), presumed to be an important mediator in asthma, has conclusively been shown to consist of LTC_4 and its two immediate metabolites LTD_4 and LTE_4 (subsequently collectively referred to as cysteinyl-containing leukotrienes, cys-LTs). Moreover, as dealt with in other chapters in this volume, several potent and selective tools have been developed for pharmacological manipulation of the release or actions of leukotrienes. In the future, clinical trials will delineate the usefulness of treatment with such agents in bronchial asthma, inflammatory and vascular diseases.

During this first decade of leukotriene research, we have investigated the formation and actions of these compounds in the human lung. This chapter serves to highlight some of our findings in a project where human lung tissue is collected at the surgery ward and immediately transferred to the laboratory for explorations.

FORMATION AND METABOLISM OF LEUKOTRIENES
IN THE HUMAN LUNG

In line with the identification by Brocklehurst of SRS-A in lung tissue of asthmatics (2), we have been able to document that challenge with specific allergen triggers the formation of cys-LTs in lung tissue of atopic asthmatics (3). The conditions for leukotriene formation in the human lung have subsequently been further characterized in a large number of lungs from non-asthmatics (4). In essence, apart from the fact that lung tissue from atopic asthmatics is sensitized and may be challenged with specific allergen, we have not detected any significant qualitative or quantitative differences in the formation and further metabolism of leukotrienes in lung tissue from non-asthmatics as compared with asthmatics. Therefore, it appears unlikely that the disease process as such changes the basic conditions for synthesis and release of leukotrienes. We rather suggest that airway hyperresponsiveness and other features of asthma reside at other levels, either at the effector cells (for example bronchial and vascular smooth muscles, mucus secreting cells, etc) or at steps prior to the activation of mediator-releasing inflammatory cells. As a corollary, lung tissue from non-asthmatics can provide us with information about leukotriene metabolism which is of relevance to the situation in asthma. The findings in such studies are summarized below.

Challenge with the calcium ionophore A23187 (0.25-2.5 µM) caused dose-dependent release of both LTB_4 and cys-LTs from the chopped human lung. During a brief 10 min incubation, approximately 300 pmol of each class of leukotrienes are formed per gram of tissue. When exogenous arachidonic acid (70 µM) was included, there was a three-fold increase in the amounts of LTB_4 formed by stimulation with A23187. In contrast, release of cys-LTs was not enhanced by exogenous arachidonic acid.

Furthermore, when the chopped lung preparation was challenged with anti-human IgE (anti-IgE, dilutions 1/30000-1/60), there was also a dose-dependent release of cys-LTs. However, LTB_4 could not be detected after this immunological activation of the preparation, even if the experiments were carried out in the presence of exogenous arachidonic acid. Since anti-IgE selectively activates those cells that carry bound IgE on the cell-surface, whereas the ionophore causes a global stimulation of all cells in the preparation, the different profiles of leukotriene release for the two stimuli suggests that LTB_4 and LTC_4 may originate from different cells.

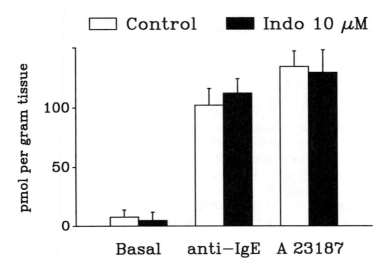

Figure 1: Lack of influence of indomethacin (Indo, 15 min preincubation) on release of cysteinyl-leukotrienes (LTC$_4$, LTD$_4$ and LTE$_4$) from chopped human lung. Results from 10 min incubations with buffer alone (basal), anti-human-IgE (titer 1/300) or ionophore A23187 (2.5 µM). Radioimmunological determinations of triplicates (SD indicated by error bar) from one subject.

The hypothesis that the initial consequence of IgE-dependent activation is release of LTC$_4$ but not LTB$_4$, is strongly supported by observations in lung tissue of atopic asthmatics (2). In this sensitized tissue, challenge with specific allergen induced the selective formation of cys-LTs, whereas A23187 triggered synthesis of both classes of leukotrienes. Moreover, challenge with anti-IgE causes a parallel release of histamine and cys-LTs from dispersed human lung cells, but the same stimulus fails to trigger formation of LTB$_4$ also in this mast cell enriched population (5). Leukotriene C$_4$ is documented to be the major leukotriene formed in lung mast cells (6). Therefore, considered together, we conclude that the pulmonary mast cell predominantly generates LTC$_4$ as a consequence of IgE-activation, whereas additional cells are responsible for the generation of LTB$_4$. The human pulmonary macrophage may be one important source of LTB$_4$ (7).

There were further differences between the two classes of

leukotrienes in the chopped human lung. Thus, metabolism of LTC_4 into LTD_4 and LTE_4 was rapid, whereas LTB_4 was metabolized slowly into Ω-oxidized metabolites. For example, LTE_4 was the major metabolite 10 min after incubation with $^3H\text{-}LTC_4$(300 nM), and only 20% of the radioactivity was associated with LTC_4. In contrast, during the same time-period, lung tissue metabolized less than 25% of $^3H\text{-}LTB_4$ (200 nM). Concerning LTE_4, we found no evidence for further metabolism of this compound in the lung during incubations up to 100 min. Therefore, bioinactivation of LTE_4 must be attributed to excretion and/or extrapulmonary metabolism.

In contrast to what has been reported for release of SRS-A from the guinea pig lung (8), we have consistently failed to document that the cyclooxygenase inhibitor indomethacin affects the release of cys-LTs in the human lung. The hypothesis has been tested with both A23187 and anti-IgE as inducer of leukotriene formation. Figure 1 shows results from one such series of experiments. The observations do not exclude the possibility that mediator release from certain individual cell-types in the human lung may be affected by cyclooxygenase products, but it is clear that there was no evidence for this type of modulation in the chopped human lung preparation as a whole. More recently, we have obtained equally negative data concerning the influence of indomethacin on leukotriene release from chopped human bronchi (unpublished).

CONTRACTION OF HUMAN BRONCHI BY LEUKOTRIENES

Soon after their discovery, it was documented that leukotrienes were potent agonists for contraction of human bronchi (9,10). Their bronchoconstrictive properties have been extensively documented in animal studies. In addition, considerable information has accumulated from bronchial provocation studies in normal subjects and asthmatics (reviewed in 11). In the main, all three cys-LTs have very similar activities on airway smooth muscle, being on a molar basis 100-1000 times as potent as histamine. In vivo, asthmatics may be hyperreactive to inhaled leukotrienes. Differences in potency and duration of action have been observed for the individual leukotrienes under in vivo conditions.

Because of the rapid metabolism of LTC_4 into LTD_4 and LTE_4, it is however difficult from data obtained in provocation studies to assess whether or not LTC_4 and LTD_4 act on the same receptor in human airways. We have therefore administered the individual leukotrienes to isolated human bronchi pretreated with reduced glutathione (10 mM), which arrested conversion of LTC_4 to LTD_4, as documented by analysis of ^{3}H-LTC$_4$ metabolism in the bronchi. Nevertheless, the relative potency and the time-course of the contraction response to LTC$_4$ did not change. Moreover, in the presence of glutathione, the LT-antagonist ICI-198,615 remained equally effective and potent as an antagonist of LTC$_4$ and LTD$_4$ (Fig.2). Therefore, the findings support and extend previous indications (12) that LTC$_4$ and LTD$_4$ act at the same receptor in human bronchial smooth muscle. Since LTE$_4$ is a full agonist for contraction in human bronchi, and since it shares with LTC$_4$ and LTD$_4$ the high potency and susceptibility to antagonism by all described LT-antagonists, we conclude that there is a homogenous population of receptors for the cys-LTs in human bronchi. In view of the rapid metabolism of LTC$_4$ and LTD$_4$ into the metabolically stable LTE$_4$, it may however be that LTE$_4$ is the individual cys-LTs that in vivo predominantly accounts for activation of the LT-receptors in the airways. It is of interest in this context that LTE$_4$ specifically can induce airways hyperresponsiveness in man (13).

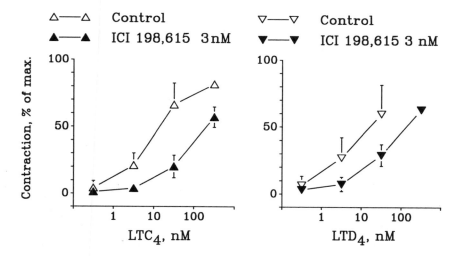

Figure 2: Influence of LT-antagonist ICI-198,615 (3nM, 5 min pretreatment) on cumulative dose-response relations for LTC$_4$ and LTD$_4$ in helical strips of human bronchi (n = 5-8). The experiments were performed in the presence of 10 mM reduced glutathione (GSH). Note the potency of the antagonist and the equal degree of antagonism versus LTC$_4$ and LTD$_4$.

LEUKOTRIENES AS MEDIATORS OF IgE-DEPENDENT CONTRACTION OF HUMAN AIRWAYS

We have previously reported that allergen challenge of bronchi obtained from atopic asthmatics produced a contraction response which by pharmacological characterization appeared to involve the cys-LTs as the major mediators (3). Due to the very limited availability of lung tissue from asthmatics for comprehensive studies with isolated bronchi, we have used the technique of challenge with anti-IgE in bronchi from non-asthmatics. In fact, we have used the same antibody as in the experiments where release of leukotrienes from the chopped lung has been characterized.

Thus, cumulative challenge with rising titers of anti-IgE (1/100000-1/300) elicits dose-dependent bronchial contractions (Fig. 3). In order to evaluate the contribution of histamine and cys-LTs to this response, a series of experiments were performed with antagonists added before the bronchi were challenged with anti-IgE.

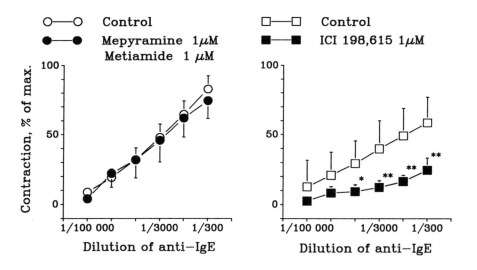

Figure 3: Influence of antihistamines (Mepyramine and Metiamide, n=8, left panel) or LT-antagonist ICI-198,615 (1 µM, n=4, right panel) on cumulative dose-response relations for anti-IgE (n=12 left panel, and n=8 right panel) in helical strips of human bronchi.
* = P<0.05; ** = P<0.01 (Student's t-test).

Initially, it was confirmed that the antihistamines (Mepyramine and Metiamide, 1 μM each) rendered the bronchi insensitive to the contractile effect of histamine. Nonetheless, the dose-response relation for anti-IgE was unaffected by the antihistamines (Fig.3). Preincubation with either the first (FPL 55712, L-648,051) or the second (ICI-198,615, SKF 104,353) generation of leukotriene receptor antagonists produced significant competitive antagonism of each of the cys-LTs (cf. Fig. 2). Moreover, these leukotriene-antagonists caused a substantial inhibition of the the contraction response to cumulative challenge with anti-IgE, as exemplified for ICI-198,615 (Fig. 3). In line with these observations with the effector-antagonists for cys-LTs, the inhibitor of leukotriene biosynthesis, piriprost (U-60,257, 100μM, 30 min preincubation) also inhibited the bronchial contraction induced by anti-IgE (anti-IgE). Therefore, the findings in this model of IgE-dependent airways anaphylaxis, strongly support the concept that the cys-LTs are the major mediators of antigen-induced contractions of human bronchi. It is likely that the same mechanism contributes to other types of mast cell-dependent bronchoconstriction, because non-immunological activation of mast cells would seem to result in the release of the same set of mediators.

CONCLUSIONS

As indicated in the introduction, ongoing and future clinical studies will ultimately evaluate the in vivo importance of the leukotrienes in different types of airway obstruction. Nevertheless, from our findings, we conclude that in human airways there exists a major leukotriene-dependent mechanism for bronchoconstriction. In fact, with respect to antigen-induced contraction of human bronchi, the cys-LTs fulfil the main classical criteria required to prove a mediator-function. Thus, (i) they are potent agonist for contraction, (ii) they are released by immunological activation of the lung, and, most important, (iii), the contraction response following immunological challenge of bronchi is substantially inhibited by agents which inhibit the release or actions of the cys-LTs.

ACKNOWLEDGEMENTS

Supported by grants from the Swedish Medical Research Council (project 14X-09071, 14X-04342, 03X-5915), the Swedish Association Against Chest and Heart Diseases, the Swedish Association Against Asthma and Allergy (RmA), the Swedish National Board for Laboratory Animals (CFN), the Scientific Council of the Swedish Association Against Use of Experimental Animals in Research, the Institute of Environmental Medicine, the Swedish Environment Protection Board (5324069-3), and Karolinska Institutet.

REFERENCES

1. Murphy, R.C., Hammarström, S., and Samuelsson, B. (1979): *Proc. Natl. Acad. Sci. USA.*, **76**:4275-4279.

2. Brocklehurst, W.E. (1960): *J. Physiol.*, **151**:416-435.

3. Dahlén, S.-E., Hansson, G., Hedqvist, P., Björck, T., Granström, E., and Dahlén, B. (1983): *Proc. Natl. Acad. Sci. USA.*, **80**:1712-1718.

4. Kumlin, M., and Dahlén, S.-E. (1990): *Biochim Biophys Acta*, in press.

5. Sydbom, A., Kumlin, M. and Dahlén, S.-E. (1987): *Agents and Actions*, **20**:198-201.

6. Schleimer, R.P., MacGlashan, D.W. Jr., Peters, S.P., Princard, R.N., Adkinson, N.F. Jr, and Lichtenstein, L.M. (1986): *Am. Rev. Respir. Dis.*, **133**:614-617.

7. Fels, A.O.S., Pawlowski, N.A., Cramer, E.B., King, T.K.C., Cohn, Z.A., and Scott, W.A. (1982): *Proc. Natl. Acad. Sci. USA.*, **79**:7866-7870.

8. Engineer, D.M., Niderhauser, U., Piper, P.J., and Sirois, P. (1978): *Br.J.Pharmacol.*, **62**:61-66.

9. Dahlén, S.-E., Hedqvist, P., Hammarström, S., and Samuelsson, B. (1980): *Nature (London)* **288**:484-486.

10. Hanna, C.J., Bach, M.K., Pare, P.D., Schellenberg, R.R. (1981): *Nature (London)* **290**:343-344.

11. Drazen, J.M. (1986): *Chest*, **89**:414-419.

12. Buckner, C.K., Krell, R.D., Laravuso, R.B., Coursin, D.B., Bernstein, P.R., and Will, J.A. (1986): *J. Pharm. Exper. Ther.*, **237**:558-562.

13. Arm, J.P., O'Hickey, S.P., Spur, B.W., Lee, T.H. (1989): *Am. Rev. Respir. Dis.* **140**:148-153.

Advances in Prostaglandin, Thromboxane, and Leukotriene Research, Vol. 20, edited by B. Samuelsson et al. Raven Press, Ltd., New York © 1990.

THE ROLE OF EICOSANOIDS IN ALLERGEN-INDUCED EARLY AND LATE

BRONCHIAL RESPONSES IN ALLERGIC SHEEP

William M. Abraham, Ph.D.

Division of Pulmonary Disease
Mount Sinai Medical Center
4300 Alton Road
Miami Beach, Florida, U.S.A.

INTRODUCTION

Certain similarities exist between the pathophysiologic responses observed in the sheep model of allergic bronchocon-striction and those observed in allergic subjects (4).

TABLE 1. Similarities between allergic sheep model
and allergic asthma

	Reference
- Natural allergy (positive skin sensitivity)	(41)
- Differential airway responsiveness between allergic and normal (non-allergic) groups	(10,41)
- Allergics bronchoconstrict to beta-blockers	(38)
- Allergics are hyperresponsive to bradykinin	(13)
- Show acute bronchoconstriction (associated with hyperinflation) to inhaled antigen; readily reversible with beta-adrenergic agents	(9,41)
- Some show late bronchial obstruction to antigen; not reversible with beta-adrenergic agents	(39)
- Early and late responses are sensitive to anti-allergic agents	(7,15)
- Late responses are sensitive to glucocorticoids	(8)
- Late responses are associated with airway inflammation (neutrophils and eosinophils)	(2,12)
- Late responses are associated with prolonged airway hyperresponsiveness	(30)

Two groups of allergic sheep are identified based on their airway responses to inhaled <u>Ascaris suum</u>. Acute responders develop only an immediate (early) bronchoconstriction to inhaled antigen, whereas dual responders develop both an early response and late bronchial obstruction (6-8 h) after antigen challenge (7). Pharmacological and biochemical evidence indicate that the 5-lipoxygenase (5-LO) and the cyclooxygenase (CO) pathways of arachidonic acid metabolism, resulting in the respective generation of leukotrienes (LT) and prostaglandins (PG)/ thromboxane (Tx), are activated in allergic sheep following allergen challenge and that the lipid mediators generated have distinct roles in pathophysiologic processes of early and late bronchial responses, airway inflammation and airway hyperresponsiveness.

Differences in Early Antigen-induced Mediator Release in Acute and Dual responders

Histamine and eicosanoids (27,31), including PGD_2, have been identified in bronchoalveolar lavage (BAL) fluid immediately after A. suum challenge in sheep, whereas, challenge with a non-specific antigen (ragweed) is not associated with mediator release or bronchoconstriction (7,40). These observations in addition to the findings that anti-allergic agents such as cromolyn sodium and nedocromil sodium, agents that can prevent mediator release from mediator containing cells in the airways, protect against allergen-induced early and late responses (7,15) suggest that antigen challenge in allergic sheep is associated with the immunologic release of mediators from mast cells/basophils. This mediator profile, however, differs between acute and dual responders, because pretreatment with the histamine H_1-antagonist chlorpheniramine almost completely blocks (~90%) the immediate antigen-induced bronchoconstriction in acute responders (9), but only partially protects (~50%) against the acute bronchoconstriction in dual responders (1). Subsequent studies using BAL fluid obtained immediately after antigen challenge from these two groups of sheep indicate that dual responders probably produce more spasmogenic LTs than do acute responders (1).

Cyclooxygenase and 5-Lipoxygenase Products and Late Responses

When glucocorticosteroids are given immediately before antigen challenge, neither histamine release nor the acute response to antigen is blocked, but the late response is abolished (8,26). This action is consistent with the ability of steroids to inhibit phospholipase A_2 an enzyme that controls arachidonic acid release from membrane phospholipids (28). To determine which arachidonic acid metabolites released/generated during the acute response to antigen are important for the development of the late response, dual responders were treated before antigen challenge with pharmacologic agents which act on either the CO or the 5-LO pathway. No blockade of the late response was observed when dual responders were pretreated with either the CO-inhibitor indomethacin (30) or the thromboxane (T_x)/endoperoxide antagonists L651,953 (6) or L670,596 (20). It should be noted, however, that the findings obtained with indomethacin and with the thromboxane antagonists are quantitatively different, probably because of the different actions of the two types of drugs. Whereas, indomethacin blocks the increase in both constrictor and dilator prostaglandins (e.g. PGE_2 and PGI_2 are elevated during the late response), the thromboxane antagonists selectively block the actions of thromboxane - a mediator associated with airway hyperresponsiveness (22,23). Thus, thromboxane antagonists can slightly reduce the severity of the late response by altering the responsiveness of the airways (22,23), whereas indomethacin can increase the severity of the late response because of the protective effects of PGE_2 and PGI_2 are removed.

When acute responders were challenged with antigen after pretreatment with indomethacin (2,21), antigen challenge produced

TABLE 2. Effect of different pharmacologic agents on antigen-induced early and late responses in allergic sheep

Drug	Dose	Route of Administration	Early[a]	Late[a]	Ref.
FPL-57231	30 mg total	Aerosol	29%	86%	(30)
LY-171883	30 mg/kg	Oral	74%	84%	(19)
WY-48,252	10 mg/kg	Oral	64%	68%	(17)
YM-16638	30 mg/kg	Oral	70%	93%	(37)
YM-16638	10 mg/kg	Oral	56%	75%	(37)
MK-571[b]	25 µg/kg/min	IV	57%	87%	(14)
MK-571	8 µg/kg/min	IV	46%	54%	(14)
MK-5711	2.5 µg/kg/min	IV	49%	34%	(14)
MK-571	5 mg	Aerosol	25%	72%	(5)
Picumast	5.0 mg total	Aerosol	63%	81%	(3)
Picumast	2.5 mg total	Aerosol	48%	55%	(3)
Picumast	1.0 mg total	Aerosol	0%	12%	(3)
WEB-2086	1 mg/kg	IV	29%	79%	(18)
YM-461	10 mg/kg	Oral	42%	82%	(36)
YM-461	3 mg/kg	Oral	38%	66%	(36)
Budesonide	2 mg total	Aerosol	41%	74%	(8)
Sch-37224	20 mg/kg	Oral	55%	78%	(16)
BI-226	10 mg	Aerosol	44%	81%	

[a]% Protection; [b]also known as L-660,711

both early and late responses. {Unmasking of late responses by indomethacin has also been reported in dogs (32).} This late response was blocked by treatment with the LT antagonist FPL-55712, a finding similar to that observed with naturally occurring late responses (35). Inhibition of CO is also associated with enhanced generation of LTC_4 and LTB_4 (recovered in BAL) immediately after local instillation of A. suum antigen in sheep (27). Thus, these results indicate that increased generation of 5-LO metabolites is likely to be associated with late responses.

Based on these observations, it is not surprising that a variety of structurally different LT-antagonists and agents which can inhibit LT generation/release are effective in blocking late responses (Table 2).

None of the treatments with the LT-antagonists completely inhibit the acute antigen-induced bronchoconstriction as would be expected, because of the contributions of histamine and PGD_2 to this response (vide supra). Data with a new 5-LO inhibitor, 226 (Boehringer Ingelheim) confirms that inhibition of the 5-LO pathway can result in the blockade of allergen-induced late responses in sheep.

Table 2 also shows that antagonists of platelet activating factor (PAF) (i.e. WEB-2086 and YM-461) inhibit late responses. These results would appear contradictory to our previous findings demonstrating the importance of 5-LO products and the late response. We subsequently showed, however, that PAF-induced responses in allergic sheep are mediated, in part, by spasmogenic LTs (18). It is not surprising, then, that both LTD_4 and PAF can induce late responses in sheep (11,18).

Inflammation and Late Response

Stimulation of the 5-LO pathway not only results in the generation of spasmogenic LTs, but also the potent chemotactic agent, LTB_4. Antigen-induced late responses in allergic sheep (12) are associated with an inflammatory response similar to that observed in man (24) as evidenced by the increase in BAL eosinophils and neutrophils at this time. Blockade of the late response with the anti-allergic agents, cromolyn sodium or nedocromil sodium, is associated with a reduction of the airway inflammation normally observed (12). Therefore, it may be that late responses can be abrogated either by antagonizing the mediators causing the response or by limiting the inflammation that ultimately results in the mediator generation.

That LTs may also be mediators of the late response is based on pharmacologic evidence that showed FPL-55712 (25) and MK-571 (20) can block the late response when given after the early response and can reverse the late response (25). These pharmacologic findings are supported by the observations that BAL fluid collected during the late response produces a bronchoconstriction that could be blocked by LT antagonists (1) and the identification of increased concentrations of immunoreactive LTC_4 and LTB_4 in BAL fluid obtained during the late response (31).

Antigen-induced Airway Hyperresponsiveness

Dual responders also develop airway hyperresponsiveness 24 h after antigen challenge (30). Pharmacologic studies indicate that this airway hyperresponsiveness is mediator dependent and can be blocked by treating animals before antigen challenge with either indomethacin; FPL-57231 (30); nedocromil sodium (15); Sch-37224 (16) and, most recently, the 5-LO inhibitor BI-226. In these studies indomethacin did not block the late response, which suggests that different mediators may be responsible for the late response, and the 24 h airway hyperresponsiveness. Similar findings have been reported in asthmatic subjects (29). Our most recent results suggest that although there are interactions between LTs and T_x in the development of airway hyperresponsiveness, there is a clear separation between the actions of these eicosanoids with T_x playing a major role in the development of airway hyperresponsiveness in the sheep model (33,34).

REFERENCES

1. Abraham, W.M. (1987). The importance of lipoxygenase products of arachidonic acid in allergen-induced late responses. Am. Rev. Respir. Dis. 135:S49-S53.
2. Abraham, W.M. (1988). The role of leukotrienes in allergen-induced late responses in allergic sheep. Annals of the New York Academy of Sciences: Biology of the Leukotrienes 524:260-270.
3. Abraham, W.M. (1988). Effect of picumast on antigen-induced early and late airway responses in allergic sheep. Drug Research
4. Abraham, W.M. (1989). Pharmacology of allergen-induced early and late airway responses and antigen-induced airway hyper-responsiveness in allergic sheep. Pul Pharm 2:33-40.
5. Abraham, W.M., Ahmed, A. and Cortes, A. (1989). The effects of a leukotriene (LT)D_4 antagonist (MK-571) on LTD_4 and antigen-induced bronchoconstriction in allergic sheep. The Faseb Journal
6. Abraham, W.M., Blinder, L., Wanner, A., Stevenson, J.S. and Tallent, M.W. (1987). Antigen-induced airway hyperresponsiveness does not contribute to airway late responses. Am. Rev. Respir. Dis. 135:A97.

7. Abraham, W.M., Delehunt, J.C., Yerger, L. and Marchette, B. (1983). Characterization of a late phase pulmonary response following antigen challenge in allergic sheep. <u>Am. Rev. Respir. Dis.</u> 128:839-844.

8. Abraham, W.M., Lanes, S., Stevenson, J.S. and Yerger, L.D. (1986). Effect of an inhaled glucocorticosteroids (budesonide) on post-antigen induced increases in airway responsiveness. <u>Bull. Europ. Physiopath. Respir. : Clin. Respir. Physiol.</u> 22:387-392.

9. Abraham, W.M., Oliver, W., Jr., King, M.M., Yerger, L. and Wanner, A. (1981). Effect of pharmacologic agents on antigen-induced decreases in specific lung conductance in sheep. <u>Am. Rev. Respir. Dis.</u> 124:554-558.

10. Abraham, W.M., Oliver, W., Jr., Welker, M.J., King, M., Wanner, A. and Sackner, M.A. (1981). Differences in airway reactivity in normal and allergic sheep after exposure to sulfur dioxide. <u>J. Appl. Physiol.</u> 51:1651-1656.

11. Abraham, W.M., Russi, E., Wanner, A., Delehunt, J.C., Yerger, L.D. and Chapman, G.A. (1985). Production of early and late pulmonary responses with inhaled leukotriene D_4 in allergic sheep. <u>Prostaglandins</u> 29:715-726.

12. Abraham, W.M., Sielczak, M.W., Wanner, A., Perruchoud, A.P., Blinder, L., Stevenson, J.S., Ahmed, A. and Yerger, L.D. (1988). Cellular markers of inflammation in the airways of allergic sheep with and without allergen-induced late responses. <u>Am. Rev. Respir. Dis.</u> 138:1565-1571.

13. Abraham, W.M., Soler, M., Ahmed, A. and Cortes, A. (1989). Pharmacology of bradykinin-induced bronchoconstriction in allergic sheep. <u>FASEB J</u> 3:275 A.

14. Abraham, W.M. and Stevenson, J.S. (1988). A new leukotriene D_4 antagonist, L-660,711, blocks allergen-induced late responses in allergic sheep. <u>Fed. Proc.</u> 2:A1057.

15. Abraham, W.M., Stevenson, J.S., Eldridge, M., Garrido, R. and Nieves, L. (1988). Nedocromil sodium in allergen-induced bronchial responses and airway hyperresponsiveness in allergic sheep. <u>J. Appl. Physiol.</u> 65(3):1062-1068.

16. Abraham, W.M., Stevenson, J.S. and Garrido, R. (1988). A leukotriene and thromboxane inhibitor (Sch 37224) blocks antigen-induced immediate and late responses and airway hyperresponsiveness in allergic sheep. <u>J. Pharmacol. Exp. Ther.</u> 247(3):1004-1011.

17. Abraham, W.M., Stevenson, J.S. and Garrido, R. (1988). The effect of an orally active leukotriene (LT) D_4 antagonist WY-48,252 on LTD_4 and antigen-induced bronchoconstrictions in allergic sheep. <u>Prostaglandins</u> 35:733-745.

18. Abraham, W.M., Stevenson, J.S. and Garrido, R. (1989). A possible role for PAF in allergen-induced late responses: Modification by a selective antagonist. <u>J. Appl. Physiol.</u> 66:2351-2357.

19. Abraham, W.M., Wanner, A., Stevenson, J.S. and Chapman, G.A. (1986). The effect of an orally active leukotriene D_4/E_4 antagonist, LY171883, on antigen-induced airway responses in allergic sheep. Prostaglandins 31:457-467.

20. Ahmed, A., Cortes, A. and Abraham, W.M. (1989). Comparative effects of a thromboxane antagonist and a leutkotriene antagonist on antigen-induced early and late airway responses in sheep. FASEB Journal 3:A438.

21. Blinder, L., Stevenson, J.S., Tallent, M.W., Jackowski, J.T., Wanner, A., Ahmed, T. and Abraham, W.M. (1987). Cyclooxygenase products of arachidonate modulate antigen-induced late responses in the airways. Am. Rev. Respir. Dis. 135:A180.

22. Chung, K.F., Aizawa, H., Becker, A.B., Frick, O., Gold, W.M. and Nadel, J.A. (1986). Inhibition of antigen-induced airway hyperresponsiveness by a thromboxane synthetase inhibitor (OKY-046) in allergic dogs. Am. Rev. Respir. Dis. 134:258-261.

23. Chung, K.F., Aizawa, H., Leikauf, G.D., Ueki, I.F., Evans, T.W. and Nadel, J.A. (1986). Airway hyperresponsiveness induced by platelet-activating factor: role of thromboxane generation. J. Pharmacol. Exp. Ther. 236:580-584.

24. de Monchy, J.G.R., Kauffman, H.F., Venge, P., Koeter, G.H., Jansen, H.M., Sluiter, H.J. and de Vries, K. (1985). Bronchoalveolar eosinophilia during allergen-induced late asthmatic reactions. Am. Rev. Respir. Dis. 131:373-376.

25. Delehunt, J.C., Perruchoud, A.P., Yerger, L., Marchette, B., Stevenson, J.S. and Abraham, W.M. (1984). The role of SRS-A in the late bronchial response following antigen challenge in allergic sheep. Am. Rev. Respir. Dis. 130:748-754.

26. Delehunt, J.C., Yerger, L., Ahmed, T. and Abraham, W.M. (1984). Inhibition of antigen-induced bronchoconstriction by methylprednisolone succinate. J. Allergy Clin. Immunol. 73:479-483.

27. Dworski, R., Sheller, J.R., Wickersham, N.E., Oates, J.A., Brigham, K.L., Roberts, L.J., III and Fitzgerald, G.A. (1989). Allergen-stimulated release of mediators into sheep bronchoalveolar lavage fluid: Effect of cyclooxygenase inhibition. Am. Rev. Respir. Dis. 139:46-51.

28. Flower, R.J. (1978). Steroidal anti-inflammatory drugs as inhibitors of phospholipase A_2. Adv. Prostaglandin Thromboxane Res. 3:105-112.

29. Kirby, J.G., Hargreave, F.E. and O'Byrne, P.M. (1987). Indomethacin inhibits allergen-induced airway hyperresponsiveness but not allergen-induced asthmatic responses. Am. Rev. Respir. Dis. 135:A312.

30. Lanes, S., Stevenson, J.S., Codias, E., Hernandez, A., Sielczak, M.W., Wanner, A. and Abraham, W.M. (1986). Indomethacin and FPL-57231 inhibit antigen-induced airway hyperresponsiveness in sheep. J. Appl. Physiol. 61:864-872.

31. Okayama, H., Aikawa, T., Ohtsu, H., Sasaki, H. and Takishima, T. (1989). Leukotriene C_4 and B_4 in bronchoalveolar lavage fluid during biphasic allergic bronchoconstriction in sheep. Am. Rev. Respir. Dis. 139:725-731.

32. Sasaki, H., Yanai, M., Aikawa, T. and Takishima, T. (1987). Indomethacin enhances late phase response to antigen challenge in dogs treated with metyrapone. Am. Rev. Respir. Dis. 135:A180.

33. Soler, M. and Abraham, W.M. (1989). The pharmacology of acute antigen-induced airway hyperresponsiveness in sheep. European Respiratory Journal 2:7545.

34. Soler, M. and Abraham, W.M. (1989). Antigen-induced airway hyperresponsiveness develops independently from late responses in sheep. Proceedings from the 8th Congress of the European Society of Pneumology

35. Soler, M., Perruchoud, A.P. and Abraham, W.M. (1988). Antigen-induced late responses unmasked by indomethacin in allergic sheep are blocked by FPL-55712. Am. Rev. Respir. Dis. 137(2):178.

36. Tomioka, K., Garrido, R., Ahmed, A., Stevenson, J.S. and Abraham, W.M. (1989). YM-461, a PAF antagonist, blocks antigen-induced late airway responses and airway hyperresponsiveness in allergic sheep. Eur. J. Pharm.

37. Tomioka, K., Garrido, R., Stevenson, J.S. and Abraham, W.M. (1988). The effect of an orally active leukotriene (LT) antagonist YM-16638 of antigen-induced early and late airway responses in allergic sheep. Prostaglandins, Leukotrienes and Essential Fatty Acids (In Press)

38. Wanner, A. and Abraham, W.M. (1982). Experimental models of Asthma. Lung 160:231-243.

39. Wanner, A., Ahmed, T. and Abraham, W.M. (1987). Drug actions on mediators. Drug therapy for asthma. In: Lung Biology and Health and Disease, edited by J.W. Jenne and S. Murphy. pp. 413-461, Marcel Dekker, Inc., New York.

40. Wanner, A., Mezey, R.J., Reinhart, M.E. and Eyre, P. (1979). Antigen-induced bronchospasm in conscious sheep. J. Appl. Physiol. 47(5)::917-922.

41. Wanner, A. and Reinhart, M. (1978). Respiratory mechanics in conscious sheep. J. Appl. Physiol. 44:479-482.

Advances in Prostaglandin, Thromboxane,
and Leukotriene Research, Vol. 20,
edited by B. Samuelsson et al.
Raven Press, Ltd., New York © 1990.

THE ROLE OF LEUKOTRIENES AND PROSTAGLANDINS IN ASTHMA: EVIDENCE
FROM CLINICAL INVESTIGATIONS

Clive Robinson and Stephen T. Holgate

Immunopharmacology Group, Clinical Pharmacology and Medicine I,
Southampton General Hospital, Southampton SO9 4XY,
United Kingdom

Structural characterization of the leukotrienes fostered great interest in the potential of compounds which are capable of inhibiting their formation or antagonising their powerful pharmacological effects. Not surprisingly, the acute bronchospasm of asthma is one potential target for such therapeutic intervention. However, in the past 10 years we have seen an explosion not only in the understanding of the complex interrelationships between the regulatory and effector systems involved in the genesis of inflammatory reactions, but also significant changes in the way in which we view the disease of asthma itself.

The view that eicosanoid mediators such as leukotrienes (LTs) and prostaglandins (PGs) are implicated in asthma is suggested by several lines of evidence which are reviewed elsewhere in this volume. Briefly summarized this evidence is based on (i) the fact that inflammatory cells implicated in the disease synthesize and release eicosanoids in response to pathophysiologically relevant stimuli (ii) the finding that certain of these eicosanoids have pharmacological effects consistent with the disease pathophysiology and (iii) that the presence of some of these agents in biological fluids correlates with exacerbations of the disease. The last of these points has traditionally been the Achilles heel of mediator pharmacology, and only recently have credible measurements of leukotrienes in biological fluids been reported (13,14).

LEUKOTRIENES AND ASTHMA

Largely as a result of the failure of the antihistamines then available to produce effective blockade of acute allergic bronchoconstriction, slow reacting substance (SRS-A) was seen as a missing link in the cascade of chemical mediators thought to be involved in asthma. Predating leukotriene characterization, the prototype SRS-A antagonist was the hydroxyacetophenone FPL 55712. This compound is poorly absorbed and has a short biological half life, but when administered by aerosolization in a small number of subjects it was reported to be of some benefit in unstable asthma. A later development, FPL 59257, which had superior in vivo properties, afforded partial protection against allergen challenge in only 2 out of 5 asthmatic subjects.

LEUKOTRIENE ANTAGONISTS AND LIPOXYGENASE INHIBITORS

Following the structural identification of SRS-A as the sulphidopeptide LTs a number of other potential LTD_4 antagonists have been developed based on the hydroxyacetophenone substructure present in FPL 55712. The principal rationale behind this approach was to produce compounds with a spasmolytic effect, although their possible ability to limit exudative inflammatory events gives them further potential. Although a number of compounds (eg LY 171,883 [Lilly]; L-648,051 and L-649,923 [Merck]), and their later developments, showed promising potency in animal models the degree of protection afforded by acute oral dosing in man against LTD_4 or allergen bronchoprovocation was generally disappointing. However, in the case of the Lilly compound LY 171,883 there was some indication of clinical benefit in a group of 138 asthmatic patients who received 400mg twice daily for six weeks and in whom FEV_1, PEFR, symptom scores and bronchodilator usage was measured. Interestingly, in this study most benefit was derived by a small sub-group of subjects with more intense symptoms.

Improvement in potency and structural divergence has been possible and a number of compounds have shown early promise in man, although there is little published evidence supporting any clinical efficacy. At the time of writing, the reported compounds of greatest interest are ICI 204,219 and MK-571 (L-660,711). Preliminary clinical results with ICI 204,219 demonstrate a 100-fold rightward shift in the dose-response curve to LTD_4-induced bronchoconstriction following a 40mg dose. This is in contrast to the smaller displacement (4-10 fold) typically seen with hydroxyacetophenones (1). The Merck quinoline MK-571 appears to have promising pharmacokoinetics. Preliminary reports of MK-571 in a double-blind, placebo-controlled study in normal subjects demonstrated impressive antagonism of LTD_4-induced bronchoconstriction when the drug was infused to achieve plasma concentrations of 1, 6, and 110 μg/ml (11). Further results from clinical studies with these compounds are eagerly awaited.

Whilst one of the theoretical advantages of an antagonist is the degree of selective intervention that can be obtained, this may be a double-edged sword when intervening in processes mediated by parallel groups of effector substances. The multiplicity of mediators derived from arachidonic acid with overlapping bronchospastic and inflammatory activities is great. For this reason there has been a concurrent interest in the development of inhibitors of 5-lipoxygenase. It has been argued that this approach would be more likely to prevent the activity of inflammatory mediators responsible for the progression of the disease. This reasoning reflects the important changes which have taken place in the understanding of asthma and the probable mechanisms of action of drugs such as corticosteroids which are already used to treat the disease.

Compounds with the ability to inhibit 5-lipoxygenase have been derived from a variety of sources (natural products and their semi-synthetic analogues as well as from synthetic organics). Many have overlapping specificities and may act to varying degrees as inhibitors of other lipoxygenases and/or cyclooxygenase as a result of possessing redox mechanisms of action. One of the first compounds to be tested in man was the cyclopentapyrrole, piriprost. Although active in vitro, this compound was without effect when tested acutely by inhalation against allergen or exercise challenge in subjects with mild asthma (12). Similar negative findings have been reported with other compounds given acutely by the oral route eg nafazatrom and the quinone AA-861 (8,9).

Other types of compound have also been investigated. In some instances eg the acetohydroxamates or the N-hydroxyurea A-64077, the precise mechanism of action is unclear, but may involve iron chelation and weak redox activity. The arylmethylphenyl ether REV 5901 is a non-redox inhibitor with LT antagonist properties, but without significant activity in man. Currently the most interesting inhibitor is the orally active Merck compound MK-886 (L-663,536) which acts by inhibiting the intracellular translocation events responsible for the activation of 5-lipoxygenase.

The disappointing findings reported above raise several important questions, not least of which is the issue of whether leukotrienes are important in asthma. However, in the majority of the early studies there was no proof that the doses delivered were in fact sufficient to produce the desired effect of enzyme inhibition or receptor antagonism. Indeed the study with nafazatrom quite clearly demonstrated this not to be the case (9). Similarly, there is apparent contradictory evidence regarding the role of leukotrienes in the allergen-induced late asthmatic reaction. The LTD_4 antagonists L-648,051 and L-649,923 are reported to be without effect (3,5) whereas ONO-1078 and nebulized SK&F 104,353 are claimed to attenuate the reaction in a proportion of subjects (7,15). With our current knowledge regarding the relative activity of these compounds it is fair to conclude that poor bioavailability and insufficient potency significantly contributed to the negative findings.

PROSTANOIDS AND ASTHMA

For many years prostaglandins and thromboxanes were dismissed from having importance in acute allergic bronchoconstriction. Two lines of argument were used to support this contention: the failure of non-steroidal anti-inflammatory compounds to provide benefit in the disease and secondly, the ability of such drugs to produce bronchoconstriction in a group of sensitive individuals, possibly as a result of the redirecting arachidonic acid metabolism into lipoxygenase pathways. However, pulmonary mast cells activated by IgE cross-linkage are a rich source of the bronchoconstrictor prostanoid PGD_2 and this can be metabolized to $9\alpha,11\beta$-PGF_2 which is also a spasmogen on airway smooth muscle (2). Other cells, such as macrophages, which are proposed to be involved in the early events following allergen challenge are also sources of bronchoconstrictor cyclooxygenase products such as TXA_2.

More recent evidence suggests that bronchoconstrictor cyclooxygenase products do participate in acute allergic bronchoconstriction, although what role they might play in the cellular infiltration and exudative events of the disease is not clear. In a group of atopic subjects flurbiprofen (150 mg daily for 3 days) produced a significant attenuation of the immediate wave of bronchoconstriction induced by allergen, although it was without effect on bronchial responsiveness to histamine (6). One of the difficulties associated with the use of cyclooxygenase inhibitors such as flurbiprofen is that they also inhibit the production of PGE_2 and PGI_2 which are deemed to be bronchoprotective. In fact, this may be a part of the basis of their ability to precipitate aspirin-sensitive asthma in certain individuals.

There is now persuasive evidence that much of the bronchoconstrictor effect of PGD_2, its metabolite $9\alpha,11\beta$-PGF_2 and thromboxane A_2 are all mediated via thromboxane TP receptors. The orally active TP receptor antagonist GR-32191 in a single 80mg dose is capable of inhibiting the airways response to inhaled PGD_2 by causing a 10 (range 1.5->30)-fold shift in the concentration-FEV_1 response curve for PGD_2 (19). This represents 70% inhibition of the response to PGD_2 under these conditions. Furthermore, as shown in Table 1, in the same atopic subjects with mild asthma it produced an inhibition of the immediate airways response to inhaled allergen.

Table 1. Inhibition of allergen-induced immediate airways response by 80mg GR-32191.

Time	Area Under FEV_1 Time Course Curve	
(min)	Placebo	GR-32191
0-60	1822	1376[*]
0-90	2384	1738[*]

Data from 9 subjects. [*]$P<0.05$ compared to placebo.

The resurgence of interest in the possible role of cyclooxygenase products as bronchoconstrictor mediators has also prompted speculation about the possible benefit which thromboxane synthase inhibitors may offer.

EICOSANOIDS AND BRONCHIAL HYPERREACTIVITY

A greater understanding of the possible cellular and molecular mechanisms of asthma has by necessity led to changes in the way in which we think about possible therapeutic intervention in the disease. The late asthmatic reaction which occurs several hours after the immediate response to inhaled allergen is usually associated with a heightened bronchial responsiveness. Exciting progress is being made in unravelling the nature of these events which are believed to be more indicative of the underlying inflammatory processes in the airways mucosa.

A number of mediators have been suggested to be involved in the genesis of this bronchial hyperresponsiveness and TXA_2 is a leading candidate. In support of this, the thromboxane synthase inhibitor OKY-046 administered orally (3000mg over 4 days) to 10 asthmatic subjects reduced the bronchial responsiveness to inhaled acetylcholine but did not affect the baseline FEV_1 or FVC. No effect was seen when the compound was administered as an inhaled dose of 30mg (8). In contrast, in a randomised and double-blind study using 7 subjects with mild asthma, the Ciba-Geigy thromboxane synthase inhibitor CGS 12970 (100mg taken 12 hours and 1 hour prior to challenge) did not produce a significant change in the bronchial responsiveness to inhaled histamine either before, or 6 hours after, allergen provocation. Furthermore it was without effect on the area under the time course-FEV_1 response curve (4). Our own studies have shown that flurbiprofen (150mg p.o.), a dose which is capable of significantly inhibiting the immediate response to inhaled allergen and which provides total inhibition of platelet thromboxane formation, has no effect on the bronchial reactivity to either histamine or bradykinin in subjects with allergic asthma (unpublished observations).

ARE THE CLINICAL MODELS RELEVANT?

The unresolved role of eicosanoids in asthma and much of the clinical data currently available makes it possible to conclude that leukotrienes are not central to the pathogenesis of asthma. Alternatively, it could be argued that the compounds that have so far been the subject of limited evaluation in man are of insufficient potency to test the hypothesis correctly. There is truth in both of these statememts; eicosanoids are but some of the many effector molecules which could participate in the events underlying asthma and the question of how just potent these inhibitors and antagonists have to be to exert

significant effects is far from clear.   These issues have much
wider significance and implications beyond the question under
consideration here.

It is apparent that in the allergen-induced early reaction
in which mast cell-derived histamine appears to be the
predominant mediator, eicosanoids play smaller roles in the
resulting bronchoconstriction.   They may be more important in
the genesis of the late reaction and associated enhanced
bronchial responsiveness which are thought to result from more
'classical inflammatory events.   Recent investigations have
shown that patients with mild, stable asthma exhibit low levels
of mucosal inflammation in the airways without exhibiting major
exacerbations of disease activity.   Patients of this type have
commonly been used in acute studies of leukotriene antagonists
and lipoxygenase inhibitors.   However, the low level of airway
mucosal inflammation present may make this an unfair test of
the activity of these compounds.   Furthermore, it is not yet
clear whether the late reactions and changes in bronchial
responsiveness which can be studied in the clinical laboratory
are predictive for efficacy in day to day asthma.   If this is
is not the case then probably the most objective way of
evaluating drug candidates of this type is by measurement of
parameters such as symptom scores and bronchodilator usage.   In
situations where we hope drugs are likely to exert anti-
inflammatory effects it may be necessary to administer drugs
for extended periods to allow inflammation to subside and
healing/repair of damaged tissue to take place.

In order to undertake such trials it is obviously essential
that the compounds have the desired effects at the doses used.
With receptor anatgonists this can be established relatively
easily irrespective of whether the compound is administered
orally or by inhalation.   Compounds showing poor efficacy in
such simple tests are unlikely to be good candidates for larger
scale trials in the general population.   However, the situation
is less clear where the compound under test is an enzyme
inhibitor, particularly if the route of administration is by
inhalation.

One way in which this issue has been addressed is to use an
ex vivo test such as the inhibition of ionophore-induced LTB_4
release in whole blood or the formation of TXB_2 during
clotting.   Although this approach is useful there are numerous
situations where the activity of drugs against blood cells
fails to mirror the degree of inhibition seen in the lung.
This strategy is also of questionable relevance when the drug
is delivered by inhalation and minimal blood concentrations are
achieved.   The true value of these tests to clinical
development will probably only become apparent when a compound
is successfully taken through development and shown to have
clinical efficacy against the disease.   The N-hydroxyurea A-

64077 may prove useful in this respect being the first lipoxygenase inhibitor to have demonstrated oral bioavailability in man.

FUTURE DIRECTIONS

The involvement of many different types of chemical mediator in the pathogenesis of asthma has been suspected for many years. Although formal proof of the participation of some of these agents is becoming available the list of other participants, at both the regulatory and effector levels, is growing. It is possible that leukotriene antagonists or 5-lipoxygenase inhibitors may be developed which offer sufficiently high potency and duration of action to demonstrate clinical efficacy against the disease, particularly if there is extensive synergy between individual mediators and inflammatory cells. However, if this is not the case then the prospects for such approaches are not good.

An obvious alternative strategem is combination therapy. Compounds may possess multiple activities and attack several points in a mediator cascade. Interesting in this respect is that a single 50mg dose of SCH 37224, an inhibitor of LT and TX release, was shown to inhibit bronchoconstriction due to cold air isocapnic hyperventilation (10). If single compounds have marginal effects, then combination with an antihistamine, PAF antagonist or other therapeutic entity may produce some benefit. The motivation to opt for this approach may be close at hand, but it does create a difficult series of problems for industry and drug regulatory bodies alike. Combination therapy is expensive because of the requirements of regulatory authorities. However, the decision to take a compound which shows only little activity in man when used alone and put it into a development programme for combination therapy will not be an easy or inexpensive option to take.

Increasing knowledge of the regulatory networks which control the activity of immunocompetent cells and their mediators will inevitably result in a switch of emphasis in the level of pharmacological intervention in asthma. Similarly, the genetic components of the disease will yield to advances in molecular biology, and this will raise the real possibility of curing asthma and other allergic diseases. However, drugs which block the effects of eicosanoids may find a place in the management of asthma until these ambitious goals are achieved.

1. **Barnes, N.C., Piper, P.J., Costello, J.F.** (1987): J.Allergy Clin. Immunol., 79:816-821.
2. **Beasley, C.R.W., Featherstone, R.L., Church, M.K., Rafferty, P., Varley, J.G., Harris, A., Robinson, C., Holgate, S.T.** (1989): J. Appl. Physiol., 66:1685-1693.
3. **Bel, E.H., Timmers, M.C., Dijkman, J.H., Sterk, P.J.** (1989): Am. Rev. Respir. Dis., 139:A460.

4. Black, P.N., Salmon, B.T., Ewan,P., Fuller, R.W. (1989):
   Am. Rev. Respir. Dis., 139:A93.
5. Britton, J.R., Hanley, S.P., Tattersfield, A.E. (1987):
   J. Allergy Clin. Immunol., 79:811-816.
6. Curzen, N.C., Rafferty, P., Holgate, S.T. (1987): Thorax,
   42:946-952.
7. Eiser N, Hayhurst, M, Denman, W. (1989): Am. Rev. Respir.
   Dis., 139:A462.
8. Fujimara, M., Sasaki, F., Nakatsumi, Y., Takahashi, Y.,
   Hifumi, S., Taga, K., Mifune, J-I, Tanaka, T., Matsuda, T.
   (1986): Thorax, 41:955-959.
9. Fuller, R.W., Maltby, N., Richmond, R., Dollery, C.T.,
   Taylor, G.W., Ritter, W., Phillip, E. (1987). Br. J.
   Clin. Pharmacol., 23:677-681.
10. Israel, E., Rosenberg, M.A., Danzig, M.R., Fourre, J.,
    Drazen, J.M. (1989): Am. Rev. Respir. Dis., 139:A65.
11. Kips, J.C., Joos, G., Margolskee, D., Delepeleire, I.,
    Rogers, J.D., Pauwels, R., Van Der Straeten, M. (1989): Am.
    Rev. Respir. Dis., 139:A63.
12. Mann, J.S., Robinson, C., Sheridan, A.Q., Clement, P.,
    Bach, M.K., Holgate, S.T. (1986): Thorax, 41:746-752.
13. Okubo, T., Takahahi, H., Sumitomo, M., Shindoh, K.,
    Suzuki, S. (1987):Int. Archs. Allergy Appl. Immunol.,
    84:149-155.
14. Taylor, G.W., Taylor, I., Black, P., Maltby, N.H., Turner,
    N., Fuller, R.W., Dollery, C.T. (1989): Lancet, i:584-588.
15. Yamai, T., Watanabe, S., Motojima, S., Fukuda, T., Makino,
    S. (1989): Am. Rev. Respir. Dis., 139:A462.

Advances in Prostaglandin, Thromboxane,
and Leukotriene Research, Vol. 20,
edited by B. Samuelsson et al.
Raven Press, Ltd., New York © 1990.

MODIFICATION OF THE ARACHIDONIC ACID CASCADE THROUGH PHOSPHOLIPASE A₂ DEPENDENT MECHANISMS

Edward A. Dennis

Department of Chemistry
University of California at San Diego
La Jolla, CA 92093-0601, U.S.A.

The biosynthesis of the eicosanoids from the prostaglandins to the leuko-trienes, including the thromboxanes, prostacyclins, HETES and lipoxins, wheth-er synthesized by the cyclooxygenase pathway or the lipoxogenase pathway, all depend on the availability of free arachidonic acid. The control step for the pro-duction of that free arachidonic acid is believed to somehow involve an as yet undefined, or clearly very poorly defined, membrane-receptor event. Presum-ably, this involves the activation of a phospholipase [Review: Dennis (3)], either directly or through secondary mediators. Presumably, this phospholipase acts in or on membranes, but other subcellular localizations are possible as well. The simplest and most logical candidate for the kind of phospholipase involved would be a phospholipase A_2 [Review: Dennis (4)], because the bulk of the ara-chidonic acid is found esterified in the sn-2 position of membrane phospholipids as shown in Figure 1. When phospholipase A_2 acts to release free arachidonic

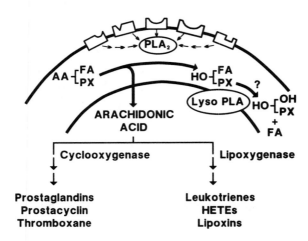

Figure 1: Role of Phospholipase A_2 in Arachidonic Acid Release. Adapted with permission from (4).

acid, the other product is a lysophospholipid. Lysophospholipids are biological detergents which are lytic to cell membranes [Review: Stafford and Dennis (12)] and they must either be reacylated or degraded further by a lysophospholipase to water soluble products as also shown in Figure 1.

Inhibitors of the cyclooxygenase pathway such as aspirin and the other non-steroidal anti-inflammatory drugs are well known, and inhibitors of the lipoxygenase pathway have been the object of active study. However, if one could inhibit the phospholipase A_2 step, one would have the potential of blocking both pathways. Indeed, the glucocorticoids such as cortisone have been suggested to act at the phospholipase A_2 step via "lipocortins", but we (2) have questioned this assumption; and we have recently considered the subject in detail elsewhere [Review: Davidson and Dennis (1)]. In summary, there is currently a great deal of interest in developing inhibitors of phospholipase A_2 not only for their obvious therapeutic potential, but also for the mechanistic insight they can provide about the enzymes mode of action at the lipid-water interface [Review: Dennis (4)].

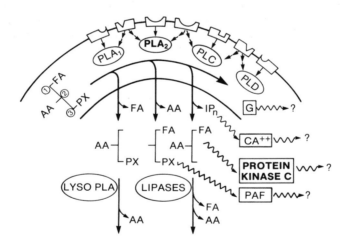

Figure 2. Role of Phospholipases in Cellular Activation. Adapted with permission from (5).

OTHER PHOSPHOLIPASES

Although a phospholipase A_2 would be the simplest and most logical candidate, other phospholipases could be possibly involved as well. Figure 2 shows the many possible ways that arachidonic acid can be liberated from the *sn*-2 position of membrane phospholipids. There are three possible first steps: a phospholipase A_1, a phospholipase A_2 or a phospholipase C. Phospholipase A_1 produces as product, a lysophospholipid, which requires a second enzyme, a lysophospholipase, to actually release the arachidonic acid. A phospholipase A_2 as described in Figure 1 releases arachidonic acid in a single step, producing as its second product a lysophospholipid. Phospholipase C produces as product a diglyceride, and this requires one or more additional lipases to actually release the arachidonic acid. If the phospholipid is an alkyl ether-containing phosphatidylcholine, and it is acted upon by phospholipase A_2, then in addition to arachidonic acid as product, the other product is an alkyl ether lysophospholipid, known as lyso-PAF, which upon acylation produces PAF or platelet activating factor, a potent cellular mediator. If the phospholipid is phosphatidylinositol or its higher phosphorylated forms and it is acted upon by PI-specific phospholipase C, then it produces as product inositol phosphate (or its higher phosphorylated forms), which mobilize intracellular Ca^{++}. The other product is diglyceride, which is an activator of protein kinase C. Exactly how these "lipid second messengers" are involved in cellular activation or just what role these play as well as phospholipase D, and/or G-proteins in the activation of the actual phospholipase A_2 leading to arachidonic acid release is unclear at this time, but is a subject of very active investigation in many laboratories (5).

PHOSPHOLIPASE A_2 STUDIES

Over the years, investigators looking at inhibitors of the phospholipases have relied almost exclusively on the study of the extracellular phospholipase A_2 either from snake venom or mammalian pancreas, because these

PHOSPHOLIPASES IN THE P388D$_1$ MURINE
MACROPHAGE-LIKE CELL LINE

Phospholipase	$[Ca^{++}]$	pH–Optimum	Localization
A_1	–	4	granules, lysosomes
A_2	– or low	7.5	cytoplasmic
A_2	+	7.5 – 9.5	membrane associated
Lyso	–	7 – 9	soluble

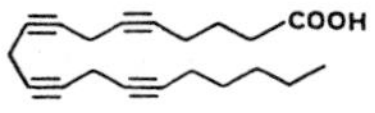

EICOSATETRAYONIC ACID (ETYA)

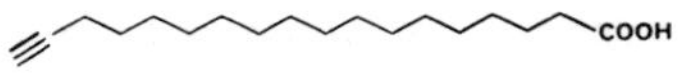

17-OCTADECYNOIC ACID (ODYA)

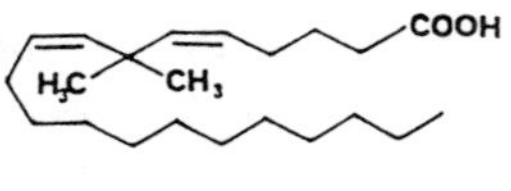

7,7-DIMETHYLEICOSADIENOIC ACID (DEDA)

Figure 3: Analogues of Arachidonic Acid.

enzymes are pure and small and could be studied mechanistically [Review: Dennis (3)]. One could develop paradigms, such as the "dual phospholipid model" (10), and develop kinetic approaches to study inhibitors. Several years ago, however, our laboratory felt that it was important to study the more relevant phospholipase A_2, the one actually involved in arachidonic acid release from relevant cells. For this reason, we turned our attention to the macrophage. We have initiated our studies on a macrophage-like cell line, P388D$_1$, as a model for the activated macrophage. This cell line has all of the characteristics of a macrophage, and most important for our purposes is that it produces arachidonic acid metabolytes in response to stimulii. When we initially examined these cells, we found that the phospholipases were ubiqitious, as they are with all cells. There are many phospholipases, and we initially separated and identified the major phospholipases in this cell (11), as summarized in Table I. Our initial focus has been on the membrane-associated, high pH-optimum

Ca^{2+}-dependent phospholipase A_2, which we (13) have solubilized and purified, and we (6) have carried out kinetic studies on this enzyme. We (14) have also purified to homogeneity a lysophospholipase, which is water-soluble, Ca^{2+}-independent, and has a neutral pH optimum and may play a role in the general metabolism of arachidonate in this cell.

INHIBITORS OF THE MACROPHAGE PHOSPHOLIPASE A_2

When we examined the affect of fatty acids on the activity of the membrane-associated macrophage phospholipase A_2, we (6) found that free fatty acids that were highly unsaturated were potent inhibitors of this enzyme. In particular, as one goes from palmitic acid to oleic acid to more unsaturated fatty acids such as arachidonic acid or eicosapentanoic acid, they are more potent as inhibitors. More careful kinetic analysis revealed that arachidonic acid is a competitive inhibitor of the enzyme with a K_I of about 5 μM. This led us to look at a number of analogs of natural fatty acids whose structures are shown in Figure 3. Interestingly, neither of the acetylenic-containing analogues inhibited the macrophage enzyme, whereas the dimethyl dienic analog of arachidonic acid (DEDA) was a potent inhibitor. DEDA had an IC_{50} of about 15 μM (7). It should be a reversible type of inhibitor.

Another inhibitor is manoalide, which is an irreversible inhibitor of the extracellular phospholipase A_2. Manoalide (Figure 4) is a natural product of sponge which has anti-inflammatory activity *in vivo* and has the interesting property of

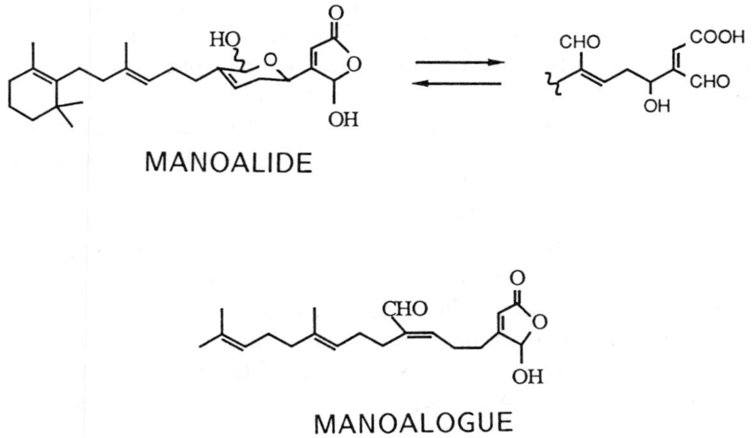

MANOALIDE

MANOALOGUE

Figure 4: Manoalide and Manoalogue.

also inhibiting phospholipase A_2 *in vitro*. It has two rings either of which can exist in an open form with alpha, beta unsaturated aldehydes which are potentially reactive groups (8). Manoalide inhibits the extracellular phospholipase A_2 in a time-dependent manner aided by Ca^{2+}, which is required for the enzyme, and protected by lysophospholipid which is a product of the enzyme. Subsequent to these studies, we have turned our attention to some synthetic analogs. The parent compound is manoalogue, which has the functionalities of manoalide, a lactone ring which can exist in the open form and an alpha-beta unsaturated aldehyde. We (9) have shown with the extracellular phospholipase that both the ability to exist in the open form and this functionality are necessary for its reaction in an irreversible manner because if one methylates the lactone ring or has an alcohol function instead of an aldehyde, manoalogue is not reactive.

With the macrophage enzyme, both manoalide and the synthetic analog, manoalogue are potent inhibitors with IC_{50}'s in the 13 and 26 μM range (7). Interestingly, they are not irreversible inhibitors of this enzyme, but rather, inhibit by a reversible mechanism. When we (7) looked at prostaglandin production by the intact $P388D_1$ cells, we found that this cell produces the usual prostaglandins in response to stimuli with the major prostaglandins being PGE_2 and PGD_2. We have focused in our initial experiments on the use of Ca^{2+} ionophore A23187 as a stimulus of PGE_2 production. When we looked specificially at the effect of manoalide and manoalogue on PGE_2 production in the presence of the ionophore, we found that both manoalide and manoalogue were potent inhibitors of prostaglandin production in the μM range.

With both manoalogue and manoalide, we have correlated the inhibition of prostaglandin generation *in vivo* with an inhibition of the release of labeled arachidonic acid from the phospholipids. This data on intact cells is correlated directly with the *in vitro* inhibition of the purified phospholipase A_2. This opens the possibility that the process being studied *in vitro* has the same inhibitory characteristics as that in the intact cell. Interestingly, DEDA which inhibits the macrophage phospholipase A_2 *in vitro* and PGE_2 production in the intact cell does not block release of labeled arachidonic acid in the intact cells suggesting that it is not acting at the phospholipase A_2 level. Also, para-bromophenacyl bromide, a potent, and irreversible inhibitor of the extracellular phospholipase A_2 neither inhibits PGE_2 production in the intact cells nor the isolated macrophage enzyme *in vitro*. Of the compounds studied, only manoalogue and manoalide showed a correlation of inhibition of arachidonic acid release in the intact cell and inhibition of a phospholipase A_2 isolated from it. Further work is underway to determine if this phospholipase A_2 is the relevant one in vivo.

ACKNOWLEDGEMENT

Financial support for our work on phospholipase A_2 has been provided by National Science Foundation grant DMB-88-17392, National Institutes of Health grants GM 20,501 and HD 26171 and the Lilly Research Laboratories. I wish to thank my students and collaborators who carried out the studies referred to herein.

REFERENCES

1. Davidson, F. F., and Dennis, E. A. (1989): *Biochem. Pharm.* In press
2. Davidson, F. F., Dennis, E. A., Powell, M., and Glenney, J. (1987): *J. Biol. Chem.*, 262: 1698-1705.
3. Dennis, E. A. (1983): *in The Enzymes, Third Edition, Vol. 16,* (Boyer, P., Edit.) Academic Press, New York, 307-353
4. Dennis, E. A. (1987): *Bio/Technology,* 5: 1294-1300.
5. Dennis, E. A. (1989): in *Cell Activation and Signal Initiation: Receptor and Phospholipase Control of Inositol Phosphate, PAF and Eicosanoid Production, UCLA Symposia on Molecular and Cellular Biology - New Series, Vol. 106,* (E. A. Dennis, A. Hunter, M. Berridge, Edits.) Alan R. Liss, New York. In press.
6. Lister, M. D., Deems, R. A., Watanabe, Y., Ulevitch, R. J, and Dennis, E. A. (1988): *J. Biol. Chem.*, 263: 7506-7513.
7. Lister, M. D., Glaser, K. B., Ulevitch, R. J., and Dennis, E. A. (1989): *J. Biol. Chem.*, 264: 8520-8528.
8. Lombardo, D., and Dennis, E. A. (1985): *J. Biol. Chem.*, 260: 7234-7240.
9. Reynolds, L. J., Morgan, B. P., Hite, G. A., Mihelich, E. D., and Dennis, E. A. (1988): *J. Am. Chem. Soc.*, 110: 5172-5177.
10. Roberts, M. F., Deems, R. A., and Dennis, E. A. (1977): *Proc. Nat'l. Acad. Sci. U.S.A.*, 74: 1950-1954.
11. Ross, M. I., Deems, R. A., Jesaitis, A. J., Dennis, E. A., and Ulevitch, R. J. (1985): *Arch. Biochem. Biophys.*, 238: 247-258.
12. Stafford, R. E., and Dennis, E. A. (1988): *Colloids and Surfaces*, 30: 47-64.
13. Ulevitch, R. J., Sano, M, Watanabe, Y., Lister, M. D., Deems, R. A., and Dennis, E. A. (1988): *J. Biol. Chem.*, 263: 3079-3085.
14. Zhang, Y., and Dennis, E. A. (1988): *J. Biol. Chem.*, 263: 9965-9972.

Advances in Prostaglandin, Thromboxane, and Leukotriene Research, Vol. 20, edited by B. Samuelsson et al. Raven Press, Ltd., New York © 1990.

ESSENTIAL FATTY ACID DEFICIENCY: PROBING THE ROLE OF ARACHIDONATE IN BIOLOGY

J. B. Lefkowith

Div. of Rheumatology, Washington University
School of Medicine, St. Louis, MO 63110 USA

INTRODUCTION

Mammals have an absolute requirement for dietary (n-6) fatty acids. In the 1930's, Burr and Burr were able to induce a state of essential fatty acid (EFA) deficiency in rats by feeding them a fat-free diet for several weeks (2,3). Several pathophysiologic effects were noted by them: in particular, growth retardation, dermatitis, caudal necrosis, reproductive inefficiency, and renal papillary necrosis. These effects were reversed or stabilized by dietary linoleate. Biochemically, EFA deficiency is characterized by a decrease in tissue (n-6) and (n-3) fatty acids and by an accumulation of (n-9) fatty acids (10). Specifically, there is an accumulation of 20:3(n-9), termed Mead acid, which is not a constituent of normal tissues (6). The ratio of the Mead acid to arachidonate has been used to define the deficiency state: a ratio of greater than 0.4 being the biochemical criterion of EFA deficiency (9).

The discovery in the 1960's that the (n-6) fatty acid, arachidonate, could be metabolized to the biologically active prostaglandin E_2 (1) linked the fields of essential fatty acid deficiency and arachidonic acid metabolism. Since then, a host of biologically active metabolites of arachidonate have been discovered (i.e. the thromboxanes, leukotrienes, and P450 metabolites) (22). Consequently, there has been a resurgence in interest in EFA deficiency as a tool to probe the role of arachidonate and its metabolites in biological phenomena.

THE BIOCHEMISTRY OF EFA DEFICIENCY

Despite long-standing recognition of the state of EFA deficiency and some of the corresponding alterations in tissue polyunsaturated fatty acids, the tenacity with which the organism can conserve arachidonate is often underestimated. Animals are able to retain arachidonate in membrane lipids in certain tissues to a remarkable degree despite maximal restriction of dietary essential fatty acids. In recent studies it has been shown that the effect of EFA deprivation on the arachidonate content of different tissues is quite different, and that the phospholipids within tissues vary markedly in their ability to retain arachidonate (16). Specifically, when mice are placed on a fat-free diet, hepatic lipids are readily depleted of arachidonate. In contrast, the renal cortex tenaciously retains arachidonate, whereas the heart actually increases its content of arachidonate. The increase in cardiac arachidonate occurs due to the selective accumulation of arachidonate within the phospholipid phosphatidylethanolamine (PE). The renal cortex retains arachidonate less selectively in PE, phosphatidylserine (PS) and phosphatidylcholine (PC). Phosphatidylinositol (PI) is unique among phospholipids in that it is invariably depleted of arachidonate regardless of the tissue.

Experiments on the mechanisms behind these tissue-specific changes in arachidonate using labelled fatty acids have elucidated a general mechanism for the conservation of arachidonic acid (16). Labelled arachidonate initially localizes to the liver following an intraperitoneal injection in EFA-deficient animals. Over a period of several days, the liver is depleted of label whereas the heart and renal cortex accumulate several times the activity of their respective control organs. In the heart, this accumulation is selective for PE. In the renal cortex accumulation is more generalized. This enhanced uptake is specific for arachidonate over 20:3(n-9). These studies suggest that the liver serves to supply other tissues with arachidonate in EFA deficiency, and that the heart and renal cortex both contain mechanisms to accumulate arachidonate selectively in certain phospholipids.

Specific enzymes which may be responsible for the conservation of arachidonate have been described. A fatty acid-CoA synthetase selective for arachidonate has been found in several different cell types and tissues (15). These cells and tissues also contain a nonspecific fatty acid-CoA synthetase; however, levels of the specific enzyme are usually equal to or greater than the nonspecific one. Only liver and adipose tissue contain significantly lower levels of the selective enzyme. Although an arachidonoyl-specific CoA synthetase might be responsible for a generalized conservation of arachidonate in EFA deficiency, such an enzyme would not explain preferential phospholipid incorporation of arachidonate within a tissue. An acyl-transferase which is selective for essential fatty acids, however, is present in cardiac cytosol (21). The preferential retention of arachidonate within PE in the EFA-deficient heart may reflect the in vivo expression of such an enzyme.

EFA DEFICIENCY AND LIPID MEDIATOR PRODUCTION

By utilizing EFA deficiency to manipulate tissue arachidonate, the availability of membrane-bound arachidonate for the production of prostaglandins is elucidated.   Despite the conservation of cardiac and renal arachidonate seen with EFA deficiency, the EFA-deficient heart and kidney when perfused ex vivo and stimulated with the receptor-mediated agonist angiotensin II produce only a fraction (25-30%) of the prostaglandin produced by the corresponding control organ (16).   When the non-specific stimulus of ischemia (11) is used, however, the EFA-deficient heart and kidney produce equal amounts of prostaglandin compared to the corresponding control organ (16).   These differences are not attributable to differences in either cyclooxygenase activity or reacylation ability.

Since PI is the only phospholipid depleted of arachidonate in the heart and renal cortex with EFA deficiency (16), these data suggest that PI is the principal source of arachidonate for metabolism in response to receptor-mediated stimulation.   It is noteworthy that PI is quantitatively a relatively minor pool of arachidonate in these organs.   Phospholipids other than PI may supply arachidonate for metabolism in response to the non-specific stimulus of ischemia.

The accumulation of 20:3(n-9) in EFA deficiency also has important implications regarding the effects of the deficiency state on eicosanoid production.   20:3(n-9) is a relatively poor substrate for cyclooxygenase, but it is metabolized in a calcium-dependent and indomethacin-inhibitable fashion by this enzyme (4).   The reaction products are several mono- and di-hydroxy eicosanoids as opposed to cyclized prostaglandin-like products. The major product is 13-hydroxy-5,8,11-eicotrienoate with small amounts of 11-hydroxy, 9-hydroxy, or dihydroxy compounds formed.   The biological effects of these metabolites have yet to be established.   20:3(n-9) is also not particularly effective in inhibiting the metabolism of arachidonate by cyclooxygenase (18).

20:3(n-9), however, is a good substrate for the 5-lipoxygenase pathway. 20:3(n-9) competes effectively with arachidonate with respect to the formation of leukotriene(LT)C (18).   Both LTC_3 and LTC_4 are formed by EFA-deficient leukocytes depending on the relative ratios of the fatty acid precursors.   In contrast, EFA deficiency markedly inhibits the formation of LTB (18)   This observation appears to be due to the fact that LTA_3, formed from 20:3(n-9), is a potent inhibitor of, but not a particularly good substrate for, LTA hydrolase (5). LTA_3 appears to bind to LTA hydrolase preventing its own conversion to LTB_3 and preventing the conversion of LTA_4 to LTB_4.

EFA deficiency has also been shown to inhibit the elaboration of platelet activating factor (PAF) by leukocytes although PAF is not directly derived from arachidonate (24).   The mechanism of this inhibition is unclear but may be due to the fact that alkylarachidonoyl-PC is the preferred substrate (as opposed to alklyacyl-PC with 20:3(n-9) in the 2 position) for the phospholipase required for the formation of lyso-PAF (25).   Thus, EFA deficiency has the capacity to inhibit lipid mediators not directly derived from arachidonate.

THE EFFECTS OF EFA DEFICIENCY ON
IMMUNOINFLAMMATORY PHENOMENA

EFA deficiency has been particularly useful in understanding the role of arachidonate and its metabolites in models of tissue inflammation. Part of the anti-inflammatory effect of EFA deficiency can be directly attributed to the marked decrease in LTB_4 generation seen in in vitro studies. In a model of acute inflammation, EFA deficiency markedly inhibited the in vivo elaboration of LTB_4 and also attenuated the subsequent influx of polymorphonuclear neutrophils (PMN) (19). A pathogenic role for LTB_4 in this model of inflammation was established by showing that BW755C, a cyclooxygenase-lipoxygenase inhibitor, also inhibited the generation of LTB_4 in vivo and led to a decrease in PMN influx comparable to EFA deficiency.

However, not all of the effects of EFA deficiency in inflammation appear to be attributable to the inhibition of LTB_4. EFA deficiency is particularly effective in ameliorating immune-mediated glomerulonephritis. EFA deficiency attenuates the glomerulonephritis seen in murine lupus leading to a dramatic prolongation in survival (12). The reasons behind this protective effect have been the subject of recent investigations. Using a model of immune-mediated glomerulonephritis in rats, nephrotoxic nephritis, it was seen that EFA deficiency markedly decreased the influx of leukocytes into the glomerulus in the context of glomerular inflammation (29). The invasion of PMNs at 3 hrs. was not affected by EFA deficiency; however, the deficiency state completely prevented the influx of macrophages later on. The influx of leukocytes into the glomerulus in this model of renal injury was accompanied by a marked enhancement in glomerular arachidonate metabolism as well as renal dysfunction (manifested as azotemia, polyuria, sodium retention, and proteinuria)(29). With EFA deficiency, the increase in glomerular arachidonate metabolism was markedly attenuated. EFA deficiency also prevented the azotemia, polyuria, and sodium retention seen in control animals and decreased the proteinuria by 70-90%.

EFA deficiency appears to provide a unique model of inhibited macrophage elicitation. This diminished influx of macrophages into a focus of inflammation occurs without the use of systemic immunosuppressive manipulations which have been used in other studies on the abrogation of glomerular inflammation (8,26). The mechanism by which EFA deficiency interferes with macrophage elicitation in the context of nephritis, however, remains to be clarified. It is clear from previous data that this effect is not a simple function of a depletion of circulating monocytes (17). It also appears that macrophage chemotactic responsiveness is not impaired by EFA deficiency (29). EFA-deficient cells are attracted to complement fragments comparably to control cells.

A possible explanation of the diminished macrophage influx is that EFA deficiency impairs a signalling mechanism attracting macrophages into the glomerulus during the course of nephritis. Although LTB_4 is a logical candidate for such a mediator since its elaboration is increased in nephritis and since EFA deficiency decreases its elaboration (29), LTB_4 is relatively inactive with respect to macrophage migration (29). Additionally, glomerular LTB_4 synthesis is increased in models of glomerular immune complex injury which do not involve the influx of leukocytes (23). Thus although LTB_4 may play a role in glomerulonephritis it is not likely to be the agent which elicits macrophages into the glomerulus. The mechanism behind the impaired elicitation of macrophages into the glomerulus in nephritis remains to be determined.

The protective effect of EFA deficiency in inflammatory renal disease is also seen in experimental hydronephrosis (30) and interstitial nephritis induced by the administration of puromycin aminonucleoside (7). In the former model, EFA deficiency impairs the influx of macrophages into the renal cortex and attenuates the enhancement in renal arachidonate metabolism as it does in glomerulonephritis (30). In the latter model the deficiency state prevents the profound decreases in renal blood flow and glomerular filtration seen acutely after the administration of puromycin aminonucleoside (7). The infiltration of macrophages into the renal interstitium seen concurrently with the decline in renal function is also prevented by the deficiency state. Thus the use of EFA deficiency may help elucidate fundamental mechanisms underlying renal inflammation and the accompanying renal dysfunction.

The striking inhibition of macrophage migration with EFA deficiency seen in glomerulonephritis may be relevant to some of the anti-inflammatory effects of the deficiency state in models of autoimmune disease not involving the kidney. EFA deficiency has been shown to prevent the insulitis and consequent diabetes in two different models of autoimmune diabetes: the low dose streptozotocin model in mice (32) and the diabetes-prone inbred BB rat (20). In the former model EFA deficiency virtually completely protected against the diabetes which resulted from the repetitive administration of low doses of streptozotocin, a beta cell toxin (32). In these studies EFA-deficient mice were also repleted with linoleate beginning 3 days after the last streptozotocin injection. These repleted animals acquired diabetes comparably to controls. These results show that EFA deficiency did not prevent the injury due to streptozotocin but rather prevented the subsequent expression of the inflammatory response. Because macrophages are the first cells to infiltrate the islets after the injection of low-dose streptozotocin (13,14), the rate of migration of macrophages into islets immediately after injection of streptozotocin could differ between the two groups and thus explain the protective effect of EFA deficiency.

The protective effect of EFA deficiency in the diabetes-prone BB rat model is also quite striking (20). EFA deficiency reduced the incidence of diabetes in these animals and delayed its onset. In this model it was possible to correlate the changes in fatty acids induced by the deficiency state with the degree of protection. These studies showed that the protective effect correlated most closely with the depletion of arachidonate rather than the accumulation of 20:3(n-9) implying that the protective effect was more likely due to a lack of arachidonate or a metabolite rather than the presence of 20:3(n-9).

EFA deficiency also has the capacity to alter tissue immunogenicity in addition to its effects on the inflammatory response. One early observation on the effects of EFA deficiency on the kidney was that the resident macrophages which reside within the glomerulus and the interstitium are depleted by the deficiency state (17). These cells have the capacity to express class II major histocompatibility antigens (Ia antigens) and stimulate allogeneic lymphocytes in a mixed lymphocyte response (27). Their depletion has profound consequences regarding the transplantation of the kidney. EFA-deficient kidneys are less immunogenic when transplanted to an unrelated donor compared to kidneys from control animals (28). This decrease in immunogenicity could be overcome by injecting the recipients with Ia-positive cells at the time of transplantation implying that the depletion of Ia-positive cells induced by EFA deficiency was responsible for the protective effect (28).

The effect of EFA deficiency on Ia-positive cells in tissues other than the kidney, however, is quite different. In the skin, EFA deficiency leads to a marked increase in Ia-bearing cells (31). This increase in Ia-positive cells appears to be due to an increase in the expression of Ia by keratinocytes rather than a change in the number of the resident dendritic cells within skin which are normally the only cell within the epidermis which expresses Ia. Epidermal cells from EFA-deficient animals are consequently more potent immunologically than cells from normal animals in the presentation of antigen to T lymphocytes and the stimulation of allogeneic lymphocytes. This increase in potency appears to result directly from the increase in Ia expression in EFA-deficient epidermal cells rather than from changes in cytokine (i.e. interleukin-1) release or decreased prostaglandin production. These results suggest that arachidonate or a metabolite may be involved in the regulation of Ia expression by keratinocytes in vivo.

SUMMARY

EFA deficiency appears to be a uniquely useful tool in probing the role of arachidonate in a variety of physiologic and pathologic processes. Recent studies have clarified the effects of the deficiency state on tissue fatty acid content and on the production of metabolites of arachidonate and related mediators such as PAF. The ability of EFA deficiency to ameliorate a variety of inflammatory states, particularly models of autoimmune disease, is striking. The central mechanism appears to be the ability of EFA deficiency to inhibit leukocyte migration into foci of inflammation. The mechanisms underlying this phenomenon are currently under investigation. Additionally EFA deficiency has the capacity to alter dramatically tissue immunogenicity by affecting the representation of Ia-bearing cells within tissues. The role of arachidonate in the regulation of Ia-bearing cells within tissues is an area of continuing interest.

ACKNOWLEDGEMENTS

This work was supported by NIH grants DK-37879 and AI-27457. Dr. Lefkowith is also the recipient of an International Life Sciences Institute award.

REFERENCES

1. Bergstrom, S., Danielsson, H. and Samuelsson, B. (1964): *Biochim. Biophys. Acta*, 90:207-210.
2. Burr, G.O. and Burr, M.M. (1929): *J. Biol. Chem.*, 82:345-367.
3. Burr, G.O. and Burr, M.M. (1930): *J. Biol. Chem.*, 86:587-621.
4. Elliott, W.J., Morrison, A.R., Sprecher, H. and Needleman, P. (1986): *J. Biol Chem.*, 261:6719-6724.
5. Evans, J.F., Nathaniel, D.J., Zamboni, R.J. and Ford-Hutchinson, A.W. (1985): *J. Biol. Chem.*, 260:10966-10970.
6. Fulco, A. and Mead, J.F. (1959): *J. Biol. Chem.*, 234:1411-1416.
7. Harris, K.P.G., Klahr, S. and Schreiner, G.F. (1989): *Clin. Res.*, 37:491.
8. Holdsworth, S.R., Neale, T.J., and Wilson, C.B. (1981): *J. Clin. Invest.*, 68:686-698.
9. Holman, R.T. (1960): *J. Nutrition*, 70:405-410.
10. Holman, R.T. (1968): *Prog. Chem. Fats Other Lipids*, 9:279-348.
11. Hsueh, W., Isakson, P.C. and Needleman, P. (1977): *Prostaglandins*, 13:1073-1091.
12. Hurd, E.R., Johnston, J.M., Okita, J.R., MacDonald, P.C., Ziff, M. and Gilliam, J.N. (1981): *J. Clin. Invest.* 67:476-485.
13. Kolb, H. (1987): *Diabetes/Metab. Rev.*, 3:751-778.
14. Kolb-Bachofen, V., Epstein, S., Kiesel, U. and Kolb, H. (1988): *Diabetes*, 37:21-27.
15. Laposata, M., Reich, E.L., and Majerus, P.W. (1985): *J. Biol. Chem.*, 260:11016-11020.
16. Lefkowith, J.B., Flippo, V., Sprecher, H., and Needleman, P. (1985): *J. Biol. Chem.*, 260:15736-15744.
17. Lefkowith, J.B. and Schreiner, G.F. (1987): *J. Clin. Invest.*, 80:947-956.
18. Lefkowith, J.B., Jakschik, B.A., Stahl, P. and Needleman, P. (1987): *J. Biol. Chem.*, 262:6668-6675.
19. Lefkowith, J.B. (1988): *J. Immunol.*, 140:228-233.
20. Lefkowith, J., Rossini, A., Mordes, J., Handler, E., Lacy, P., Wright, J., Cormier, J., and Schreiner, G.F. (1989): *FASEB J.*, 3:300.
21. Needleman, P. Wyche, A., Sprecher, H., Elliott, W.J. and Evers, A.S. (1985): *Biochim. Biophys. Acta*, 836:267-273.

22. Needleman, P., Turk, J., Jakschik, B.A., Morrison, A.R. and Lefkowith, J.B. (1986): *Ann. Rev. Biochem.*, 55:69-102.
23. Rahman, M.A., Nakazawa, M., Emancipator, S.N., and Dunn, M.J. (1988): *J. Clin. Invest.*, 81:1945-1952.
24. Ramesha, C.S. and Pickett, W.C. (1986): *J. Biol. Chem.*, 261:7592-7595.
25. Ramesha, C.S. and Pickett, W.C. (1987): *J. Lipid Res.*, 28:326-331.
26. Schreiner, G.F., Cotran, R.S., Pardo, V., and Unanue, E.R. (1978): *J. Exp. Med.*, 147:369-384.
27. Schreiner, G.F., Kiely, J.M., Cotran, R.S. and Unanue, E.R. (1981): *J. Clin. Invest.*, 68:920-931.
28. Schreiner, G.F., Flye, W., Brunt, E., Korber, K. and Lefkowith, J.B. (1988): *Science*, 240:1032-1033.
29. Schreiner, G.F., Rovin, B. and Lefkowith, J.B. (1989): *J. Immunol.*, 143:3192-3199.
30. Spaethe, S.M., Freed, M.S., De Schryver-Kecskemeti, K., Lefkowith, J.B., and Needleman, P. (1987): *J. Pharmacol. Exp. Ther.*, 245:1088-1094.
31. Udey, M.C., Peck, R.D., Schreiner, G.F. and Lefkowith, J.B. (1989): *Clin. Res.*, 37:687.
32. Wright, J., Lefkowith, J.B., Schreiner, G.F., and Lacy, P. (1988): *Proc. Natl. Acad. Sci. USA*, 85:6137-6141.

Advances in Prostaglandin, Thromboxane,
and Leukotriene Research, Vol. 20,
edited by B. Samuelsson et al.
Raven Press, Ltd., New York © 1990.

THE MODIFICATION OF THE ARACHIDONIC ACID CASCADE BY n-3 FATTY ACIDS

Peter C. Weber

Universität München, Institut für Prophylaxe und
Epidemiologie der Kreislaufkrankheiten,
Pettenkoferstr. 9, 8000 München 2, F.R.G.

Eicosanoids, the oxygenation products of
arachidonic acid (AA; C20:4n-6) or related 20-carbon
polyunsaturated fatty acids are involved in the
physiology and pathophysiology of haemostasis, the
immune response, atherothrombotic, allergic and chronic
inflammatory disorders. Interference with eicosanoid
formation is a characteristic of steroidal and non-
steroidal antiinflammatory agents, antiplatelet and
other cardiovascular drugs, and - in conjunction with
the design of eicosanoid receptor blockers - a target
of refined pharmacological intervention strategies. A
change of the arachidonic acid cascade and eicosanoid-
dependent cellular functions may, however, also be
achieved by a nutritional modification of the eicosanoid precursor fatty acid pool.

Eicosanoids' Role in Cell Function

Eicosanoids and related lipid mediators, such as
1,2 DAG or PAF, function as a modulatory device in
stimulus-response coupling and for cell to cell
communication. Some eicosanoids, like TXA2 and LTB4,
might amplify an initial (Ca++-related) signal for
cell activation by stimulating specific membrane
receptors coupled to phospholipases (PLC, PLA2),
thereby further increasing intracellular Ca++-
concentrations. Other eicosanoids, such als PGI2 or
PGD2 - via an increase of cAMP - might, on the
contrary, blunt an initial signal for cell activation
by decreasing intracellular Ca++ release. A pharmacological modification of phospholipases, cyclooxygenase and lipoxygenase activities or eicosanoid
receptors and/or nutritional manipulation of membrane
fatty acid composition and the eicosanoid precursor
pool, leading to a qualitative change in the spectrum
of eicosanoids formed might, therefore, act by
modifying this modulating system of cell function; see
Figure 1. During the last couple of years the bio-

chemistry of marine long-chain n-3 fatty acids and their eicosanoids and their influence on the arachidonic acid cascade and related cellular function has attracted increasing attention (4,19, 35,38).

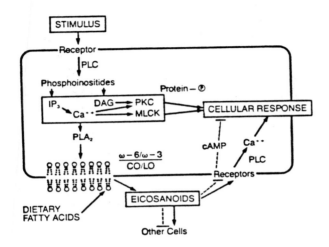

Fig.1. Scheme of the putative role of n-6 and n-3 eicosanoid precursor fatty acids in membrane phospholipids as determined by dietary intake and their eicosanoids for the modulation of stimulus-response coupling and cell communication. PLC, phopholipase C; IP3, inostitol trisphosphate: DAG, 1,2 diacylglycerol; PKC, protein kinase C; MLCK, myosin light chain kinase; PLA2, phospholipase A2; CO, cyclooxygenase; LO, lipooxygenase: Protein-P, phosphorylated protein.

Dietary Fatty Acids and the Eicosanoid System

Under our "Western" dietary conditions, arachidonic acid is by far the dominant direct precursor fatty acid for eicosanoid formation. In the mammalian organism fatty acids belonging to different families, such as n-3 and n-6 fatty acids, cannot be interconverted . Nutritional intake, therefore, determines the fatty acid composition in plasma and in cell membranes (Figure 2). In vivo in the adult organism the formation of the eicosanoid precursor fatty acids from their respective short-chain parent fatty acids, C18:2n-6 or C18:3n-3, is a slow process. This implies that the long-chain eicosanoid precursor fatty acids in the diet might have a more direct and actual effect

on the eicosanoid precursor pool (32). In the marine
food chain there is accumulation of the long-chain n-3
derivatives of 18:3n-3, that is eicosapentaenoic (EPA
C20:5n-3) and docosahexaenoic (DHA C22:6n-3) acids in
the lipids of zooplankton and fishes. Several independent lines of evidence suggest that an increased
intake of those long-chain n-3 fatty acids leads to a
reduction of atherothrombotic, inflammatory and proliferative disorders (3,4,5,16,17,27).

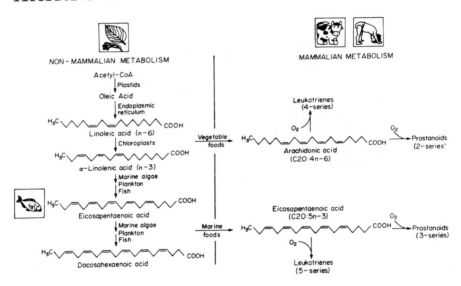

Fig.2. Origin and metabolism of n-6 and n-3 polyunsaturated fatty acids and biosynthesis of eicosanoids from arachidonic acid (C20:4n-6) and eicosapentaenoic acid (C20:5n-3).

Functional Effects of n-3 Fatty Acids

n-3 fatty acid enriched diets induce a series of
functional alterations that may unterlie its
beneficial effects: they reduce blood pressure and
decrease vascular reactivity (24), they reduce
platelet aggregability (31,32,35) and increase
platelet survival (22), reduce chemotaxis and inflammatory potential of white blood cells (7,11,10,33,36)
and reduce vascular cell proliferation (20,37).
Although the causative factors for these effects have
only partially been identified , alterations by n-3
fatty acids of the arachidonic acid cascade and
related cellular functions are assumed to play a major
role (39).

Biochemical Effects of n-3 Fatty Acids

n-3 fatty acids in the diet are rapidly absorbed and incorporated into plasma lipids over a period of hours (32). Incorporation of these fatty acids into cellular membrane phopholipids takes longer and appears to occur during cell formation, at least under in vivo conditions in the not stimulated cell (31,32). Dietary EPA and DHA, which partially replace (24,35) and redistribute (13) arachidonic· acid (AA) in a specific time- and dose-dependent manner lipids (24, 31,35) induce a series of biochemical events, summarized in Table 1.

Once incorporated into cellular membranes, EPA and DHA are less readily released upon cell stimulation (9), reducing substrate availability for eicosanoid generation and decreasing potent amplification mechanisms (e.g. oxygen free radicals (11)), to which AA metabolites contribute, e.g. as a cellular response to injury. In addition to reducing AA levels (24,35) and most of its eicosanoid derivatives (31,35), n-3 fatty acids EPA and also DHA, which can be rapidly retroconverted to EPA (10), serve as precursors to a class of eicosanoids (8,31,36) with an attenuated and desirable spectrum of biological activity: TXA3 formed in small quantities in n-3 fatty acid enriched platelets in addition to a significantly reduced TXA2 formation is almot inactive as platelet aggregator and vasoconstrictor (4,35). LTB5 formed from EPA in neutrophils and monocytes/macrophages (36) is one order of magnitude less active as a chemotactic agent as compared to LTB4, which in addition, is reduced after prolonged dietary n-3 fatty acids. In contrast, PGI3, which is formed from dietary n-3 fatty acids in amounts of up to 50% of an unchanged synthesis of PGI2 (8,31), is biologically as active as PGI2 to inhibit platelet aggregation and adhesion and to reduce vascular tone, thereby increasing the thrombo- resistance of endothelial cells.

Formation of platelet activating factor, PAF, is also reduced by n-3 fatty acids through interference with the turnover of the PAF precursor pool (30,40). In addition, the formation and action of endothelial derived relaxation factor, EDRF, is increased by n-3 fatty acids (25,29) thereby decreasing vasospastic responses, e.g. of coronary arteries, to vasoconstrictors. Recently, other important factors involved in atherosclerosis and inflammation have been found to be profoundly affected by n-3 fatty acids. The formation of the cytokines, interleukin 1, Il1 and tumor necrosis factors, TNF, in mononuclear cells is

Table 1
Effects of n-3 Fatty Acid (n-3 FA) on Factors involved
in Atherothrombosis and Inflammation.

Factor	Effect of n-3 FA	Function	Ref.
Arachidonic Acid, AA	↓	eicosanoid precursor; aggregates platelets; inhibits retinoic acid binding	(35) (24) (28)
Thromboxane, TXA2	↓	platelet aggregation; vasoconstriction; increase of i.c.Ca++	(31)
Leukotriene, LTB4	↓	neutrophil chemoattractant; increase of i.c.Ca++	(36)
Prostacyclin, PGI2/3	↑	prevent platelet aggregation; vasodilatation; increase cAMP;	(8)
PAF	↓	activates platelets and WBL	(30)
Oxygen free Radicals	↓	cellular damage; enhance LDL uptake via scavenger pathway; stimulate arachidonic acid metabolism	(11)
Lipid Hydroperoxides	↓	stimulate eicosanoid formation	(19)
EDRF	↑	reduces arterial vasoconstrictor response	(29)
PDGF	↓	chemoattractant and mitogen for smooth muscles and macrophages	(12)
Interleukin 1, Il1 and Tumor necrosis factor, TNF	↓	stimulate neutrophil O2 free radical formation; stimulate lymphocyte proliferation; stimulate SMC proliferation; stimulate PAF; express intercellular adhesion molecule-1 on endothelial cells; inhibit plasminogen activator - thus procoagulants	(7)
TPA	↑	increases endogenous fibrinolysis	(2)
Fibrinogen	↓	blood clotting factor	(15)

significantly suppressed in human volunteers 6 weeks
on and as long as 10 weeks after cessation of fish
oil supplementation (7). As well, the production in
bovine endothelial cell cultures of PDGF - like
protein is significantly suppressed by n-3 fatty acids
(12). In conjunction with their modulatoy effects on
the arachidonic acid cascade n-3 fatty acids exert an
antiatherothrombotic and anti-inflammatory effect that
will interfere at several steps e.g. in the
pathogenesis of atherosclerosis; see Figure 3.

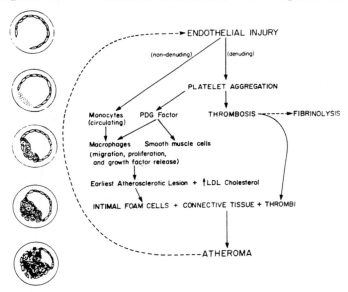

Fig.3. Sequential steps in the pathogenesis of atherosclerosis. Note that n-3 fatty acids interfere in
several places with the atherosclerotic process
(compare Table 1).

In addition, n-3 fatty acids influence other
factors which are of pathophysiological significance
in atherothrombotic disorders: n-3 fatty acids increase tissue plasminogen activator, TPA (2), thereby
increasing endogenous fibrinolytic activity of blood
and decrease fibrinogen levels (15), thereby
reducing the coagulation potential. n-3 fatty acids,
furthermore, decrease the synthesis and secretion,
and thereby blood levels of VLDL and triglycerides in

volunteers and patients (14). Although total or LDL cholesterol concentrations are not significantly affected by n-3 fatty acids (14), LDL-particle size, which is directly correlated to its atherogenicity, may be reduced, possibly through inhibition of LCAT activity by n-3 fatty acids (26).

Future studies

The further evaluation of the relationship of n-6 versus n-3 fatty acids and their eicosanoids to membrane receptor function, the modulation of transmembrane signaling mechanisms, phospholipase activation, formation of 1,2 DAG and PAF, Ca++-release (1), inositol phosphate turnover (1,23) and gene expression (34) should contribute to a better understanding of the role of these fatty acids in cell function. Some interesting areas for future research include the study of the reabsorption, organ distribution, cellular and lipid species incorporation of these fatty acids and their potential role in the modification of the proliferative and inflammatory response as it relates to cell injury and cell repair. Importantly, the clinical promise (6) of n-3 fatty acids and their biological significance deduced from biochemical and functional studies needs to be evaluated in carefully conducted clinical trials.

References

1. Bankey, P.E., Billiar, T.R., Wang, W.Y., Carlson, A., Holman,R.T., Cerra, F.B. (1989). J Surgical Res, 46:439-444.
2. Barcelli, U., Glas-Greenwalt, P., Pollack, VE. (1985). Thromb Research, 39:307-312.
3. Bittiner, S.B., Tucker, W.F., Cartwright I., Bleehen S.S.(1988) Lancet, 1:378-380.
4. Dyerberg, J., Bang, H.O.,, Stoffersen, E., Moncada, S., Vane, J.R. (1978). Lancet, 1:117-119.
5. Davis, H.R., Bridenstine, R.T., Vesselinovitch, D. Wissler, R.W. (1987). Arteriosclerosis, 7:441-449.
6. Dehmer, G.J., Popma, J.J., v.d.Berg, E.K.,Eichorn, E.D., Prewitt, J.B., Campbell, W.B., Jennings, L., Willerson, J.T., Schmitz, J.M. (1988). N Engl J Med, 319:733-740.

7. Endres, S., Ghorbani, R., Kelley, V.E., Georgilis, K., Lonnemann, G., v.d.Meer, J.W., Cannon, J.G., Rogers, T.S.,Klempner M, Weber, P.C., Schaefer, E.J., Wolff, S.M., Dinarello, C.A. (1989): N Engl J Med, 320:265-271.
8. Fischer, S. and Weber, P.C. (1984). Nature, 307:165-168.
9. Fischer, S., v.Schacky, C., Siess, W., Strasser, T., Weber, P.C. (1984). Biochem Biophys Res Commun, 120:907-918.
10. Fischer, S., Vischer, A., Preac-Mursic, V., Weber,P.C.(1987). Prostaglandins, 34:367-375.
11. Fisher, M., Upchurch, K.S., Levine, P.H., Johnson, M.H., Vaudreuil, C.H., Natale, A., Hoogasian, J.J. (1986): Inflammation, 10:387- 391.
12. Fox, P.L. and DiCorleto, P.E. (1988). Science, 241:453-456.
13. Garg, M.L., Wierzbicki, A.A., Thomson, A.B. and Clandinin, M.T. (1989). Biochem J, 261:11-15.
14. Harris, W.S. (1989). J Lipid Research, 30:785-807.
15. Hostmark, A.T., Bjerkedal, T., Kierulf, P., Flaten, H. and Ulshagen, K. (1988). Br Med J 297:180-181.
16. Kremer, J.M., Jubiz, W. and Michalek A., Rynes R.J., Bartholomew, L.E. Bigaoette, J., Timchalk, M., Beeler, D., Lininger, L. (1987). Ann Intern Med 106:497-503.
17. Kromhout, D., Bosschieter, E.B., de Lezenne, Coulander C. (1985). N Engl J Med, 312:1205-1209.
18. Kelley, V.E., Kirkman, R.L., Bastos, M., Berrett, L.V., Strom, T.B. (1989). Transplantation, 48: 98-102.
19. Lands, W.E., Miller jr., J.F. and Rich, S. (1987). Advances in Prostaglandin, Thromboxane and Leukotriene Res, 17:p.876-879. B.Samuelsson, R.Paoletti and P.W.Ramwell. Raven Press, N. Y.
20. Landymore, R.W., Mc.Aulay, M., Sheridan, B. and Cameron, C. (1986). Ann Thorac Surgery, 41:54-57.
21. Mc.Lennan, P.L., Abeywardena, M.Y. and Charnock J.S. (1987). Prostaglandins, 27:183-195.
22. Levine, P.H., Fisher, M., Schneider, P.B., Whitten, R.H., Weiner, B.H., Ockene, I.S., Johnson, B.F., Johnson, M.H., Doyle, E.M., Riendeau, P.A. and Hoogasian,J.J. (1989). Arch Intern Med, 149:1113-1116.

23. Locher, R., Sachinidis, A., Steiner, A., Vogt, E. and Vetter, W. (1989). Biochim Biophys Acta, 1012:279-283.
24. Lorenz, R., Spengler, U., Fischer, S., Duhm, J. and Weber, P.C. (1983). Circulation, 67:504-511.
25. Malis, C., Varadarajan, G.S., Force, T., Weber, P.C. and Leaf, A.(1988): A H A, abstract No.860.
26. Parks, J.S., Bullock, B.C. and Rudel, L.L. (1989). J Biol Chem, 264:2545-2551.
27. Prickett, J.D., Robinson, D.R. and Steinberg A.D. (1981). J Clin Invest 68:556-559.
28. Sani, B.P., Allen, R.D., Moorer, C.M. and Mc.Gee, B.W. (1987). Biochem Biophys Res Commun 147:25-30.
29. Shimokawa, H., Lam, J.Y.T., Chesebro, J.H., Bowie, E.J.W. and Vanhoutte, P.M. (1987). Circulation, 76:898-905.
30. Sperling, R.I., Robin, J.L., Kylander, K.A., Lee, T.H.,Lewis,R.A.and Austen, K.F (1987). J Immunology, 139:4186-4191.
31. v.Schacky, C., Fischer, S., Weber, P.C. (1985). J Clin Invest, 76:1626-1631.
32. v.Schacky, C., Weber, P.C. (1985). J Clin Invest, 76:2446-2450.
33. Schmidt, E.B., Pedersen, J.O., Ekelund, S., Grunnet, N., Jersild, C. and Dyerberg, J. (1989). Atherosclerosis, 77:53-57.
34. Sellmayer, A., Weber, P.C., Bonventre, J. (1989). Abstract, ASN-Meeting, Washington.
35. Siess, W., Roth, P., Scherer, B., Kurzmann, I., Böhlig, B., Weber, P.C. (1980). Lancet, 1:441-444.
36. Strasser, T., Fischer, S., Weber, P.C. (1985). Proc Natl Acad Sci, 82:1540-1543.
37. Weiner, B.H., Ockene, I.S., Levine, P.H., Cuenoud, H.F., Fisher, M., Johnson, B.F., Daoud, A.S., Jarnolych, J., Hosmer,D., Johnson M.H., Natale, A., Vaudreuil, C.H., Hoogasian, J.J. (1986). N Engl J Med, 315:841-846.
38. Weber, P.C., Fischer, S., v.Schacky, C., Lorenz, R. and Strasser, T. (1986). Progr Lipid Research, 25:273-276.
39. Weber, P.C. (1989). J Intern Med 225, Suppl.1:61-68.
40. Yeo, Y.K., Philbrick, D.J. and Holub, B.J. (1989). Biochem Biophys Res Commun, 160:1238-1242.

*Advances in Prostaglandin, Thromboxane,
and Leukotriene Research,* Vol. 20,
edited by B. Samuelsson et al.
Raven Press, Ltd., New York © 1990.

MODIFICATION OF ARACHIDONIC ACID METABOLISM

VIA THE CYTOCHROME P450-RELATED MONOOXYGENASE SYSTEM

Michal Laniado Schwartzman

Department of Pharmacology
New York Medical College
Valhalla, New York   10595

INTRODUCTION

The microsomal cytochrome P450 enzymes are a family of hemo-
proteins that serve as the terminal acceptor in the NADPH-
dependent mixed function oxidase system. This enzyme system, in
the presence of NADPH and molecular oxygen, metabolize arachidonic acid to several oxygenated metabolites including 1) four
regioisomeric EETs (5,6; 8,9; 11,12; 14,15), which can be hydrolyzed by epoxide hydrolase to the corresponding diols (DHTs); 2)
six regioisomeric cis-trans-conjugated HETEs; and 3) w and w-1
alcohols (8). It is becoming evident that the status of
cyclooxygenase and lipoxygenase derived arachidonate metabolites
as modulators of cell function is to be shared with compounds of
the newly discovered branch of the arachidonic acid cascade.
Thus, several studies by our laboratory and others demonstrated
that the EETs and their hydrolytic metabolites DHTs possess a
wide range of biological activities. These include stimulation
of peptide hormone release (2) inhibition of Na^+-K^+-ATPase (21),
vasodilation (3,18), mobilization of microsomal Ca^{++} (14) and
inhibition of platelet aggregation (9). In addition, the w and
w-1 alcohols of arachidonic acid, are also biologically active;
20-HETE is a potent vasoconstrictor (15) and 19-HETE is a
stimulator of Na^+-K^+-ATPase activity (7). The biological effects
implicate a role for these compounds in physiological and
pathophysiological processes.
In this chapter, the cytochrome P450 metabolism of arachidonic acid in rat kidney and bovine cornea will be described
with their possible contribution to the development and/or
regulation of hypertension and inflammation.

CORNEAL CYTOCHROME P450 ARACHIDONATE METABOLISM

Incubation of bovine corneal epithelial microsomes with ^{14}C-
arachidonic acid in the presence of NADPH resulted in the
formation of four major metabolites; A, B, C and D (Figure 1).
Metabolites formation was not affected by indomethacin or by

BW-755C (23). Preincubation with SKF-525A, or with carbon
monoxide, both are known inhibitors of cytochrome P450 enzymes
resulted in a 50% to 70% inhibition of product formation. These
results together with the demonstration of an active cytochrome
P450 system in the cornea (24) provided the evidences that these
metabolites are cytochrome P450 dependent.

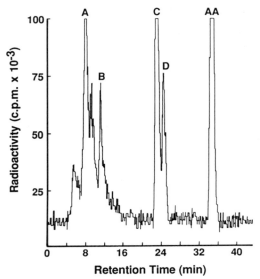

FIG. 1. Reverse
phase HPLC separation
of ^{14}C-arachidonic
acid metabolites
formed by corneal
epithelial microsomes
in the presence of
NADPH.

In view of previous reports that some cytochrome P450-
arachidonic metabolites are biologically active compounds, the
discovery of this pathway in the cornea is important. Epithelial
cells of the thick ascending limb of Henle's loop of rabbit
kidney generate a cytochrome P450-arachidonate metabolite that
inhibits Na^+-K^+-ATPase (21). Since the corneal epithelium has
transport properties that are similar to those of the renal
cells, metabolites of the cytochrome P450 in the cornea may have
an important role in the modulation of active ion transport
mechanisms. We determined the Na^+-K^+-ATPase activity of membrane
fractions from the corneal epithelium in the presence and
absence of metabolites A, B, C, and D using ouabain as a
reference standard. We found that only metabolite C inhibited
Na^+-K^+-ATPase activity with a potency 1000-fold greater than
ouabain. The UV absorbance at 236 nm and the results of GC/MS
analysis of compound C were indicative of a 12-hydroxy-5,8,10,14-
eicosatetraenoic acid (12-HETE) structure (25). When comparing
the effects of the chemically synthesized isomers of 12-HETE, we
found that 12(R)-HETE but not 12(S)-HETE inhibited Na^+-K^+-ATPase
to the same degree as the purified compound C from the corneal
epithelium. Both compound C and synthetic 12(R)-HETE demonstrated similar dose-dependent inhibition with an EC_{50} at 10^{-7}M.
Thus, compound C corresponds to 12(R)-HETE.

Deturgescence of the cornea, mediated by the corneal endo-
thelium and secretion of aqueous humor by the ciliary epithelium
are examples of basic physiological transport functions dependent
upon Na^+-K^+-ATPase-based metabolic pumps that are readily
inhibited by digitalis glycosides such as ouabain. 12(R)-HETE,
as an endogenous inhibitor of Na^+-K^+-ATPase, may modulate these
and other important functions in the eye. This compound may be
important for normal aqueous humor formation, a determinant of
ocular hypertension. We therefore, examined the effect of 12(R)
HETE on intraocular pressure (IOP) of the rabbit eye and
compared it to its isomer 12(S)-HETE.

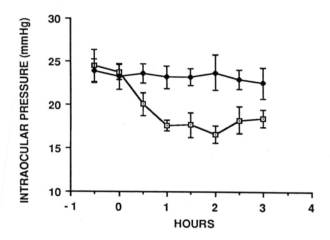

FIG. 2. Effect of topically applied 12(R)-HETE on intraocular
pressure (IOP) of the rabbit eye. 12(R)-HETE (1 µg) was applied
to both eyes of the experimental rabbits. Control rabbits
received a drop of the vehicle. Results are mean ± SEM, n=6 in
each group. Closed squares-control; open squares experimental.

As seen in figure 2, topical application of 1 µg of 12(R)HETE to
both eyes of the rabbit resulted in a marked reduction in IOP of
4-7 mmHg within 30 to 120 min. Lowering of IOP by a single
application of 12(R)HETE was long lasting, i.e. 9 days and was
not associated with any signs of inflammation. No effect on IOP
was found for the control vehicle or 12(S)HETE. Furthermore,
the 12(R)-HETE effect was not associated with any signs of
inflammation. These results arise the possibility of 12(R)HETE
being an endogenous corneal modulator of aqueous humor dynamics
and implicate its role in pathophysiological states such as
glaucoma and cataracts.
    The other biologically active cytochrome P450 metabolite
compound D, is eluted after 24.8 minutes on reverse-phase HPLC
(Figure 1). Purification of this metabolites and further GC/MS

analysis identified its structure as 12-hydroxy-5,8,14-
eicosatrienoic acid(12-DiHETE) (17). This compound is a powerful
vasodilator of several smooth muscle preparations (16).
Comparison of the vasodilatory effects of the two synthetic
isomers, 12(R) and 12(S)DiHETE, demonstrated that the biological
effect is restricted to the (R) configuration. In addition to
its vasodilatory properties in isolated blood vessels, the
12(R)DiHETE had pronounced effects on the eye. Topical application of small amounts (10 ng) of this compound to the rabbit eye
resulted in local ocular vasodilation. Injection of as little
as 5 ng of 12(R)DiHETE into the anterior chamber caused a 7-fold
increase in protein concentration of the aqueous humor, indicative of a breakdown of the blood aqueous barrier (16). Vasodilatation and breakdown of the blood aqueous barrier are well
known consequences of ocular injury and inflammation. We hypo-
thesize that ocular inflammation which typically occurs following corneal surfaces injury is partially mediated by 12(R)DiHETE
which is produced by the corneal epithelium and released into
the tear film.

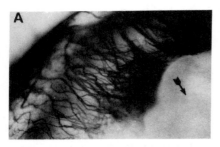
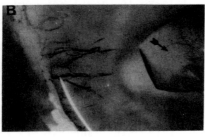

FIG. 3A. Neovascular-
ization induced by 12-
(R)-DiHETE. Pictures
were taken 7 days
after implantation.
Arrow indicates loca-
tion of pellets.
A) 1 ug of 12(R)DiHETE
B) Control pellet.

    Since neovascularization is one of the manifestations of
chronic inflammation, we tested the ability of 12(R)DiHETE to
stimulate angiogenesis. 12(R)DiHETE (0.5 - 12 µg) was combined
with a polymer (Elvax 40P) to form a pellet. The pellet was
then surgically implanted into the rabbit corneas. Neovascularization occurred in all cornea implanted with 12(R)DiHETE.
Increased numbers of limbal vessels in the region of the implant
were seen within 2-4 days depending on the amount of 12(R)DiHETE.

By the fourth day, blind-ending sprouts originating from the limbal vessels advanced toward the implant site. These sprouts reached the implants in 6-8 days and formed extensive anastomoses with active blood flow (Figure 3A). Histological examination of the corneas removed 7 days after implantation of the compound, confirmed the slit-lamp observation of a rich proliferation of new vessels. A dense infiltration of poly-morphonuclear leukocytes surrounded the new blood vessels in the stroma of corneas that received 12(R)DiHETE. No vessels nor leukocyte infiltration were observed in corneas in the absence of 12(R)-HETE or corneas implanted with 12(S)DiHETE (Figure 3B).

Since chemoattraction of blood elements (especially neutro-phils) could account for the angiogenic activity of 12(R)DiHETE, we measured the chemotactic activity of this compound on human neutrophils. Significant stimulation of neutrophil migration was observed in all experiments with 12(R)DiHETE at concentra-tions ranging between 10^{-6}M and 10^{-11}M. Significant responses were observed at doses as low as 10^{-11}M, a concentration at which LTB_4 does not exhibit significant chemotactic activity (10). The maximum response, 815% over control, was achieved at 10^{-10}M. 12(S)DiHETE showed a significant stimulation (210%) only at the highest concentration tested (10^{-6}M). Thus, the neovascular effect of 12(R)DiHETE could be due to its chemo-tactic properties. Eliason and Elliott demonstrated that corneal epithelial homogenates contain heat stable factor(s) which stimulate the proliferation of endothelial cells in vitro and vascularization in the cornea in vivo (6). These authors conclude that the corneal epithelium is the source of a secreted stimulant(s) for the growth of vascular endothelial cells. 12(R)DiHETE, which is an endogenous metabolite of arachidonic acid in the corneal epithelium, has the characteristics of such a factor. It possesses proinflammatory properties, and has very potent angiogenic capabilities. Thus, it may qualify as the intrinsic corneal angiogenic factor proposed by Eliason and Elliott. In association with other inflammatory mechanisms 12(R)DiHETE may account for the neovascularization in the cornea which occurs frequently in chronic inflammation or in the reparative stages of an acute injury.

RENAL CYTOCHROME P450 ARACHIDONATE METABOLISM

The cytochrome P450-arachidonate metabolism is expressed in both the cortex and the outer medulla of rat and rabbit kidneys (23,26). In the renal cortex, arachidonic acid is converted mainly by w/w-1 hydroxylases to 19- and 20-HETEs and in the rabbit this activity is located primarily in the proximal tubules (13). The highest concentration of cytochrome P450 arachidonate metabolism in rabbit renal medulla is found in the thick ascending limb of Henle's loop (TALH) where arachidonate is mainly converted to two major metabolites, a Na^+-K^+-ATPase inhibitor and a vasodilator (21). The formation of these

metabolites in the TALH is stimulated by arginine vasopressin
and salmone calcitonin and demonstrates a large change when
challenged by either elevated blood pressure or increased salt
intake (4). The latter finding prompted us to search for
similar products generated in the renal tissues of the spontan-
eously hypertensive rats (SHR). The SHR have been extensively
studied as an animal model of human essential hypertension.
Between ages of 5 to 13 weeks, blood pressure increases most
rapidly. Elevation of blood pressure in the SHR can be
partially suppressed by renal transplant from a normotensive
donor (21,22). The resetting of renal function appears to occur
early in the SHR and may be necessary for the development of
hypertension (1). For example, fractional sodium and water
excretion were significantly less in the SHR when compared to
the age-matched WKY, a difference which disappeared by 8 weeks
of age (5).

We previously demonstrated that total cytochrome P450
metabolism of arachidonic acid is increased in kidney of SHR
during the rapid elevation of blood pressure (20). The cytochrome P450 metabolites of renal microsomes can be separated by
HPLC into 3 major peaks. The GC/MS analysis of these peaks is
summarized in Table 1 and demonstrates that they are derived
from at least two different types of enzyme activities: 1) the
epoxygenase which metabolized arachidonate mainly to 11,12-EET
(peak III) which is further hydrolased to 11,12 DHT (peak I) and
2) w- and w-1 hydroxylases which generate the 20-HETE and
19-HETE (peak II). The 20-HETE is further oxidized by alcohol
dehydrogenase to the 1,20 dioic acid (peak I).

TABLE 1: GC/MS analysis of the cytochrome P450-arachidonate
metabolites formed renal microsomes of SHR

Peak	RP-HPLC Retention time (min)		GC/MS (m/z) me-TMS (+H$_2$)	Structure
I	17.5	Ia)	496, 486, 465, 406, 385, 315 295, 213	11,12 DHT
		Ib)	362, 331, 299, 261, 215, 180	1,20 dioic acid
II	19.0	IIa)	406, 391, 375, 117	19 HETE
		IIb)	406, 391, 375, 103	20 HETE
III	27.0	IIIa)	334, 316, 303 (340, 322, 309, 227, 155)	11,12 EET
		IIIb)	----- -----	unknown

We have recently shown that a selective depletion of cytochrome P450 in SHR kidney by tin markedly reduced the blood

pressure of 7-week-old SHR (20). Tin is a potent and specific
inducer of renal heme oxygenase, the rate limiting enzyme in
heme degradation. Hence, an increase in its activity corresponds
to a decrease in available heme for incorporation into
cytochrome P450 apoprotein (13). The reduction of blood
pressure was correlated therefore with a decrease in cytochrome
P450- dependent arachidonate metabolism. We found that tin
treatment caused a specific reduction of 50% in the w/w-1
hydroxylase activities (peak II) whereas the activity of the
epoxygenase(s) (peak I and III) was not affected.

The question arose concerning which metabolites may contribute to the pathogenesis of hypertension in SHR? We had some
evidence to suggest that the w/w-1 hydroxylated compounds were
the ones. This was supported by the fact that only peak II was
reduced by tin treatment with a corresponding reduction of blood
pressure in young SHR. Our hypothesis was that these metabolites
formed in the kidney of SHR possesses biological activities that
promote hypertension. When the three HPLC peaks were tested for
their effects on Na^+-K^+-ATPase and vascular tone of rat aortic
rings, the only peak that had an effect, i.e. stimulation of the
Na^+-K^+-ATPase and vasoconstriction, was peak II. We found that
19(S)HETE but not 19(R)-HETE is a potent stimulator of partially
purified Na^+-K^+-ATPase of rat kidney with an EC_{50} of 3×10^{-7}M.
Both 19(R)- and 20-HETEs did not have any significant effect
whereas 12(R)HETE at 10^{-6}M inhibit Na^+-K^+-ATPase by 56% (7).

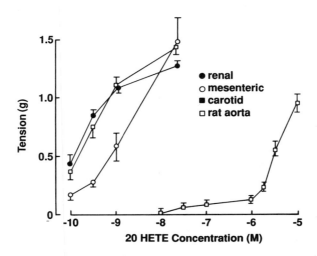

FIG. 4. Effect of 20-HETE on the basal tone of isolated
vascular smooth muscle preparations.

The ability of these compounds to affect vascular reactivity was first determined on the basal tone of rat aortic rings. Both 19- and 20-HETEs constricted the rat aorta. 20-HETE was the most potent vasoconstrictor among these arachidonate w/w-1 metabolites; i.e., it induced the contractions in rat aortic rings at a threshold dose of 10^{-7}M and an estimated EC_{50} of 3.8 ± 0.1 x 10^{6}M. When testing the vasoreactivity of 20-HETE in more muscular arteries a greater response was found. 20-HETE was a powerful vasoconstrictor of rabbit mesenteric, renal and carotid arteries with estimated EC_{50} values of 1.5 ± 0.5 x 10^{-10}M and 4.6 ± 0.2 x 10^{-10}M, respectively (Figure 4). The 20-HETE induced vasoconstriction was indomethacin dependent suggesting that its effect is mediated via further metabolism by cyclooxygenase. In recent study, we demonstrated the formation of vasoconstrictor endoperoxide analogues of 20-HETE by cyclooxygenase enzyme (15).

Hypertension may be induced and exacerbated by a large sodium intake and frequently can be treated by limiting sodium intake and/or by administrating natriuretics (19). Thus the activity of Na^+-K^+-ATPase is an important determinant of renal functions. 19(S)-HETE by stimulating Na^+-K^+-ATPase, may serve as an endogenous regulator of salt and water excretion by the kidney and, therefore contribute to the maintenance of body fluid and circulatory hemeostasis. Changes in vascular resistance are also events that lead to changes in blood pressure. 20-HETE may increase renal vascular resistance possibly leading to an increase in blood pressure either directly or by decreasing renal blood flow. Thus 19(S)-HETE and 20-HETE formed in large quantities in the kidney may play a role in the pathogenesis of hypertension in SHR by regulating regional blood flow and extracellular fluid volume.

ACKNOWLEDGEMENTS

This work was supported by NIH grants, EY06513 and HL34300 and by the Mathers Foundation. Michal Laniado Schwartzman is a recipient of Irma T. Hirschl Career Scientist Award.

REFERENCES

1. Beierwaltes, W.H., Arendshorst, W.J., and Klemmer, P.J. (1982) Hypertension 4:908-915.
2. Capdevila, J., Chacos, N., Falck, J.R., Manna, S., Negro Vilar, A. and Ojeda, S. (1981) Endocrinology 113:421-432.
3. Carroll, M.A., Schwartzman, M., Capdevila, J., Falck, J.R., McGiff, J.C. (1987) Eur. J. Pharmacol. 138:281-283.
4. Carroll, M.A., Schwartzman, M.L., Baba, M., Miller, M.J.S. and McGiff, J.D. (1988) Am. J. Physiol. 255:F151-F157.
5. Dilley, J.R., Stier, C.T., Jr., and Arendshorst, W.J. (1986) Am. J. Physiol. 246-F12-F20.
6. Eliason, J.A. and Elliot, J.P. (1987) Invest. Ophthal. Vis. Sci. 28:1963-1969.

7. Escalante, B., Falck, J.R., Yadagiri, P., Sun, L. and Laniado-Schwartzman, M. (1988) Biochem. Biophys. Res. Commun. 152:1269-1274.
8. Estabrook, R.W., Chacos, N., Marlin-Wixtrom, C. and Capdevila, J. (1982): In: Oxygenases and Oxygen metabolism. Edited by M. Nazake, S. Yamamoto, Y., Ishimura, M.J. Coon, L. Ernste and R.W. Estabrook, pp. 371-384. Academic Press, New York.
9. Fitzpatrick, F.A., Ennis, M.D., Baze, M.E. Wynalda, M.A., McGee, J.E., and Liggett, W.F. (1986) J. Biol. Chem. 261: 15334-15338.
10. Ford-Hutchinson, A.W., Braz, M.A., Doig, M.V., Shipley, M.E. and Smith, M.J.H. (1980) Nature 260:264-265.
11. Former, C.H. and Klontworth, G.K (1976) Am. J. Pathol 82: 157-167.
12. Kappas, A. and Maines, M.D. (1976) Science 192:60-62.
13. Koop, D., Morrison, A. and Duglas, J. (1988) Kidney Int. 33:162.
14. Kutsky, P., Falck, J.R., Weiss, G., Manna, S., Chacos, N. and Capdevila, J. (1983) Prostaglandins 26:13-21.
15. Laniado Schwartzman, M., Falck, J.R., Yadagiri, P., and Escalante, B. (1989) J. Biol. Chem. 264:11658-11662.
16. Masferrer, J.L., Murphy, R.C., Pagano, J.P., Dunn, M.W. and Laniado Schwartzman, M. (1989) Invest. Ophthal. Vis. Sci. 30:454-460.
17. Murphy, R.C., Falck, J.R., Lumin, S., Yadagiri, P., Zirrolli, J.A., Balazy, M., Masferrer, J.L., Abraham, N.G. and Schwartzman, M.L. (1988) J. Biol. Chem 263:17197-17202.
18. Proctor, K.G., Falck, J.R. and Capdevila, J. (1987) Circ. Res. 60:50-59.
19. Roman, R.J. (1987) Hypertension 9 (Suppl. III): 11-130.
20. Sacerdoti, D., Escalante, B., Abraham, N.G., McGiff, J.C., Levere, R.D. and Schwartzman, M.L. (1989) Science 243:388-390.
21. Schwartzman, M., Ferreri, N.R., Carroll, M.A., Songu-Mize, E. and McGiff, J.C. (1985) Nature (Lond) 314:620-622.
22. Schwartzman, M.L., Abraham, N.G., Masferrer, J.L., Dunn, M. W. and McGiff, J.C. (1985) Biochem. Biophys. Res. Commun. 132:343-348.
23. Schwartzman, M.L., Abraham, N.G., Carroll, M.A., Levere, R.D. and McGiff, J.C. (1986) Biochem. J. 238-283-290.
24. Schwartzman, M.L. Masferrer, J., Dunn, M.W., McGiff, J.C. and Abraham, N.G. (1987) Curr. Eye. Res. 6:623-630.
25. Schwartzman, M.L., Balazy, M., Masferrer, J.L., Abraham, N. G., McGiff, J.C. and Murphy, R.C. (1987) Proc. Natl. Acad. Sci., USA 84:8121-8124.
26. Zenser, T.V., Mattammal, M.B. and Davis, B.D. (1978) J. Pharmacol. Exp. Ther. 207:719-725.

Advances in Prostaglandin, Thromboxane,
and Leukotriene Research, Vol. 20,
edited by B. Samuelsson et al.
Raven Press, Ltd., New York © 1990.

PHARMACOLOGIC MODULATION OF THE
CYCLOOXYGENASE PATHWAY IN THE HUMAN KIDNEY

Carlo Patrono

Department of Pharmacology, Catholic University
School of Medicine, Largo F. Vito 1, 00168 Rome, Italy

BACKGROUND

A link between long-term use of non-narcotic analgesics and renal damage has been suspected since the early fifties (9). This was largely based on epidemiological evidence and substantiated by animal studies. The prevalence of analgesic-associated renal papillary necrosis shows a striking variation in geographic distribution, with values as low as <1% in USA and England and as high as 21% in Australia (9). Even though phenacetin present in analgesic combinations was initially implicated as the single agent responsible for papillary necrosis, it is now well established that aspirin and other nonsteroidal antiinflammatory drugs (NSADs) can cause similar lesions in man as they do in rats. Two major mechanisms have been proposed to explain the development of renal papillary necrosis in human and experimental studies: a) medullary ischemia, possibly due to inhibition of renal prostaglandin (PG) synthesis; b) a direct toxic effect on the papilla by drugs concentrating in the medulla at higher concentrations than in plasma (9). While the former can account for similar effects of structurally unrelated NSADs, the latter has been suggested to contribute to nephrotoxicity induced by aspirin, phenacetin and paracetamol (9).

A cause-effect relationship has been more clearly established between the short-term administration of a variety of NSADs and acute, usually reversible changes in renal function. Although the prevalence of these functional changes in the general patient population is difficult to assess, several risk groups have been identified (e.g. patients with chronic glomerular disease) in which NSADs almost invariably depress renal function in a transient fashion.

Studies in this area were stimulated by the observations of Donker et al. (2) in The Netherlands and of Kimberly and Plotz

(8) in the USA, suggesting a causal link between indomethacin- and aspirin-induced suppression of renal prostaglandin synthesis and depression of renal function in patients with miscellaneous kidney disease.

Other groups of patients experiencing similar adverse effects were soon identified i.e. patients with severe liver (22) or heart (12) failure. Some insight into the mechanism(s) underlying the prostaglandin-dependence of renal function in such diverse clinical conditions was provided by experimental studies in related animal models (7) and by in vitro studies of isolated rat glomeruli and cultured mesangial cells (10). The elegant in vitro studies of Dunn and his associates in Cleveland have indicated mesangial cell contraction as a possible cause of reduction in filtration surface area of the glomerulus. This contractile response to various agonists (e.g. angiotensin II, thromboxane A_2) is enhanced by pretreatment of mesangial cells with NSADs and is attenuated by exogenously added or endogenously synthesized vasodilator prostaglandins (e.g. PGE_2, PGI_2) (10).

By the mid-eighties, it was apparent that NSAD administration can be associated with various renal syndromes, including salt retention and oedema, hyperkalemia, acute renal failure, acute interstitial nephritis and the nephrotic syndrome (5).

The discovery by Ciabattoni et al. (4) that one particular NSAD, sulindac, had no measurable effect on renal prostaglandin synthesis and haemodynamics provided additional impetus for looking more closely at the biochemical and functional effects of different NSADs. This has resulted in a number of studies that were reviewed by Patrono and Dunn in 1987 (15). Furthermore, the availability of NSADs with variable effects on renal vs extra-renal prostaglandin synthesis has provided an investigative tool to understand the mechanism(s) underlying NSADs-induced loss of blood pressure control in treated hypertensive patients (15,3).

CURRENT STATUS

Short-term administration of NSADs to healthy individuals has little measurable consequence, if any, on renal function. This is likely to reflect the redundance of regulatory mechanisms controlling glomerular and tubular functions, that can compensate for partially suppressed prostaglandin synthesis.

In contrast, the same drugs given at currently employed antiinflammatory doses can acutely impair renal function in a variety of clinical circumstances characterized by either a reduction in the effective circulatory volume or preexisting renal disease. This occurs within the first 24 hours after dosing and is consistent with its being related to reduced biosynthesis of a mediator(s) contributing to maintenance of renal function in that setting. PGs produced within the kidney, both in cortical and medullary compartments (18), can indeed fulfill such a regulatory role by virtue of their relaxant effects on vascular smooth muscle and glomerular mesangial cells (10,15). Why is maintenance of renal function critically dependent upon the integrity of PG synthesis only under the above pathophysiologic conditions? A tentative answer is represented in Fig.1 and can be rationalized as follows.

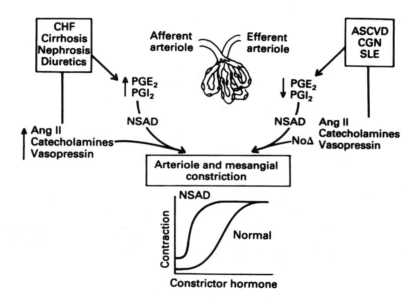

FIG. 1. Scheme depicting the balance between vasoconstriction and vasodilation existing in the pre- and post-glomerular circulation, and the glomerular mesangium. Abbreviations include: arteriosclerotic cardiovascular disease (ASCVD); chronic glomerulonephritis (CGN); systemic lupus erythematous (SLE); congestive heart failure (CHF); angiotensin II (ANG II); nonsteroidal antiinflammatory drugs (NSAD). The graph schematically depicts the enhanced arteriolar and mesangial contraction to constrictor hormones after inhibition of prostaglandin synthesis. Reproduced from Patrono and Dunn, (1987): Kidney Int., 32:1-12, with permission.

The contraction/dilation status of glomerular arterioles and mesangium is physiologically under the influence of systemic as well as locally generated agonists, interacting with specific receptors that transduce opposing signals for the intracellular ionic milieu. These include angiotensin II, arginine-vasopressin, catecholamines, and a variety of lipid mediators (e.g. eicosanoids) synthesized at or near the cell membrane. Increased circulating levels of contractile agonists, as seen in patients with congestive heart failure, or locally decreased biosynthesis of relaxant eicosanoids (e.g. PGI_2) as seen in chronic glomerular disease will create the setting for enhanced vascular and mesangial contraction in the face of acutely decreased renal PG synthesis following NSAD administration (15).

Several factors have been identified that predispose patients with congestive heart failure to the development of functional renal insufficiency after treatment with cyclooxygenase inhibitors: a) marked renal hypoperfusion, b) vigorous diuretic therapy, c) diabetes mellitus, and d) intensity of intrarenal hormonal release (12). In patients with chronic glomerular disease, the severity of ibuprofen-induced impairment of renal hemodynamics was inversely related to the basal rate of intrarenal PGI_2 production (4).

Clinically, this will be reflected in a 20 to 50% reduction in renal blood flow and glomerular filtration rate, that is promptly reversible upon discontinuing the offending NSAD. Although there may be pathogenetic links between these acute hemodynamic changes attributed to NSADs and the major chronic lesion of renal papillary necrosis, such a relationship remains elusive because of lack of properly controlled prospective studies.

In conflict with a commonly held view that long-term suppression of renal PG synthesis by NSADs may have deleterious effects on renal functional and structural integrity, two distinct lines of evidence have suggested potential long-term benefits (6,21). The first is related to the use of indomethacin for reducing proteinuria in patients with the nephrotic syndrome (21). A major limitation in the study of Vriesendorp et al. suggesting better preservation of renal function in indomethacin-treated patients than controls is related to its retrospective nature.

The second line of evidence is represented by the findings of Donadio et al. (6) in patients with membranoproliferative glomerulonephritis treated with aspirin (325 mg tid) plus dipyridamole (75 mg tid). As discussed in greater detail elsewhere (16), the slower deterioration of renal function demonstrated in aspirin- vs placebo-treated patients is likely to be due to the antiplatelet effect of the drug rather than to its trivial effect (at this particular dosage) on renal PG synthesis. Thus, it is only at full antiinflammatory dosage (4 to 5 gr/day) that appreciable suppression of renal PG synthesis has been demonstrated following aspirin administration in patients with systemic lupus erythe natosus (8). This is associated with similar reductions in renal 1 :nction as seen after other NSADs (16).

Aspirin provides an interesting example of tissue-selective inhibition of cyclooxygenase activity, with substantial sparing of extra-platelet PG synthesis at doses (30-50 mg/day) fully suppressing platelet TXA_2 biosynthesis (13). Limited "sensitivi-ty" of the renal cyclooxygenase(s), coupled with rapid (ie within a few hours) re-synthesis of the enzyme following irre-versible acetylation by aspirin, provides a reasonable explana-tion for such biochemical selectivity.

Selective sparing of renal cyclooxygenase activity and pres-ervation of PG-dependent renal fucntion has been demonstrated following the short-term administration of sulindac at antiinfl-ammatory dosage in patients with chronic glomerular disease (4). This finding has been substantially confirmed, though conflicting results have appeared in the literature (see ref. 15 for a detailed review of these studies).

Interestingly, corticosteroids have not been associated with a similar spectrum of renal syndromes as described for NSADs. Although it would be logical to expect reduced renal PG synth-esis, because of corticosteroid-induced reduction in arachidonate release through a protein inhibitor of phospholipase A_2 (vari-ously re-ferred to as macrocortin, lipomodulin, renocortin, and lipocortin: see ref.17), no evidence can be found in the litera-ture for in vivo suppression of renal PG synthesis following anti-inflammatory doses of glucocorticoids. Perhaps, limited reduction in substrate availability, as presumably induced by corticosteroids in man, has but trivial consequences on eicosa-noid production in vivo because of the very substantial capacity of cells to oxygenate arachidonate released fron membrane phospholipids, a capacity largely in excess of the very low biosynthetic rate under physiological circumstances (14).

In patients with rheumatoid arthritis, long-term treatment with aurothiomalate and penicillamine does not affect renal PG synthesis or function (19). In contrast, at least one recent report from Unsworth et al. (20) suggests that asymptomatic, reversible impairment of renal function is common in patients with rheumatoid arthritis who have been treated with NSADs for at least six months.

Long-term use of aspirin, for the primary or secondary pr-ophylaxis of thrombotic events (ie at daily doses equal to or lower than 300 mg), is unlikely to pose a serious threat to renal function of healthy individuals or patients with cardio-vascular or cerebrovascular disorders.

FUTURE DIRECTIONS

Previous studies attempting to define the effects of NSADs on renal function fall under three headings. The first, and most common in the recent literature, usually involves the monitoring of urinary PG excretion and renal function for a period of a few days to a few weeks in patients at risk who have been randomized to receive one of two NSADs and/or placebo (5,7,15). The second examines the incidence of previous NSAD use in patients presenting with renal failure to a dialysis unit (1). The third assesses renal function in patients routinely admitted to a rheumatology ward, in whom long-term NSAD therapy was withdrawn and compares this group to a population in whom NSADs were maintained (20). Each type of investigational approach suffers from inherent limitations and looks at a different subset of the patient population exposed to NSADs, within a highly variable time-frame.

What we clearly need to define the long-term consequences of renal cyclooxygenase inhibition are properly controlled large-scale prospective studies with end-points related to kidney biochemistry and function. Because the nature of the patients to be involved in such studies (ie those who clearly require long-term antiinflammatory therapy) would severely limit the feasibility of a placebo control, one could envisage randomizing patients to a non-selective cyclooxygenase inhibitor or to sulindac. Selective sparing of renal PG synthesis by the latter would presumably allow the definition of those long-term consequences, if any, that are dependent upon suppression of renal cyclooxygenase activity by the former.

In addition, short-term mechanistic studies of selective TX-synthase inhibitors, TXA_2-receptor antagonists, 5-lipoxygenase inhibitors and leukotriene antagonists (11) might help to dissect out the contribution of individual eicosanoids to maintenance or deterioration of renal function under specific experimental and clinical settings.

REFERENCES

1. Adams, D.H., Michael. J., Bacon, P.A., et al. (1986) Lancet, I:57-59.

2. Aristz, L., Donker, A.J.M., Brentjens, J.R.H., Van der Hem, G.K. (1976): Acta Med. Scand., 199:121-25.

3. Brown, J., Dollery, C., Valdes, G. (1986): Am. J. Med., 81(2B):43-57.

4. Ciabattoni, G., Cinotti, G.A., Pierucci, A., et al. (1984): N. Engl. J. Med., 310:279-83.

5. Clive, D.M., Stoff, J.S. (1984): N. Engl. J. Med., 310:563-71.

6. Donadio, J.V., Anderson, C.F., Mitchell, J.C., et al. (1984): N. Engl. Med. J., 310:1421-1426.

7. Dunn, M.J., Zambraski, E.J. (1980): Kidney Int. 18:609-22.

8. Kimberly, R.P., Plotz, P.H. (1977): N. Engl. J. Med., 296:418-24.

9. Kinkaid Smith, P. (1988): Drugs, 32:109-28.

10. Menè, P., Dunn, M.J. (1988) Circulation Res., 62:(5)916-925.

11. Nicosia, S., Patrono, C. (1989): FASEB J., 3:1941-1945.

12. Packer, M. (1988): Circulation, 77(Suppl.I):64-73.

13. Patrignani, P., Filabozzi, P., Patrono, C. (1982): J. Clin. Invest., 69:1366-1372.

14. Patrono, C., Ciabattoni, G., Pugliese, F., et al. (1986): J. Clin. Invest. 77:590-598.

15. Patrono, C., Dunn, M.J. (1987): Kidney Int. 33:1-12.

16. Patrono, C., Pierucci, A. (1986): Am. J. Med., 81(2B):71-83.

17. Rothhut, B., Russo-Marie, F., Wood, J., et al. (1983): Biochem. Biophys. Res. Commun., 117(3):878-84.

18. Schlondorff, D. (1986): Am. J. Med., 81(2B):1-11.

19. Seppälä, E., Lehtinen, K., Isomäki, H., et al. (1988): Int. J. Clin. Pharm. Res., VIII(3):149-156.

20. Unsworth, J., Sturman, S., Lunec, J., Blake, D.R. (1987): Ann. Rheum. Dis., 46:233-236.

21. Vriesendorp, R., Donker, A.J.M., De Zeeuw, D., et al. (1986): Am. J. Med., 81(2B):84-94.

22. Zipser, R.D. (1986): Am. J. Med., 81(2B):95-103.

Subject Index

Subject Index